Library of Congress Cataloging in Publication Data
Main entry under title:

Immune complexes and the pathogenesis of various
    diseases.

    1. Immune complexes. 2. Immune complex diseases.
I. Branca, Margherita. [DNLM: 1. Immunology--
Collected works. 2. Pathology--Collected works.
QW 504 I28 1972]
QR181.I39   616.07'9'08   72-10434
ISBN 0-8422-7058-2

TABLE OF CONTENTS

CREDITS & ACKNOWLEDGMENTS

Andres, G. A.; L. Accinni; S. M. Beiser; C. L. Christian; G. A. Cinotti; B. F. Erlanger; K. C. Hsu; and B. C. Seegal, "Localization of Fluorescein-labeled Antinucleoside Antibodies in Glomeruli of Patients with Active Systemic Lupus Erythematosus Nephritis," *The Journal of Clinical Investigation*, 1970, 49:2106-2118.

Blomgren, Stephen E.; John J. Condemi; and John H. Vaughan, "Procainamide-induced Lupus Erythematosus: Clinical and Laboratory Observations," *The American Journal of Medicine*, 1972, 52:338-3348.

Branca, Margherita; S. De Petris; A. C. Allison; Jennifer J. Harvey; and M. S. Hirsch, "Immune Complex Diseases: I. Pathological Changes in the Kidneys of Balb/c Mice Neonatally Infected with Moloney Leukaemogenic and Murine Sarcoma Viruses," *Clinical and Experimental Immunology*, 1971, 9:853-868.

Cochrane, Charles G., "Mechanisms Involved in the Deposition of Immune Complexes in Tissues," *The Journal of Experimental Medicine*, 1971, 134:75-89.

Glenner, George G.; Daniel Ein; and William D. Terry, "The Immunoglobulin Origin of Amyloid," *The American Journal of Medicine*, 1972, 52:141-147.

Gocke, David J.; Konrad Hsu; Councilman Morgan; Stepheno Bombardieri; Michael Lockshin; and Charles L. Christian, "Vasculitis in Association with Australia Antigen," *The Journal of Experimental Medicine*, 1971, 134:330-339.

Gutman, Robert A.; Gary E. Striker; Bruce C. Gilliland; and Ralph E. Cutler, "The Immune Complex Glomerulonephritis of Bacterial Endocarditis," *Medicine*, 1972, 51:1-25.

Henson, Peter M., "Interaction of Cells with Immune Complexes: Adherence, Release of Constituents, and Tissue Injury," *The Journal of Experimental Medicine*, 1971, 134:114-135.

Hotchin, John, "Virus, Cell Surface, and Self: Lymphocytic Choriomeningitis of Mice," *A. J. C. P.*, 1971, 56:333-349.

Lindqvist, K. J.; and C. K. Osterland, "Human Antibodies to Vascular Endothelium," *Clinical and Experimental Immunology*, 1971, 9:753-760.

Lindstrom, F. D., "Urinary Immunoglobulins in Rheumatoid Arthritis and Other Connective Tissue Diseases," *Annals of Clinical Research*, 1971, 3:39-45.

Morton, Jane I.; and Benjamin V. Siegel, "Radiation Sensitivity of New Zealand Black Mice and the Development of Autoimmune Disease and Neoplasia," *Proceedings of the National Academy of Sciences*, 1971, 68:124-126.

Waller, Marion; R. J. Duma; E. D. Farley, Jr.; and Jane Atkinson, "The Influence of Infection on Titres of Antiglobulin Antibodies," *Clinical and Experimental Immunology*, 1971, 8:451-459.

Weissmann, Gerald, "Lysosomal Mechanisms of Tissue Injury in Arthritis," *New England Journal of Medicine*, 1972, 286:141-147.

Zabriskie, John B., "The Role of Streptococci in Human Glomerulonephritis," *The Journal of Experimental Medicine*, 1971, 134:180-192.

PREFACE

Recent studies have implicated immune complexes in many connective tissue diseases, such as rheumatoid arthritis and systemic lupus erythematosus. Other snydromes, including glomerulonephritis and various cardiomyopathies, are also often the result of immune complexes. The pathogenesis of these diseases is due to the interaction of a specific antibody with its respective antigen. Although this is a normal process in the immune defense against infectious agents, antigen-antibody complexes which form in the presence of excess antigens are usually soluble. These soluble complexes remain in the circulation and can be deposited in such sites as the glomeruli, the walls of small vessels, the skin, and the synovial tissues. Once deposited, the immune complexes readily fix complement, in turn tirggering the release of several factors which establish a foci of inflammation. Tissue damage then occurs as a result of the severe inflammatory reaction.

The etiological agents of these diseases have long eluded investigators, whose observations were that antibodies apparently interact with various tissues, thereby bringing about the lesions. However, experiments with laboratory animals--particularly the New Zealand Black (NZB) strain of mice--have provided additional insight into this category of disease. The most important model to date, the NZB mice present a hemolytic-renal-lymphomatous disease complex which is clinically related to idiopathic glomerulonephritis, lupus, and other connective tissue diseases as well as to malignant lymphoma in man. Since these animals were shown to have autoantibody responses to a variety of autologous tissue antigens, they were originally defined as having "autoimmune" disease. Subsequent investigations have implicated wild type Gross leukemia virus in the etiology and pathogenesis of the disease. The significance of this finding has gained increasing recognition as viral antigens have recently been observed in human cases of nephritis, artheritis, and arthritis.

Thus, the pathological sequel in these diseases, associated with the formation of immune complexes, can be regarded as a consequence of an underlying infection, presumably viral. Therefore, a more appropriate term for these syndromes would be "immune" diseases rather than "autoimmune", since the pathological process in NZB mice--and often in humans--can be altered by agents which suppress the immune response. From these same studies it is also becoming apparent that, by themselves, some viral diseases are not necessarily harmful to the host, but that the pathology results from the immune mechanism trying to deal with the infection. These observations have provided exciting new information on the relationship between the immune mechanism and certain diseases.

Reflecting the current enthusiasm in the field, this collection brings together the literature on recent investigations of the diseases resulting from immune complexes. Studies using both animal and human models are included. Also provided are several articles which describe various diseases not previously classified as involving immune complexes but which now appear to be candidates for this category.

Ronald T. Acton, Ph.D.
September, 1972

Diseases of Experimental Animals
Which Implicate Immune Complexes

IMMUNE COMPLEX DISEASES

I. PATHOLOGICAL CHANGES IN THE KIDNEYS OF BALB/c MICE NEONATALLY INFECTED WITH MOLONEY LEUKAEMOGENIC AND MURINE SARCOMA VIRUSES

MARGHERITA BRANCA , S. DE PETRIS, A. C. ALLISON, JENNIFER J. HARVEY AND M. S. HIRSCH

INTRODUCTION

Certain viruses, such as lymphocytic choriomeningitis (LCM) and murine and avian leukaemogenic viruses, produce lifelong infections and are regularly transmitted from mothers to offspring. For many years it was accepted that such vertical transmission (VT) can occur because when mice are infected with these viruses in the immediate postnatal period tolerance to virus antigens is induced (Burnet & Fenner, 1949; Hotchin, 1962; Volkert & Hannover-Larsen, 1965; Axelrad, 1965; Klein & Klein, 1966). However, this interpretation has been challenged recently, largely because of the findings of Oldstone & Dixon (1967, 1969) that mice neonatally infected with LCM virus are not completely tolerant but form some antibodies which are deposited in the renal glomeruli in the form of virus antigen–antibody complexes. The presence in the circulation of virus-antibody complexes retaining infectivity had been demonstrated by Notkins *et al.* (1966) in the case of the lactate dehydrogenase elevating virus; the infectivity of these complexes can be abolished by treatment with appropriate antisera against homologous immunoglobulins.

Many mouse strains carry leukaemogenic viruses which are potentially pathogenic in terms of induction of leukaemias, lymphomas or immune complex diseases. Thus the renal disease and neoplasias of NZB mice may be related to the presence of a leukaemogenic virus in this strain (Mellors, Aoki & Huebner, 1969). Hence detailed investigations of these viruses and the immune responses which they can elicit under different conditions are of interest. We have studied BALB/c mice infected neonatally with Moloney leukaemogenic virus (MLV) or with the lymphocytic component of murine sarcoma virus (MSV-H) which is so far indistinguishable antigenically from MLV. The advantage of this system are the rapidity with which leukaemias and renal pathological changes, due apparently to immune complex formation, develop (5–7 months) and the availability of a satisfactory assay for neutralizing antibodies (Hirsch & Harvey, 1969). The presence of immune complexes in the kidneys of mice neonatally infected with MLV has already been reported (Hirsch, Allison & Harvey, 1969). We now give a description of the renal pathological changes in the mice observed by light and electron microscopy and a discussion of the role of immune complexes in their development.

MATERIALS AND METHODS

Animals

BALB/c mice were infected with 0·1 ml of Moloney leukaemogenic virus (MLV) intraperitoneally within the first 18 hr of life or were in the 3rd to 9th generation receiving vertically-transmitted milk-borne MLV or the lymphocytic leukaemogenic virus separated from MSV-H ('late' MSV, see Harvey & East, 1969). In all, twenty-two infected mice were studied in detail and fifteen normal, untreated BALB/c mice housed in the same room were studied as controls.

Pathology

Groups of virus-infected and control mice were killed at the age of 2, 3, 4, 5, 6 and 7 months by ether anaesthesia, and total body and kidney weights recorded. For light microscopy kidneys were fixed in formol-acetic-alcohol for 24 hr and embedded in paraffin; they were serially sectioned at 5 μ and stained with haematoxylin and eosin and with periodic-acid-Schiff (PAS). For electron microscopy samples of kidneys cortex were fixed by immersion in 2% cold glutaraldehyde in 0·1 M phosphate buffer for 2½ hr or for 17–30 days. Prolonged fixation preserved the tissue better. They were washed in phosphate buffer, postfixed with 1% Osmium tetroxide in the same buffer for 2 hr, dehydrated through a graded series of alcohols and embedded in Araldite. Thin sections were stained with uranylacetate and lead citrate and examined with a 6EMB-AEI electron microscope.

Immunofluorescence

Kidneys were rapidly frozen in liquid nitrogen and isopentane. Frozen 4 μ sections were mounted on clean coverslips, thoroughly dried and repeatedly washed at room temperature with phosphate-buffered saline (pH 7·1) to remove unbound globulin. They were stained for 30 min with fluorescein-conjugated goat antimouse-γ-globulin (Hyland or Nordic), washed repeatedly and mounted in buffered glycerol. Similar sections were examined for the presence of MLV antigens by an indirect immunofluorescence technique, using hyperimmune rabbit anti-MLV serum and fluorescein isothiocyanate-conjugated horse anti-rabbit-γ-globulin serum (Hyland).

Elution of antibody

Gamma-globulin was eluted from immune complexes in kidneys of 3–4-month-old MLV-infected animals and age-matched controls. Glomerular basement membrane fractions were prepared by standard procedures (Unanue & Dixon, 1967), washed four times in phosphate-buffered saline and once in unbuffered saline to remove unbound globulins, and antigen–antibody complexes dissociated in 0·2 M sodium citrate buffer, pH 3·2, for 2 hr at room temperature. After centrifugation the supernatant containing the eluates was brought back to neutrality and tested for antibody against MSV–MLV antigens. Equal volumes of eluates and an undiluted stock preparation of MSV-H were mixed and incubated at 37°C for 1 hr. Newborn Parkes mice were inoculated intraperitoneally with 0·1 ml of the virus eluate mixtures and killed 21 days later for a spleen weight assay of MSV infectivity (Hirsch & Harvey, 1969).

Neutralization of circulating virus-antibody complexes

Samples of serum from MSV- and from MLV-infected mice were mixed with equal amounts of either unconjugated rabbit anti-mouse globulin, normal rabbit serum (NRS) or saline for 1 hr at 37°C. They were then inoculated intraperitoneally (0·1 ml) into newborn mice. To determine which immunoglobulin class was complexed with circulating virus, samples of serum from infected mice were mixed with equal amounts of specific rabbit antisera against mouse immunoglobulins IgG, IgM and IgA, as well as with saline, for 1 hr at 37°C and inoculated intraperitoneally (0·1 ml) into newborn mice. Spleen weight assays were carried out at 21 days.

RESULTS

No significant difference in kidney weight has been found between controls and experimental animals.

Light microscopy

Control BALB/c mice show some renal glomerular abnormalities. In one control aged 2 months, and more obviously in others aged 7 months, patchy mesangial thickening with PAS-positive material was observed. Nevertheless, from comparison of control and MLV-infected mice it is clear that additional glomerular changes are present in the latter. In the experimental animals no difference is noted between groups receiving neonatal inoculation of MLV and those receiving vertically transmitted MLV or 'late' MSV. The histopathological glomerular changes are first clearly discernible at 3 or 4 months of age and are more consistent and obvious in older animals (5–7 months) or when a renal interstitial leukaemic infiltration was present.

Early and characteristic structural features are enlargement of the intercapillary or mesangial matrix and hypertrophy of the endothelial and mesangial cells. In some cases an obvious increase in the PAS positivity of the intercapillary membranous material is present. Both the endothelial and mesangial hypertrophy are due to an increase in the amount of cytoplasm, while the nuclei are also larger and less densely stained than usual. In particular, the endothelial cells project into the lumina of the capillaries and sometimes appear to occlude them (Figs 1 and 2). The general pattern of the changes described corresponds to that of a 'membranous glomerulitis'.

In 5-month infected animals, the changes are more severe and the glomeruli are usually enlarged. The enlargement of the mesangial areas is conspicuous, with heavy patchy deposition of strongly PAS-positive material, while a lobular pattern of capillaries can be discerned (Fig. 3). In such cases the Bowman's space is nearly or completely obliterated.

At 7 months the enlargement of the glomerulus can be very obvious with increase in the number of nuclei, while a remarkable dilation and distortion of the glomerular capillaries and collapse of the structures are common and prominent (Fig. 4). All these features correspond to the picture of proliferative, membranous, or lobular glomerulonephritis.

When an interstitial leukaemic infiltration is present in the renal parenchyma, the glomeruli are often severely affected. In fact, at 3 months the glomeruli can already show interstitial sclero-hyalinosis with partial obliteration and distortion of the tuft and some cellular degenerative changes (karyorrhexis, karyolysis or atrophy). The increase in number of nuclei and cellular distortion are also obvious and some wire-loop capillaries are very prominent (Fig. 5). This picture of chronic glomerulonephritis is more evident in older animals where the glomeruli appear remarkably enlarged and heavily affected (Fig. 6). Usually the changes are generalized, the majority of glomeruli throughout the kidney being affected to about the same degree. Occasionally in some animals only a few glomeruli or part of them show clear changes.

In conclusion, the histopathological findings suggest that the earliest event in all experimental groups is the alteration occurring in the mesangial area; later a variety or lesions develop also elsewhere in the kidney. Initially the histological pattern corresponds to that expected in a membranous glomerulitis; later they resemble those of a chronic, proliferative glomerulonephritis, with variable degrees of sclerosis. Tubular changes are slight initially, but later casts are prominent and there are some associated tubular cell degenerative changes.

Immunofluorescence

Kidneys of mice infected neonatally with MLV showed no detectable bound immunoglobulin before they were 70–90-days old. At this age bound immunoglobulin was demonstrable in the form of fine granular deposits mainly in the mesangial region. In mice aged 100–120 days the deposits were relatively coarse and lumpy and quite widely distributed in the glomeruli (Fig. 7). All glomeruli were involved to a greater or lesser extent, but there was no fluorescence of tubular cells. Viral antigens were found to have a similar distribution in the glomeruli but were observed also in the form of less intense, fine focal areas of fluorescence elsewhere in the kidney (Fig. 9). Kidneys of control BALB/c mice of comparable age did not contain immunoglobulin or viral antigens demonstrable by immunofluorescence (Fig. 8). Sections of kidneys of infected mice treated for 30 min in citrate buffer, pH 3·2, and washed in phosphate-buffered saline before staining lost the specific glomerular fluorescence.

Fig. 1–6 Light microscopy. Sections of kidney of mice infected with MLV or MSV. Fig. 1–4 and Fig. 6, PAS staining; Fig. 5, haematoxylin-eosin. (× 540.)

Fig. 1. Glomerulus of 4-month-old mouse vertically infected with MSV, showing some early alterations, i.e. increase in the number of endothelial and mesangial cells with partial obliteration of capillary lumina.

Fig. 2. Glomerulus of 4-month-old mouse neonatally infected with MLV, showing enlargement of the glomerular body with increased numbers of endothelial and mesangial cells. The prominent cuboidal cells, bordered by microvilli are tubular cells which in the mouse line part of the Bowman's capsule (Crabtree, 1940). In electron microscope preparations the microvilli appear to reach the surface of epithelial cells of the capillaries.

Fig. 3. Glomerulus of 5-month-old mouse vertically infected with MSV, showing marked mesangial thickening with a lobular pattern and nearly complete obliteration of Bowman's capsule.

Fig. 4. Enlarged glomerulus of 7-month-old mouse neonatal'y infected with MLV, showing increase in the number of endothelial and mesangial cells and some peripheral prominently dilated capillaries.

Fig. 5. Glomerulus of 3-month-old mouse neonatally infected with MSV, showing heavy mesangial thickening, partial obliteration and distortion of the tuft, signs of cellular degeneration and very prominent wire-loop capillaries. A light parenchymal lymphocytic infiltration is present.

Electron microscopy

Observations were made on kidneys of control animals and on kidneys of experimental animals, which under the light microscope showed slight to fairly severe glomerular alterations (like those illustrated in Figs 1–4). No study was made of cases corresponding to the most marked glomerular changes, which were usually associated with interstitial leukaemic infiltrations.

Glomeruli of 2 and 4-month-old *control* animals had a normal appearance. The basement membrane alongside the mesangial cells showed some irregularity but elsewhere it was thin and smooth with only a very occasional projection on the epithelial side. Although the endothelial cells formed the usual thin lining of glomerular capillaries, the cell bodies were prominent and had many reticulated extensions in some regions. Epithelial cells showed moderate amounts of cytoplasm, few vacuoles and many polysomes and microtubules. Foot processes were discrete except in very occasional restricted areas.

Kidneys from mice aged 3 and 4 months infected with MLV by vertical transmission and showing *initial* alterations under the light microscope (i.e. moderate mesangial, epithelial and endothelial proliferation with relatively slight PAS-positive membrane thickening) at the electron microscopical level had an overall appearance similar to the controls. The most prominent change noted in these kidneys was in the endothelial cells, which were large, with more abundant and less dense cytoplasm than in the controls. In many places, the endothelial cell cytoplasm swelled into the capillary lumina and reticulated extensions were common (Figs 10 and 11). Sometimes only a marked reticulation was noted, but no swelling. Epithelial cells were normal, but with a larger number of small and large vacuoles,

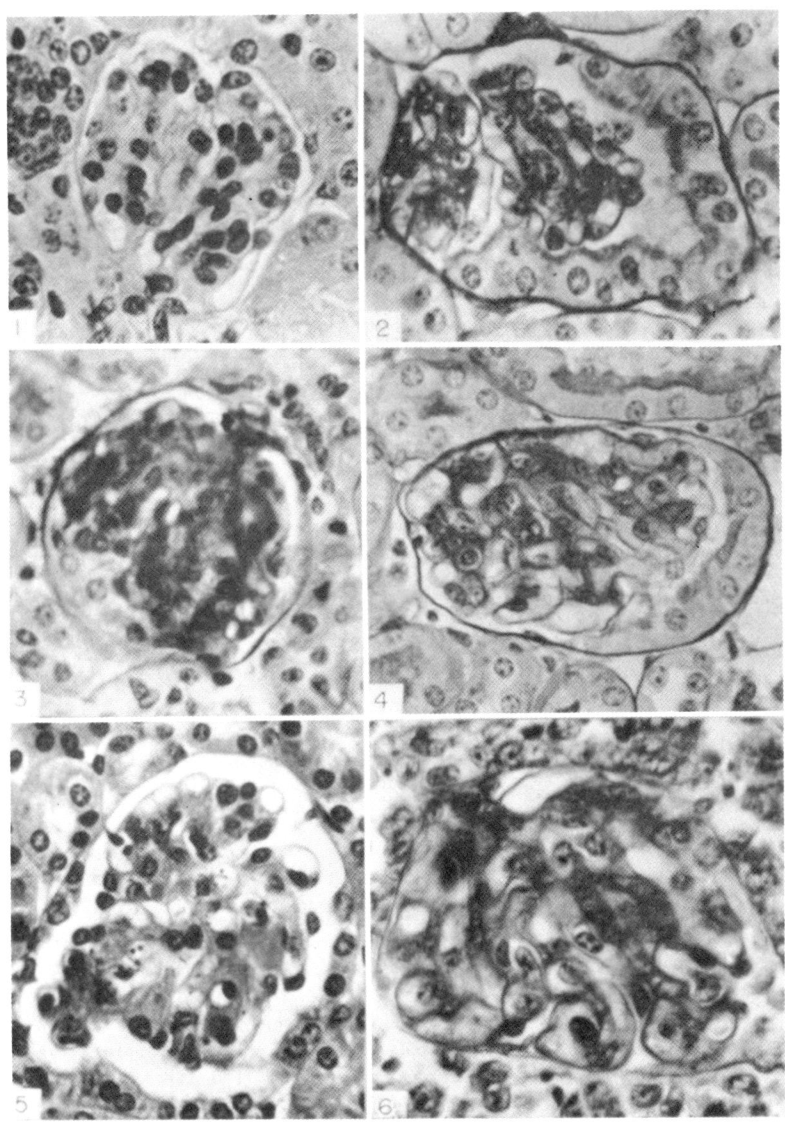

FIG. 6. Remarkably enlarged glomerulus of a more than 1-year-old mouse neonatally infected with MLV, showing increased numbers of endothelial and mesangial cells, dilated capillaries and patchy mesangial thickening. A massive parenchymal lymphocytic infiltration is present.

including multivesicular (or 'multigranular') bodies (Fig. 14). In some glomeruli they appeared to have increased in number and filled most of the capsular space, but they still maintained a normal ultrastructure. Fusion of epithelial foot processes was seen in some areas. Irregularity of the basement membrane was observed near the mesangial cells. Along the capillaries the basement membrane was generally normal; only in occasional areas it was markedly thickened with formation of subepithelial bulges (Fig. 13).

In a more advanced stage of the disease (corresponding to that illustrated in Fig. 3), in which light microscopy showed more obvious PAS-positive thickening of the basement membrane, marked alterations were detected by electron microscopy. The mesangial area was enlarged and the mesangial matrix had an irregular texture formed by material of

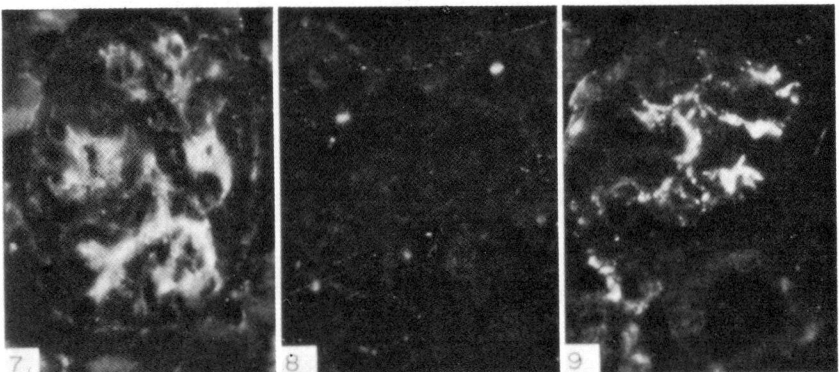

FIG. 7. Glomerulus of a 3-month-old mouse, vertically infected with MSV, stained with fluorescein-conjugated anti-immunoglobulin antiserum. Strong specific granular fluorescence is localized mainly in the mesangium. The pale fluorescence of some tubules is blue auto-fluorescence. (× 540.)
Fig. 8. Glomerulus of a 3-month-old uninfected (control) BALB/c mouse, stained with fluorescein-conjugated anti-immunoglobulin antiserum. A small glomerulus, which by ordinary light microscopy appeared located in the centre of the photograph, does not show any fluorescnce. (× 540.)
FIG. 9. Glomerulus of a 3-month-old BALB/c mouse vertically infected with MSV, stained with rabbit anti-MLV antibody and then fluorescein-conjugated anti-rabbit immunoglobulin serum. Virus-specific antigen appears as granular fluorescence in the mesangium and glomerular capillaries. (× 540.)

variable density (Fig. 16). In many places the basement membrane was obviously thickened and irregular, convoluted and in places duplicated (Figs 17 and 18). In several regions moderately dense subepithelial projections were observed (Fig. 15). At other points these projections corresponded to areas of reduced density (Fig. 18). The foot processes of epithelial cells were fused in many regions, mostly near the dome-like projections of the basement membrane, and the proliferative changes in the epithelial and especially endo-thelial cells described in the previous paragraph were again present, although the cytoplasmic swelling was not marked.

A few particles consistent in appearance with type C viruses were occasionally observed

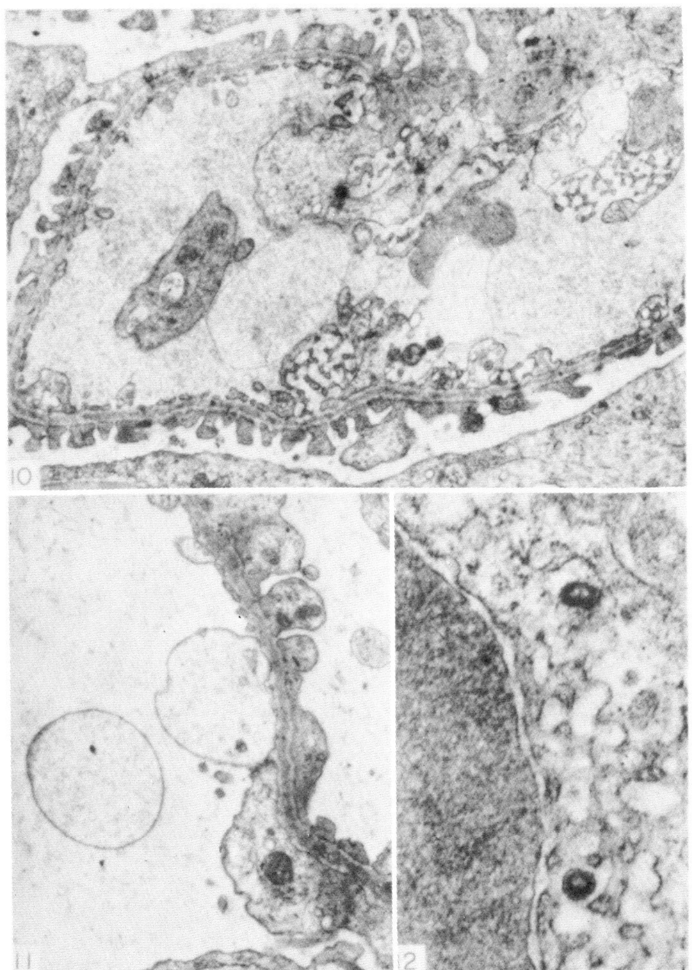

FIG. 10. Glomerular capillary of a 3-month-old mouse neonatally infected with MLV, showing marked swelling and reticulation of the endothelial cells. The basement membrane is normal. ($\times$ 13,600.)

FIG. 11. Same mouse as in Fig. 10. Detail of the process of swelling and blebbing of an endothelial cell. ($\times$ 16,000.)

FIG. 12. Two virus particles present in the fenestrated area of an endothelial cell of a 3-month-old mouse neonatally infected with MLV. The upper particle is possibly budding from the cell membrane (suggestion for the presence of a stalk is more evident in underexposed prints). ($\times$ 47,760.)

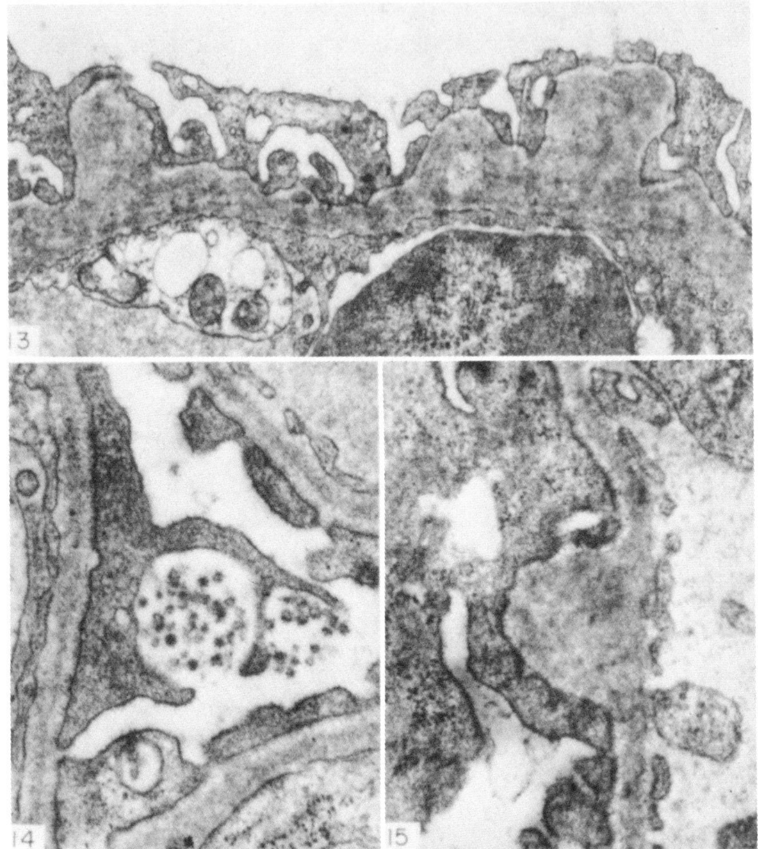

FIG. 13. Glomerulus of a 4-month-old mouse, vertically infected with MSV, showing a thickened basement membrane with marked subepithelial projections. (× 20,340.)
FIG. 14. Same mouse as in Fig. 12. Detail of 'multigranular' vacuoles of an epithelial cell in the process of releasing their contents into the capsular space. (× 38,250.)
FIG. 15. Typical local thickening of the basement membrane, with partial fusion of the foot processes of epithelial cells in a glomerulus of a 5-month-old mouse vertically infected with MSV (same mouse as in Fig. 3). (× 38,700.)

in cytoplasmic vacuoles or, extra-cellularly, in the fenestrations of endothelial cells of some mice. In one case an image possibly representing a particle budding from the cell membrane of an endothelial cell was found (Fig. 12). Owing to the scarcity of virus particles in our samples, we have been unable to confirm more conclusively this finding. No viruses were seen in the basement membrane.

Characterization of eluted antibody

Eluates of kidneys from mice neonatally infected with MLV had the capacity to neutralize MSV. As shown in Table 1, the spleen weights of inoculated animals were in the normal range, significantly less than those of animals inoculated with MSV mixed with eluates from uninfected animals. Undiluted eluates were tested by Outcherlony immuno-diffusion in agarose against specific rabbit anti-mouse IgG, IgM and IgA sera. Eluates from kidneys of mice carrying MLV showed well-defined precipitation with antisera against IgM, a weaker reaction with anti-IgG, but no reaction with anti-IgA.

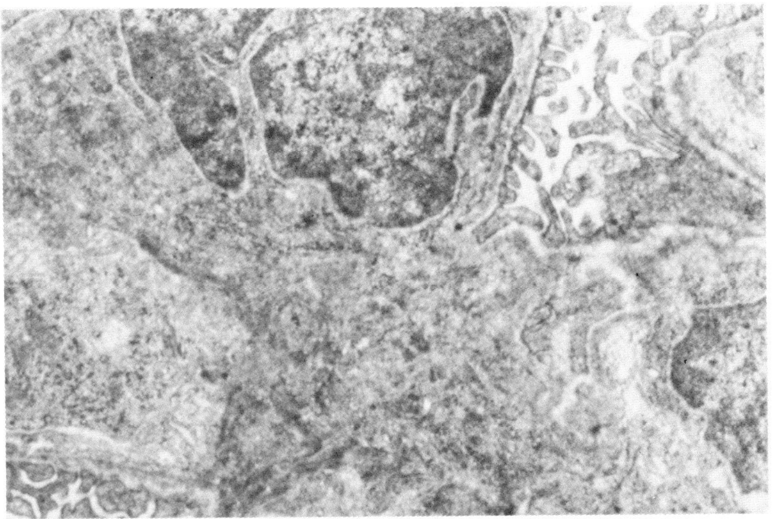

FIG. 16. Mesangial area from the same mouse as in Fig. 12, showing the considerable thickening and irregular dense texture of the intercellular matrix. ($\times$ 13,500).

Presence of non-neutralized virus-antibody complexes in serum

All twenty inoculated with MSV-NRS or MSV-saline mixtures developed tumours and fatal splenomegalic disease characteristic of MSV-H between 14 and 21 days later. Only one of twelve mice inoculated with MSV plasma-anti-mouse-immunoglobulin mixture developed a local tumour and splenomegalic disease, and none developed late lymphocytic leukaemia. Similarly, only one out of thirteen animals inoculated with the MLV plasma-anti-mouse-immunoglobulin mixtures developed characteristic lymphocytic leukaemias whereas this was observed in nine out of ten animals receiving MLV plasma NRS mixtures during a 6-month period of observation. The results in Table 2 suggest that most of the antibody associated with the circulating infectious MSV complexes is in the IgM class. Significant reduction in splenomegaly was observed after exposure to specific anti-IgM sera, but not anti-IgG or IgA sera.

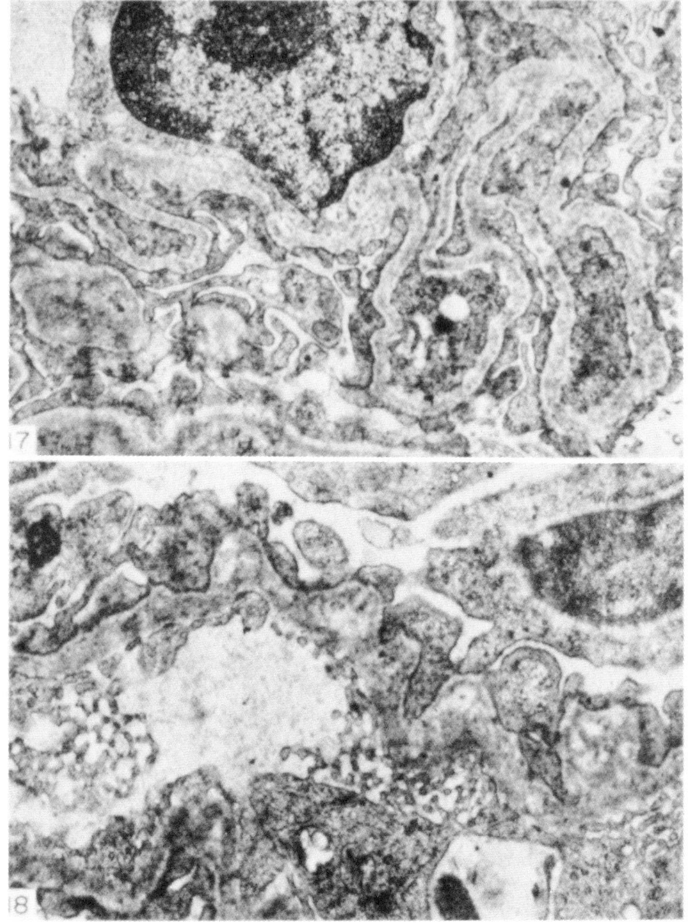

FIG. 17. Convoluted and distorted basement membrane with partial fusion of the foot processes in a glomerulus of the same mouse as in Fig. 12. (× 12,000.)

FIG. 18. Glomerulus from the same mouse as in Fig. 12, showing bulging and distortion of the basement membrane. The endothelial cells present extensive reticulation, but no swelling. (× 18,400).

DISCUSSION

The observations here presented show that BALB/c mice infected neonatally with MLV and 'late' MSV, by inoculation of virus or vertical transmission from the mother, develop conspicuous renal glomerular changes by the age of 4–5 months. These abnormalities precede the appearance of overt leukaemia, although they are increased in severity when the

TABLE 1. Effects of citrate eluates from saline washed kidney homogenates on MSV-H induced splenomegaly of newborn mice

Group	No.	Mean spleen weights $\pm$ S.E. (g)
Neonatally infected MLV	19	0·100* ± 0·015
Control BALB/c	16	0·149 ± 0·008

Equal amounts of eluates and undiluted sarcoma inducing preparations of MSV-H were mixed and incubated at 37°C for 1 hr. Newborn Parkes mice were inoculated intraperitoneally with 0·1 ml of the mixtures and were killed 21 days later.

* Mean significantly less than control mean ($P<0.05$; Dunnett's procedure).

leukaemia becomes manifest. The initial glomerular abnormalities observed by light and electron microscopy include proliferation of mesangial, endothelial and epithelial cells; later there is marked thickening and deposition of PAS-positive material in the basement membrane, localized necrosis and variable degrees of glomerulosclerosis, with formation of PAS-positive casts and secondary tubular cell degenerative changes. The pathology is characteristic of chronic, proliferative glomerulonephritis.

Several observations suggest that the glomerular pathology results from the deposition of immune complexes rather than being due to a direct effect of MLV on the kidney or to autoimmunity. The virus does not have any known cytopathic effects and the electron microscopic evidence suggested that virus replication in renal glomerular cells was slight or absent. The granular pattern of deposition of bound immunoglobulin in the glomerular capillary walls, and its release by mild acid treatment, provides strong evidence for the presence of immune complexes. Part at least of the bound antibody is directed against viral antigen, as shown by the capacity of eluates to neutralize MSV. The glomerular lesions observed by electron microscopy, in particular the swelling of endothelial cells in early

TABLE 2. Effects of anti-immunoglobulin sera on splenomegaly induced by MSV from serum of neonatally infected mice

Groups	No.	Mean spleen weights $\pm$ S.E. (g)
Anti-IgM	15	0·107* ± 0·010
Anti-IgA	8	0·176 ± 0·015
Anti-IgG	14	0·159 ± 0·015
Saline control	23	0·159 ± 0·011

Equal amounts of infectious serum and rabbit anti-mouse immunoglobulin serum were mixed and incubated at 37°C for 1 hr. Newborn Parkes mice were inoculated intraperitoneally with 0·1 ml of the mixtures and were killed 21 days later.

* Mean significantly less than control mean ($P<0.05$; Dunnett's procedure).

stages and the thickening of the basement membrane with formation of subepithelial projections and fusion of the foot processes of the epithelial cells in more advanced lesions, are
similar to the glomerular changes induced by immune complexes (Dixon, Feldman &
Vazquez, 1961; Feldman, 1964). No typical dense localized deposits (presumably antigen–
antibody aggregates) (see, for example, Feldman, 1963) were evident in the cases examined
by us, which included only early and intermediate stages of the disease The presence of the
discrete deposits may not necessarily be a constant characteristic of an immune complex
disease, since their formation probably depends on the rate of deposition and the nature of
the antigen–antibody complex.

The presence of infectious MSV and MLV virus-antibody complexes in the circulation
was strongly suggested by the observed neutralization of virus in plasma by antisera against
mouse immunoglobulins, specifically mouse IgM. This result is not inconsistent with the
finding of neutralizing antibody in kidneys. Notkins and his collaborators (Notkins *et al.*,
1966; Ashe & Notkins, 1966; Notkins, 1968) have shown with lactate dehydrogenase virus
and herpes simplex virus that antibody can neutralize the great majority of virus exposed to
it, leaving a small fraction of residual infectivity. This residual fraction cannot be eliminated
by addition of further antibody, but is neutralized by exposure to anti-immunoglobulin
serum. Similarly, the anti-viral antibody in our mice may have been sufficient to neutralize
virus used in the *in vitro* tests but failed to neutralize all the virus liberated into the circulation *in vivo*. Probably much of the antibody *in vivo* is complexed with non-virion 'soluble'
virus-specific antigens known to be present in sera of animals infected with leukaemogenic
viruses (Aoki, Boyse & Old, 1968).

The results we have obtained show that newborn animals exposed to MLV are capable of
producing some antibody. It is nevertheless clear that the antibody responses of newborn
and older mice to MLV are not the same. Klein & Klein (1965, 1966) have reported that
mice inoculated neonatally with MLV showed a deficient or delayed antibody response,
measured by the indirect fluorescent antibody test against Moloney lymphoma cells, in
comparison with mice infected as adults. In neonatally infected mice there was a correlation
between the development of antibodies and the length of the preleukaemic latency period. A
remarkable feature of the antibody response in our mice neonatally infected with MLV
was the relationship to IgM, as shown by neutralization of virus in plasma by specific
antisera. Fink (1970) has also found that the antibody against MLV, measured by indirect
haemagglutination, is in the IgM fraction. There is a possible analogy with the prolonged
production of IgM antibody observed in human newborns congenitally infected with
rubella virus (Soothill *et al.*, 1966). Other antibodies produced by newborn mice are also
found in the macroglobulin fraction (Boraker & Hildemann, 1965). Perhaps the usual
switch from IgM to IgG antibody production does not take place in these neonatally
virus-infected animals.

The question then arises whether our observations are isolated and exceptional or provide
an example of a relatively common immunopathological reaction in experimental animals.
The findings of similar glomerular lesions in rats neonatally infected with MLV shows that
the response is not confined to one strain of mice. Dunn & Green (1966) and Recher *et al.*
(1966) mention the occurrence of an unusual kidney lesion consisting of hyalinization of the
glomeruli and hyaline tubular casts, not staining for amyloid, in BALB/c mice infected with
Rauscher leukaemogenic virus or MLV. When survival of infected mice was prolonged by
administration of propylthiouracil or repeated blood transfusions, the glomerular lesions

were more pronounced (Dunn *et al.*, 1966). The aetiology of the lesions they observed was not explained, but it seems clear that they are very similar to those we now describe.

One of the most striking renal lesions spontaneously occurring in mice is the glomerulonephritis of conventional (Helyer & Howie, 1963; Holmes & Burnet, 1963) and germ-free (East & Branca, 1969) New Zealand black (NZB) mice and their hybrids (Howie & Helyer, 1968). The pathology and electron microscopy of this condition strongly suggests an immune complex aetiology (Manaligod *et al.*, 1967; Lambert & Dixon, 1968). The NZB carry a virus serologically related to the Gross leukaemogenic virus and evidence for the presence of group specific murine leukaemia virus antigen (MULV) in the kidneys has been presented by Nowinski *et al.* (1968) and Mellors *et al.* (1969). The antigen was localized in the mesangium. In mice aged 3–9 months G soluble type-specific viral antigen was found by Mellors *et al.* (1969) in the circulation; later the antigen disappeared from the plasma but specific antibody appeared. Membranous glomerulonephritis became increasingly prevalent in mice at the time of elimination of antigen from the plasma. These observations may implicate complexes of virus-specific antigen and antibody in the glomerular disease of NZB mice, although the lupus-like nephritis observed in NZB/NZW hybrids and associated with antibodies against DNA (Lambert & Dixon, 1968) may have a more complicated aetiology.

Deposition of virus-specific antigen–antibody complexes in the kidneys of mice neonatally infected with lymphocytic choriomeningitis virus (LCM) has been described by Oldstone & Dixon (1967, 1969). These may account for the glomerulonephritis of late onset observed in mice congenitally infected with LCM (Hotchin & Collins, 1964). This is seen also in 'germ-free' mice carrying LCM (Pollard, Kajima & Sharon, 1968).

Recher *et al.* (1966) reported the presence of glomerulonephritis in AKR and BALB/c mice developing spontaneous lymphatic leukaemia or inoculated with Gross passage A, Friend or Rauscher leukaemogenic viruses. Their electron microscopic studies of AKR mice showed mature virus particles in the renal lesions (unlike those in the animals we studied). Possibly a higher level of viraemia, with secondary deposition of virus in the kidney, occurs in the AKR mice. Recher *et al.* suggest that glomerulonephritis may be the result of an autoimmune reaction to a tissue antigen altered by viral infection. From inspection of their electron micrographs, an immune complex disease seems more likely. In irradiated AKR mice receiving syngeneic bone marrow, a manipulation preventing leukaemia prolongs life and survivors die of renal disease (Uphoff, 1969); again, an immune complex aetiology seems probable.

Several strains of mice, including BALB/c, develop renal lesions as they grow old, and these are intensified by radiation (Guttman & Kohn, 1960). Such lesions were observed in our BALB/c controls, although they were much less conspicuous than in those neonatally infected with MLV. Evidence is also accumulating that most strains of mice, including BALB/c, carry a leukaemogenic virus, even when in the 'germ-free' state (Kajima & Pollard, 1965; Hartley *et al.*, 1969). Perhaps all of these viruses are able to elicit some antibody response in the hosts, with the possible development of immune complex disease. As a rule the complexes accumulate slowly, so that they are seen only in ageing animals. However, when the balance is disturbed by irradiation, by introducing a new virus, e.g. MLV or LCM, into hosts, or when there is an unusual immune response—as in NZB mice—immune complex diseases, such as glomerulonephritis, are intensified and appear earlier. The existence of similar glomerular lesions in other species of ageing experimental animals, including rats and hamsters (Guttman & Kohn, 1960), suggests a comparable aetiology, although further observations are required to establish the point. A comparable but more extreme manifestation is the glomerulonephritis accompanying Aleutian mink disease (Henson *et al.*, 1968), which is associated with the deposition of virus antigen–antibody complexes in the renal glomeruli (Porter *et al.*, 1969).

ACKNOWLEDGMENTS

We acknowledge the skilful technical assistance of Mrs Maureen Bedford. We are grateful to Mr B. Auger of the Imperial Cancer Research Fund for kindly preparing the light micrographs.

REFERENCES

AOKI, T., BOYSE, E.A. & OLD, L.J. (1968) Wild-type Gross leukaemia virus. I. Soluble antigen (GSA) in the plasma and tissues of infected mice. *J. nat. Cancer Inst.* **41**, 89.

ASHE, W.K. & NOTKINS, A.L. (1966) Neutralization of an infectious herpes simplex virus-antibody complex by anti-γ-globulin. *Proc. nat. Acad. Sci. (Wash)*, **56**, 447.

AXELRAD, A. (1965) Antigenic behaviour of lymphoma cell populations in mice as revealed by the spleen colony method. *Prog. exp. Tumor Res. (Basel)*, **6**, 30.

BORAKER, D.K. & HILDEMANN, W.H. (1965) Maturation of alloimmune responsiveness in mice. *Transplantation*, **3**, 202.

BURNET, F.M. & FENNER, F. (1949) *The Production of Antibodies* 2nd ed. Macmillan, Melbourne.

CRABTREE, C.E. (1940) Sex differences in the structure of Bowman's capsule in the mouse. *Science*, **91**, 299.

DIXON, F.J., FELDMAN, J.D. & VAZQUEZ, J.J. (1961) Experimental glomerulonephritis. The pathogenesis of a laboratory model resembling the spectrum of human glomerulonephritis. *J. exp. Med.* **113**, 899.

DUNN, T.B. & GREEN, A.W. (1966) Morphology of BALB/c mice inoculated with Rauscher virus. *J. nat. Cancer Inst.* **36**, 987.

DUNN, T.B., MALMGREN, R.A., CARNEY, P.G. & GREEN, A.W. (1966). Propylthiouracil and transfusion modifications of the effects of the Rauscher virus in BALB/c mice. *J. nat. Cancer Inst.* **36**, 1003.

EAST, J. & BRANCA, M. (1969) Autoimmune reactions and malignant changes in germ-free New Zealand Black mice. *Clin. Exp. Immunol.* **4**, 621.

FELDMAN, J.D. (1963) Pathogenesis of ultrastructural glomerular changes induced by immunological means (Ed. by P. Grabar & P. Miescher), *Immunopathology*, vol. 3, p. 263. Benno Schwabe, Basel.

FELDMAN, J.D. (1964) Ultrastructure of immunological processes. *Adv. Immunol.* **4**, 175.

FINK, M.A. (1970) *Proc. 4th Quadrennial Cancer Conference*, p. 211. University Press, Perugia.

GUTTMAN, P.H. & KOHN, H.I. (1960) Progressive intercapillary glomerulosclerosis in the mouse, rat and Chinese hamster, associated with ageing and X-ray exposure. *Amer. J. Path.* **37**, 293.

HARTLEY, J.W., ROWE, W.P., CAPPS. W.I. & HUEBNER, R.J. (1969) Isolation of naturally occurring viruses of the murine leukaemia group in tissue culture. *J. Virol.* **3**, 126.

HARVEY, J.J. & EAST, J. (1969) Biological activity and separation of a leukaemogenic virus from murine sarcoma virus-Harvey (MSV-H). *Int. J. Cancer*, **4**, 655.

HELYER, B.J. & HOWIE, J.B. (1963) Spontaneous auto-immune disease in NZB/BL mice. *Brit. J. Haematol.* **9**, 119.

HENSON, J.B., GORHAM, J.R. TANAKA, Y. & PADGETT, G.A. (1968) The sequential development of ultrastructural lesions in the glomeruli of mink with the experimental Aleutian disease. *Lab. Invest.* **19**, 153.

HIRSCH, M.S., ALLISON, A.C. & HARVEY, J.J. (1969) Immune complexes in mice neonatally infected with Moloney leukaemogenic and murine sarcoma viruses. *Nature (Lond.)* **223**, 739.

HIRSCH, M.S. & HARVEY, J.J. (1969) A spleen weight assay for murine sarcoma virus Harvey (MSV-H). *Int. J. Cancer.* **4**, 440.

HOLMES, M.D. & BURNET, F.M. (1963) The natural history of autoimmune disease in NZB mice. *Ann. intern. Med.* **59**, 265.

HOTCHIN, J. (1962) The biology of lymphocytic choriomeningitis infection: virus induced immune disease. *Cold. Spr. Harb. Symp. quant. Biol.* **27**, 479.

HOTCHIN, J. & COLLINS, D.N. (1964) Glomerulonephritis and late onset disease of mice following neonatal virus infection. *Nature (Lond.)* **203**, 1357.

HOWIE, J.B. & HELYER, B.J. (1968) The immunology and pathology of NZB mice. *Advan. Immunol.* **9**, 215.

KAJIMA, M. & POLLARD, M. (1965) Detection of virus-like particles in germ-free mice. *J. Bacteriol.* **90**, 1448.

KLEIN, E. & KLEIN, G. (1965) Antibody response and leukaemia development in mice inoculated neonatally with the Moloney virus. *Cancer Res.* **25**, 851.

KLEIN, E. & KLEIN, G. (1966) Immunological tolerance of neonatally infected mice to the Moloney leukaemia virus. *Nature (Lond.)* **209**, 163.

LAMBERT, P.H. & DIXON, F.J. (1968) Pathogenesis of the glomerulonephritis of NZB/W mice. *J. exp. Med.* **127**, 507.

MANALIGOD, J.R., PIRANI, C.L. MIYASATO, F. & POLLAK, V.E. (1967) The renal changes in NZB/B1 and NZB-NZW F_1 hybrid mice. Light and electron microscopic studies. *Nephron,* **4**, 215.

MELLORS, R.C., AOKI, T. & HEUBNER, R.J. (1969) Further implication of murine leukaemia-like virus in the disorders of NZB mice. *J. exp. Med.* **129**, 1045.

NOTKINS, A.L. (1968) Neutralization of sensitized virus by anti-γ-globulin. *Perspect. Virology,* **6**, 189.

NOTKINS, A.L., MAHAR, S., SCHEELE, C. & GOFFMAN, J. (1966) Infectious virus-antibody complex in the blood of chronically infected mice. *J. exp. Med.* **124**, 81.

NOWINSKI, R.C., OLD, L.J., BOYSE, E.A., DE HARVEN, E. & GEERING, G. (1968) Group-specific viral antigens in the milk and tissues of mice infected with mammary tumour virus or Gross leukaemia virus. *Virology,* **34**, 617.

OLDSTONE, M.B.A. & DIXON, F.J. (1967) Lymphocytic choriomeningitis: production of antibody by 'tolerant' infected mice. *Science,* **158**, 1193.

OLDSTONE, M.B.A. & DIXON, F.J. (1969) Pathogenesis of chronic disease associated with persistent lymphocytic choriomeningitis viral infection. I. Relationship of antibody production to disease in neonatally infected mice. *J. exp. Med.* **129**, 483.

POLLARD, M., KAJIMA, M. & SHARON, N. (1968) LCM Virus-induced Immunopathology in Congenitally infected Gnotobiotic mice. *Perspect. Virology,* **6**, 193.

PORTER, D.D., LARSEN, A.E. & PORTER, H.G. (1969) The pathogenesis of Aleutian disease of mink. I. *In vivo* viral replication and the host antibody response to viral antigen. *J. exp. Med.,* **130**, 575.

RECHER, L., TANAKA, T., SYKES, J.A., YUMUTO, T., SEMAN, G., YOUNG, L. & DMOCHOWSKI, L. (1966) Further studies on the biological relationship of murine leukaemia viruses and on kidney lesions of mice with leukaemia induced by these viruses. *J. nat. Cancer Inst. Monogr.* **22**, 459.

SOOTHILL, J.F., HAYES, K. & DUDGEON, J.A. (1966) The immunoglobulins in congenital rubella. *Lancet,* **i**, 1385.

UNANUE, E.R. & DIXON, F.J. (1967) Experimental glomerulonephritis: immunological events and pathogenetic mechanisms. *Advan. Immunol.* **6**, 1.

UPHOFF, D.E. (1969) Longevity of AKR mice increased by reduced incidence of thymic lymphomas. *Transplantation,* **8**, 203.

VOLKERT, M. & HANNOVER-LARSEN, J. (1965) Immunological tolerance to viruses. *Progr. med. Virol.* **7**, 160.

Virus, Cell Surface, and Self:
Lymphocytic Choriomeningitis of Mice

John Hotchin, M.D., Ph.D.

The name "arenovirus"[83] has been proposed to include the LCM group, Machupo,[68] Lassa,[15] and similar viruses. They are pleomorphic virions, 50 to 200 mμ in diameter, usually spherical or cup-shaped, containing several ribonuclease-sensitive electron dense granules.[18] The particles are formed by budding and are covered by spiked processes; their nucleic acid appears to be RNA.[14, 22, 74] The virus grows *in vitro* in many kinds of mammalian tissue, *e.g.,*

Supported in part by grant 5-RO1-A1-03846-06 from the National Institutes of Health.

mouse,[36] monkey,[3] and human,[9, 71] usually
without CPE, which when present is only
partial and temporary. The ability of tissue
cultures to become persistently infected
with LCM virus after temporary CPE is
probably responsible for conflicting reports
concerning LCM-CPE in mouse strain L
cells.[9, 41, 72, 97] The synthesis of viral antigens *in vitro* can be visualized by immunofluorescent staining with anti-LCM serum.[10]

The Effects of Acute LCM Infection Upon the Mouse

Although LCM virus induces disease in
the rat, guinea pig, and monkey, mice (the
natural host) have proven to be the most
useful laboratory animals. Several other
species, including chicks, dogs, rabbits, and
hamsters, develop inapparent infection. Intracerebral (IC) inoculation of mice has
been the classical method of propagating
the virus; acute disease begins 5 to 7 days
later. The mice are hunched and ruffled
and have blepharitis and facial edema.
Fatal convulsions are likely to occur at 6
to 8 days. The convulsions frequently can
be initiated by disturbing the mice, especially when vertigo is induced by spinning
affected animals by the tail. High doses of
virus sometimes induce lower mortality
than lower doses,[44] and the mice that re-
cover are persistently infected. Some (viscerotropic) LCM strains cause few or no
convulsions, but tend to induce a wasting
disease with death at 10 to 20 days.[44] Intra-
nasal (IN) or subcutaneous (SC) inoculation produces mild illness with low mortality, followed by immunity. Intraperi-
toneal (IP) inoculation causes fatal disease,
sometimes convulsive, but often with the
formation of peritoneal and pleural exu-
dates which may be severe enough to cause
obvious respiratory distress.[80] Inoculation
of the footpad causes well-marked swelling
8 to 15 days later.[42] Detailed clinical and
pathologic effects of LCM have been reviewed by Farmer and Janeway,[21] Maurer,[64]
and Lillie and Armstrong.[60] Most organs of
the animal are affected, including CNS,
lungs, liver, and kidneys, and these show
severe cellular infiltration and destruction.
The CNS changes include meningitis and
mild encephalitis. Familiarity with the extensive cellular destruction in acute murine
LCM makes the complete protection which
is afforded by immune suppressants seem
very remarkable, particularly when it is
realized that in the presence of immune
suppression virus multiplication continues
in an unabated but harmless manner.

Immunofluorescent studies by several
groups[10, 13, 66, 67, 79] have shown generalized virus replication in almost all organs
and cell types beginning 24 hr. after LCM
infection of the mouse. In the brain, antigen is found mainly in the choroid plexus,
ependyma, and leptomeninges, with relatively little antigen in brain parenchyma.
Antigen has been found in peripheral leukocytes[5] from the seventh day onwards.

The Effects of Chronic LCM Infection on the Mouse

After inoculation of mice with LCM
virus by various routes, a proportion of
animals survive. These fall into two categories, according to whether they are persistently infected with virus or have suppressed the infection. Persistently infected
survivors of LCM inoculation into adult
mice are more numerous following high
inoculum doses; for this reason the effect
was initially termed high dose immune
paralysis (HDIP).[44] In newborn[35, 38] or congenitally[90] infected mice, inoculation of
most mouse strains results in a very high
proportion of survivors, all of which remain persistently infected for their entire
life spans. The proportion of survivors is
directly related to the viscerotropic qualities of the virus strain.[43, 56, 57, 94] Neuro-
tropic strains tend to kill newborn mice.[43]
After neonatal inoculation some mice (depending on mouse and virus strain) become

Table 1. The Chief Features of Different Types of Murine LCM Infection*

Age of Mouse	Inoculum Size ID_{50}	Route	Type of Infection	Time of Appearance of Antibody			Duration of Virus Persistence in	
				FAB†	CF	N	Blood	Kidney
One day	All	All	PTI	M—8 days I—36 days	—	—	Lifelong	Lifelong
Six weeks	$>10^4$ 10^1–10^3	IC,IP,IV All	HDIP Acute	6–7 days 6–7 days	7–8 d 7–8 d	6–12 mo. 6–12 mo.	6–10 mo. 2–4 weeks	10–12 mo. 2–4 mo.
Two to six mo.	$>10^5$ $>10^5$	IC,IP,IV All	HDIP Acute	6–7 days 6–7 days	7–8 d 7–8 d	6–12 mo. ?	3–6 mo. 2–3 weeks	6–9 mo. 2–4 mo.

* These figures are approximate and are based on results using the WE strain of LCM and Albany strain albino mice.

† M = maternal; I = infant.

runted [36, 38, 93] for a few weeks, whereas others show no illness. All survivors weigh a few Grams less than control mice throughout their remaining life spans.

A summary of the main differences between the various types of LCM infection in mice is shown in Table 1. All of these types can be viewed as basically similar host–virus interactions in which the main variable is the intensity of the host immune response to the virus. Acute infection results in the most intense response which, if not fatal, normally results in rapid virus suppression. The immune response in chronic HDIP infection is much less severe, and although fluorescent and complement-fixing antibody is demonstrably present,[49] there appears to be a severe impairment of the cellular homograft rejection component. The duration of viremia is dependent on many host and virus-controlled variables of which a very significant one is host age at the time of inoculation. Younger animals exhibit more severe impairment of their immune response and apparently have greater difficulty in suppressing the infection.

The slow disease manifestations of persistent murine LCM include chronic glomerulonephritis,[13, 16, 34, 41, 45, 69, 75, 76, 93, 100] pyelonephritis,[16] splenic hyperplasia, hepatitis, and hypergammaglobulinemia.[75, 76] Immunofluorescent study has shown [13, 66, 100] that almost all tissues of neonatally and congenitally LCM-infected mice contain viral antigen for many months. Older animals show a relative disappearance of antigen.[66, 100] Some strains of mice and LCM virus do not produce slow disease after congenital infection.[66, 67, 95]

The Pathogenesis of LCM Lesions

The role of the immune response in the causation of lesions in acute LCM has been clarified by a wide variety of different immunosuppressive measures. X-irradiation of the host prior to inoculation with LCM was found [81] to confer protection and to prevent the pathologic histology previously attributed to a direct effect of the virus [17, 35–37, 39, 99] (Fig. 1). The x-irradiation severely reduced the peripheral leukocyte count and abolished virus-induced lesions but had no effect on virus growth or titer. A similar ameliorative effect on virus-induced tissue lesions has been noted with St. Louis encephalitis [25] and Langat viruses.[98] The use of other immune suppressive agents has confirmed the original concept that the major part of clinical LCM disease is caused by a homograft rejection of virus-infected tissue.[41] This conclusion

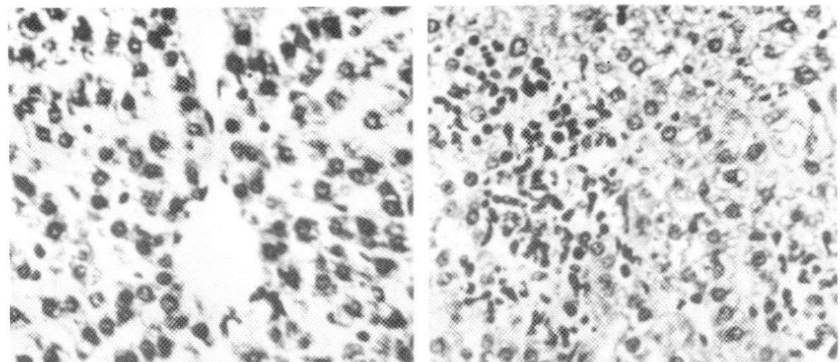

FIG. 1. The histology of mouse hepatic tissue 6 days after IP inoculation with LCM virus. Sections are from different mice, both of which received similar virus inoculations; the mouse from which the section on the left was taken received 350 r. of whole-body x-irradiation 24 hr. prior to virus. This section lacked the pathologic changes caused by LCM virus and was essentially normal. Virus titers in the two livers were the same.

has been based on a considerable volume of work with amethopterin,[6, 8, 27, 28, 41, 58, 59] myleran,[7] cortisone,[36] BCNU,[84] neonatal thymectomy,[19, 20, 46, 82, 85] antilymphocytic serum (ALS),[24, 61, 96] and antimouse thymocyte serum (AMT).[32-34] All of these agents conferred protection against the virus without interfering with its multiplication. They all interfered with the cellular immune response to the virus, but in the case of antilymphocyte or antithymocyte serum, allowed the humoral antibody response to "soluble" viral products to continue unchecked. This situation has been referred to as "split tolerance,"[34] and the antibody formation was believed to be the cause of chronic glomerulonephritis. A similar "split tolerance" can also be caused by high virus doses alone, and has been called the "high dose immune paralysis," or HDIP phenomenon.[12, 44] Several variations of this effect have been described[53, 55] with different levels of viremia and antibody.

The Mechanism of LCM Virus Tolerance and Disease

In general, the concept propounded by the author[35, 41]—that LCM disease in the mouse is due mainly to an immunologic conflict—appears to have gained general acceptance from workers in the field.[57, 82, 91, 92] The concept is summarized in Figure 2. The virus is seen as an agent capable of modifying the infected cell surface in an immunologically recognizable way by the insertion of new antigen in the outer cell membrane. The new antigen is recognized by the immunologic surveillance mechanism of the host, and a cellular immune response is initiated by the thymus-dependent lymphoid system. The resulting sensitized lymphocytes are capable of lysing the infected cells with which they come in contact. This constitutes a homograft rejection by the host of its own virus-infected tissue. The resulting tissue damage may be lethal, and in any event results in the liberation of large amounts of host and viral antigens into the tissue fluids. These antigens are then free to stimulate a powerful humoral antibody response. At the present time it seems likely that this mechanism may be a general phenomenon with many (but not all) of the persistent viruses and slow virus diseases. There is good evidence[77] that it holds true for Aleutian mink disease. It seems safe to predict that the same mechanism will prove to be operative for several other agents, perhaps including equine infectious anemia, African swine fever, and conceivably, human serum hepatitis.

Does Persistent Tolerant Infection of Mice with LCM Cause Generalized Disease?

In the foregoing section it was pointed out that some workers have reported the absence of disease in mice with lifelong persistent LCM virus infection, although others report multiple pathologic lesions. These variations can probably be explained by genetic differences in the mouse and virus strains used. However, the question remains as to how much the observed lesions, which are mainly vascular, can be explained on the basis of secondary effects of capillary blockage by antigen–antibody precipitates. Therefore, a quantitative study of parameters of control and LCM-infected mice was made over a two-year period, to establish whether significant changes occurred. This study had the advantage of quantitative (weight) measurements which eliminated the "background noise" inherent in a pathologic study of mice which develop multiple lesions in the control population, during a prolonged experiment.

Variables measured consisted of weight changes of liver, kidney, spleen, and thymus, leukocyte count, hematocrit, and renal function. The experimental animals con-

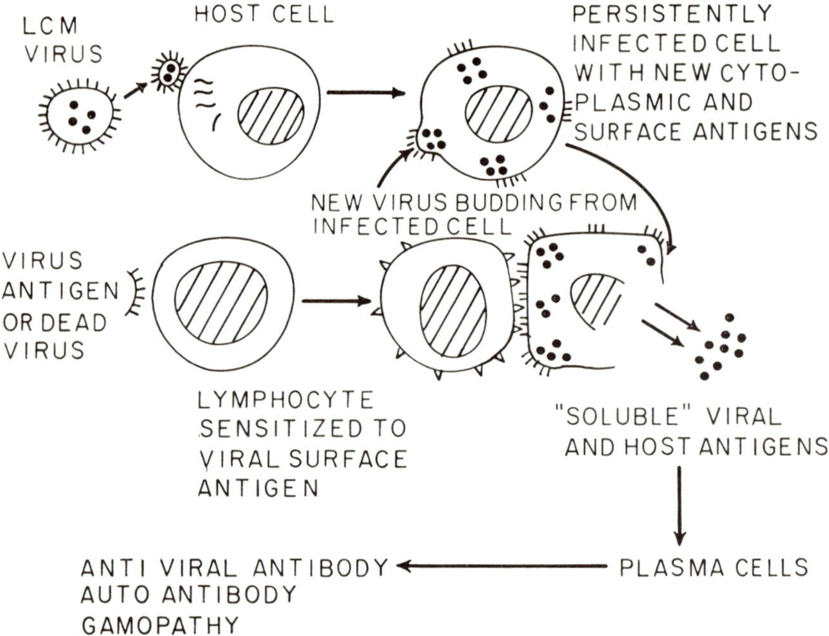

Fig. 2. Diagram of the pathogenetic mechanism of LCM virus infection. After infection of a host cell, a new antigen appears in the surface and virus particles bud from the surface. Thymus-dependent lymphocytes become sensitized to the new antigen, possibly *via* dead virus particles, and are then able to cause the lysis of infected cells. Soluble host and viral antigens are then released into the circulation and stimulate the formation of humoral antibodies.

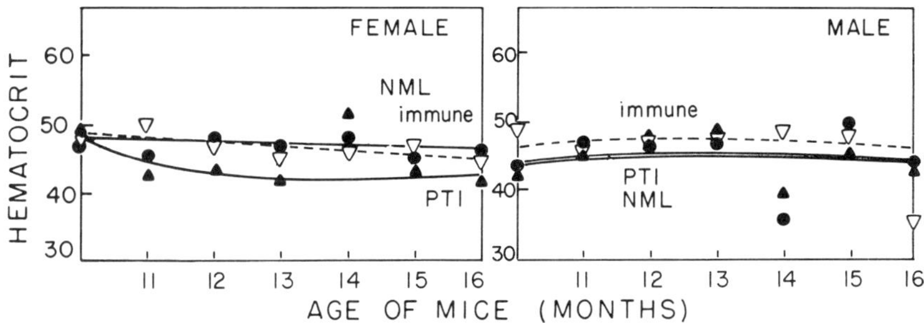

FIG. 3. The changes in hematocrits of the blood of mice. PTI = mice with persistent tolerant LCM virus infection following IC inoculation at birth. Immune = mice which received SC LCM inoculation at 1 month of age. NML = control mice which received an IP injection of normal mouse liver suspension at birth.

sisted of groups of mice inoculated with LCM virus or control normal mouse tissue.

Materials and Methods

Virus

The strain of LCM virus was the same as that used in previous experiments.[41] It was a "docile" strain with a high tolerance-inducing capacity.[40] Virus was stored at −90 C. as 20% liver suspension, and a 10^{-3} dilution in GTH diluent (gelatin 0.05% in Hanks' saline buffer with Tris in place of bicarbonate) was used as inoculum in all experiments. Normal mouse liver (NML) suspension (20%) was used for the control animals at the same dilutions.

Mice

The strain of mice used was the "Albany" albino strain from a colony developed 20 years ago in this laboratory. Mice were used at 12 hr. of age except where indicated. All offspring were used on the same day and randomized before allocation into groups. Collection of mice of known age was carried out according to the method previously described.[40]

Inoculation

Intracerebral (IC) and subcutaneous (SC) inoculations were made with 0.02 ml. inoc-

ula. Dilutions were made in GTH throughout and kept at 0 C. before use. Each newborn mouse's tail was clipped after inoculation to ensure later elimination of any additional (uninoculated) mice born during the experiments.

Weight Measurements of Mice

All mice were checked daily after initial inoculations for any acute deaths. Approximately 28 to 35 days postinoculation mice were sexed and pooled into separate groups, males and females. They were weighed monthly and checked weekly for any unusual signs, such as late disease, ruffled fur, hunched back, and tumors.

Bleeding

Orbital bleeding of the mice under ether anesthesia was performed using a Pasteur pipette. Leukocyte counts were made using the Becton-Dickinson Unopette technic. Hematocrit values were determined by centrifugation of blood samples in an Adams Readocrit and the per cent based on the length of packed erythrocytes divided by the length of erythrocytes plus serum.

Creatinine Clearance

Mice were starved overnight and then given 1,850 mg. creatinine per kg. intraperitoneally (IP) and 1½ hr. later bled orbitally. Analysis of the plasma (0.1 ml.) was performed according to the Jaffy reaction[2] and expressed as milligrams of creatinine per 100 ml. plasma.

Experimental Design

Time and Route of Inoculation

The inoculation routines were the following:

(1) IC inoculation into 12-hour-old mice of a 20% suspension of NML diluted 10^{-3}.

(2) No inoculation; normal controls.

(3) IC inoculation of LCM (UBC, M/B_6L_{11}, Pool A-319 mouse liver) diluted to 10^{-3} into 12-hour-old mice (persistently infected group).

(4) SC inoculation of LCM (UBC, M/B_6L_{11}, Pool A-319 mouse liver) diluted to 10^{-3} into one-month-old mice (immune group, which had suppressed the virus infection).

For each of these groups, 20 litters of Albany mice were used. Each litter, with the mother, was kept in a small individual cage for 21 days postinoculation, after which they were weaned and pooled—40 mice to one large cage.

Tissue Sampling

Four mice (two males and two females) were removed monthly from each group. Two representative mice, one male and one female, were photographed. All mice were weighed individually and then bled out under anesthesia; a portion of the blood was taken for leukocyte count and hematocrit estimation. In addition, the liver, kidneys, spleen, and thymus of each mouse were dried and weighed separately.

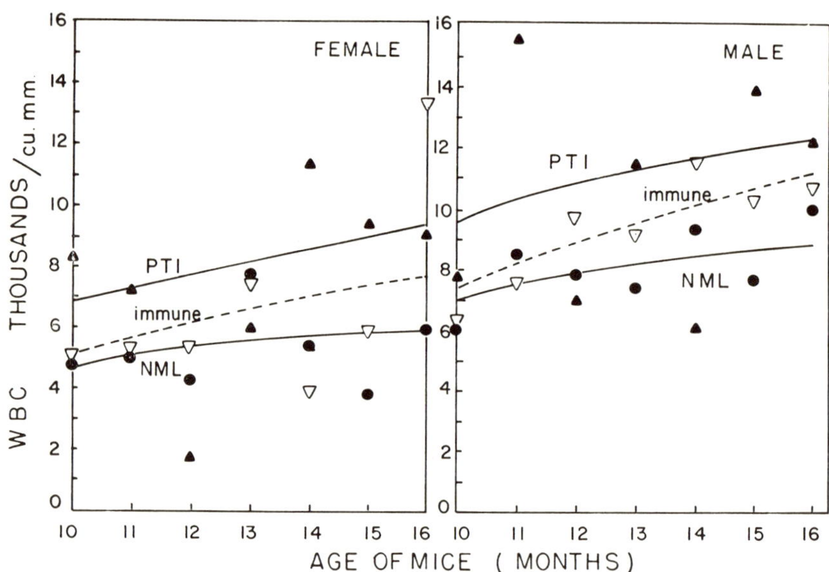

Fig. 4. The changes in leukocyte counts of mice with and without LCM infection. Key to abbreviations is given in Figure 3.

Results

Effects of Persistent Tolerant LCM Infection

Appearance. The previously described clinical features of late disease [41] were confirmed, with particular emphasis on the hunched position, wasting, and the unkempt appearance of the mice. In addition, considerable weakness was often evident, particularly of the hind limbs of the animals. Observation of the various control groups indicated that kinking of the tail was not confined to old persistent tolerantly infected (PTI) mice as previously thought, but was also present in other groups. This may be a reaction to frequent handling of the animals *via* the tail with forceps.

The comparison of weight-gain curves for the various groups showed a consistent progressive relative loss in the weights of PTI mice.

Hematocrit and Leukocyte Count. Observation of PTI mice with clinical disease gave an impression of pallor, as judged by the color of the ears, skin, and tail vein of the infected mice. Previous work [47] had shown that PTI mice have lower erythrocyte counts than immune mice. To test for the occurrence of anemia or leukopenia, hematocrits and leukocyte counts were performed on groups of PTI, immune, and NML control mice at monthly intervals. Slightly lower hematocrit values were observed in the female PTI mice compared with the control groups (NML and immune), as can be seen in Figure 3. The male mice showed very little difference between groups. The female PTI mice had slightly lower values, on the borderline of significance. For adult mice normal hematocrit is 42% and leukocyte count 4,000 to 12,000 cells per cu. mm.[86] In Figure 4, higher leukocyte counts are evident in the PTI groups, especially in the males, since four of the seven values lie on or above the 11,000 mark; however, the overall analysis of each group over the 10 months indicates no significant differences in count between immune and PTI groups, although both are higher than the NML control.

Harvesting of Organs from PTI, Immune, and NML Mice. Four mice (two males and two females) from each inoculum type (LCM-PTI, NML, and LCM immune) were removed and sacrificed each

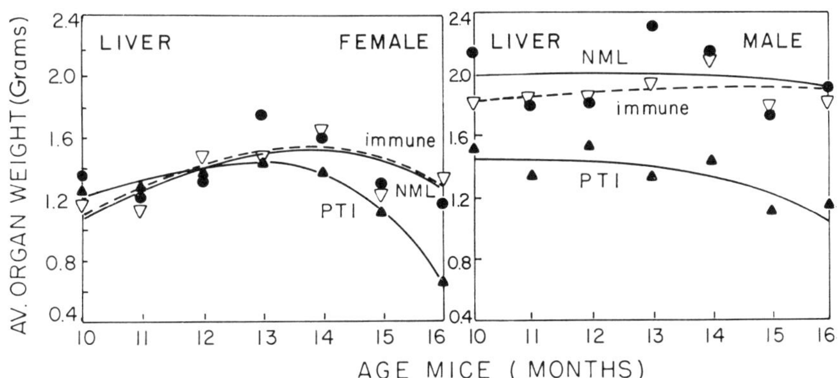

Fig. 5. Hepatic weight changes in mice with and without LCM infection. Key to abbreviations is given in Figure 3.

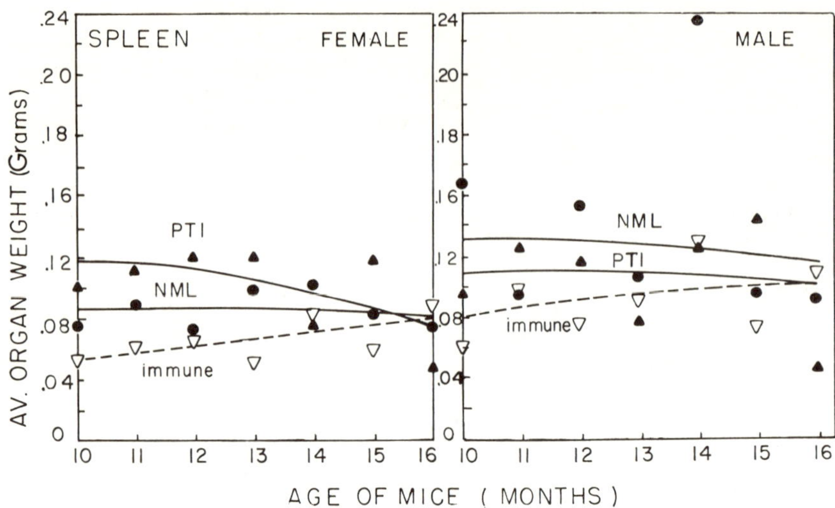

FIG. 6. Splenic weight changes in mice with and without LCM infection. Key to abbreviations is given in Figure 3.

month; the liver, spleen, kidneys, and thymus were harvested, blotted on filter paper, and then weighed. The monthly weights for each organ were averaged and plotted for each sex (Figures 5 through 8). Comparison with the average weights showed that the PTI mice have small kidneys (Fig. 7) particularly the males, which had fairly gross differences in comparison with NML and immune mice. The liver (Fig. 5) also showed some diminution in size in the PTI mice, particularly males, but this was less marked than the diminution of the kidneys. Spleens (Fig. 6) showed a mixed response, the females exhibiting some increases in size in the PTI animals, whereas males' spleens were the same size as the controls, although among the NML male mice, there were three spleens with unusually high weights, which tended to make the PTI male spleen weight seem low. The thymus (Fig. 8) showed a fairly consistent diminution in weight in PTI animals, both male and female.

Creatinine Clearance. Due to the apparent localization of the LCM late disease process in the kidneys of the affected animals,[4, 45] additional studies were carried out to determine the levels of creatinine clearance in PTI animals of various ages. The results of such an experiment can be seen in Figure 9. In the control animals a slight slope does occur over the range from 3 months to 26 months; however, the slope of the line of this group is less obvious than that in the PTI group, in which a marked decrease in creatinine clearance can be seen, starting from nine months of age and increasing substantially to 18 months of age.

The main conclusion from these results was that persistent LCM infection caused:

(1) A diminution in size of the kidney.

(2) A similar, but less marked, diminution in size of the liver.

(3) Elevation of the leukocyte count.

(4) All of these effects (1–3) were more marked in **male mice.**

(5) Inoculation of the same amount of virus at one month of age did not cause these effects, *i.e.*, the PTI state was necessary.

(6) The infection did not cause anemia.

(7) The rate of creatinine clearance from LCM–PTI mice for a standardized period of time was much less than that of controls.

From these experiments it was clear that the LCM virus inoculation was responsible for the late onset of disease previously described [41, 47] and that the disease occurred only when the virus was inoculated close to the time of birth under conditions which induce a persistent tolerant infection. Apparently the protracted infection, with continuous high levels of virus multiplication made possible by the tolerant state of the host, is necessary in order to produce this disease. The main macroscopic changes were confirmed to be in the kidney, and consisted of marked diminution in size, particularly in the male. Normally, even in advanced wasting, the undamaged kidney does not change in size.[73] These changes are accompanied by similar but less marked

shrinkage of the liver. Thus, the major lesion of the virus-induced disease appears to be in the kidney, but it may be significant that the liver also is involved; further investigation may show a pathogenic feature common to both organs. These changes do not constitute evidence of a gross generalized disease process, and could be secondary manifestations of impaired capillary circulation. It is well known[26, 87–89] that LCM virus is excreted by the kidney in acute and chronic LCM infection; however, in the acute disease, there is no evidence of any pathologic process[3, 21] comparable to late-onset glomerulonephritis or experimental chronic glomerulonephritis.[23] The low creatinine values of the 18-month PTI mice may be due to the high mortality rate of the sick animals and the fact that the animals tested were not a true representation of this group, the more severely affected ones having died. The commencement of impaired kidney function coincides with the onset of clinical disease, suggesting a correlation between the two. Low creatinine values for the five- and seven-month

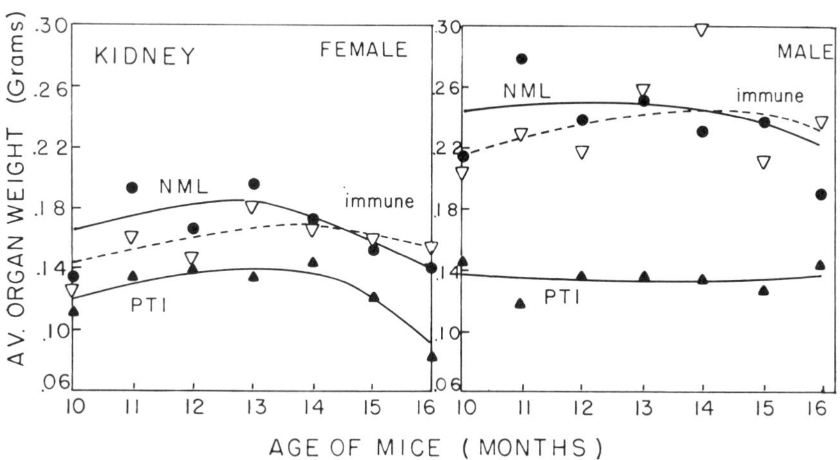

Fig. 7. Renal weight changes in mice with and without LCM infection. Key to abbreviations is given in Figure 3.

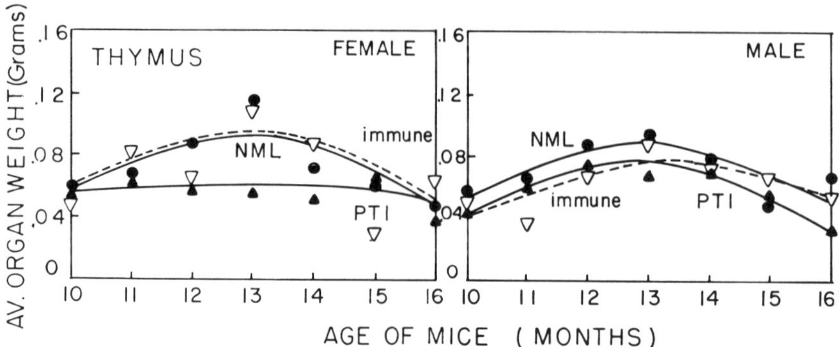

FIG. 8. Thymic weight changes in mice with and without LCM infection. Key to abbreviations given in Figure 3.

PTI mice may be a consequence of the early phase of the pathogenetic process, conceivably causing a compensatory increase in glomerular filtration rates.

Similar glomerular lesions are also found in viral leukemic mice,[78] NZB mice,[30, 63, 65] and mice with Aleutian mink disease.[31, 52] In these diseases a comparable mechanism is plausible, involving the production of antigen–antibody complexes and consequent glomerular blockage. In the LCM model, a gradual loss of tolerance would provide a logical explanation for the slow production of such immune complexes. The finding of low levels of antibody to LCM antigens in these mice[12] indicates that this type of declining tolerance may be the rule for neonatal LCM infection. Animals made tolerant when adult have higher levels of antibody and lose tolerance more rapidly. Until recently it was generally believed that mice do not normally produce neutralizing antibody to LCM virus. However, studies have shown[48] that mice can readily make high titers of this antibody, but that this occurs only many months after infection. These two facts render a gradual immune response against previously tolerated LCM infection a plausible explanation for an immune complex origin for LCM glomerulonephritis, but

this may be only a part of a subtle pathogenetic mechanism beyond the resolution of these experiments. Complement-fixing antibody has been reported to be eluted from LCM glomerulonephritic kidneys[69]; however, this report did not mention control of the anticomplementary substances reported[29] to be present in large amount in eluates made by comparable procedures.

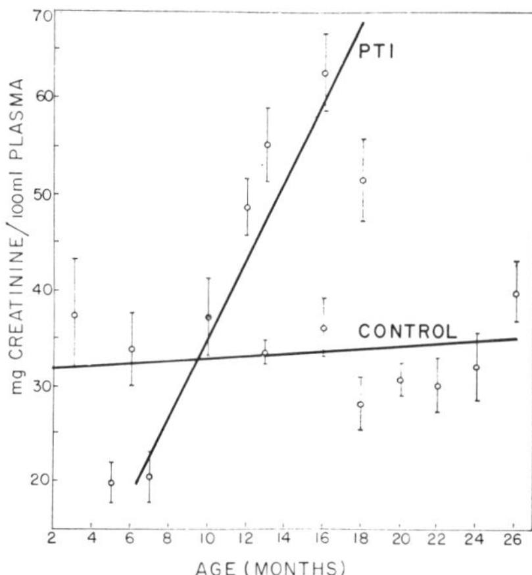

FIG. 9. Creatine values of mouse blood after a standard injection of creatinine. High values indicate impaired kidney function. PTI = mice with persistent tolerant LCM infection following neonatal inoculation. Control = normal mice.

FIG. 10. Diagram illustrating the complex nature of the LCM antigen–antibody-containing elements of the kidney in mice with persistent LCM infection. Glomeruli contain deposits of possible antigen–antibody complexes; the cortex and medulla also contain infiltrated round cells capable of making antibody. Both cortex and medulla contain cells rich in soluble antigen and both contain free virus at titers of 10^3–10^7 ID_{50} per Gm. The blood contained in the kidney carries virus (of average titer 10^5), variable levels of CF antibody, "fluorescent" antibody, and anticomplementary antigen–antibody complexes. Antibody extracted from kidneys of this type may have come from blood or plasma cells, which constitute a much greater section area than the glomeruli.

It is clear (Fig. 10) that other interpretations for the origin of antigen–antibody complexes reported in kidney eluates are possible, and a cautious interpretation appears to be prudent at the present time. The round cell infiltration found in the renal lesions [4] indicates a cellular immune response of considerable magnitude. The possibility remains that much of the tissue damage in these mice is caused by a prolonged, very low level cellular immune response. The presence of circulating virus–antibody complexes in the murine circulation apparently does not necessarily cause significant glomerulonephritis, as is shown by the example of lactic dehydrogenase virus.* Some of the earliest lesions in acute LCM occur in the reticuloendothelial system and capillary endothelium.† It seems quite possible

---

* Notkins, A., personal communication.
† Niven, J., and Hotchin, J., unpublished observations.

that LCM causes a generalized endothelial infection with production of antigen in the endothelial cell surface. In this event, the glomerulonephritis and arteritis may be local manifestations of a generalized vascular infection. A final resolution of the mechanism involved must await more delicate immunologic methods for investigating tissue damage.

The Key Role of the Cell Surface in LCM Virus-Induced Autoimmune Disease

Several aspects of the foregoing pathogenetic mechanisms are of special importance. These include the ability of the virus to induce membrane change and the host cellular response. The virus has recently been characterized by electron microscopy [18, 51] and the presence of immunologically specific antigens in the surface of infected cells has been demonstrated by the same technic.[1] Immunofluorescent methods have been used in my laboratory to demonstrate (Fig. 11) that LCM infected BHK21 cells have a surface antigen which is virus-induced, and which reacts with specific

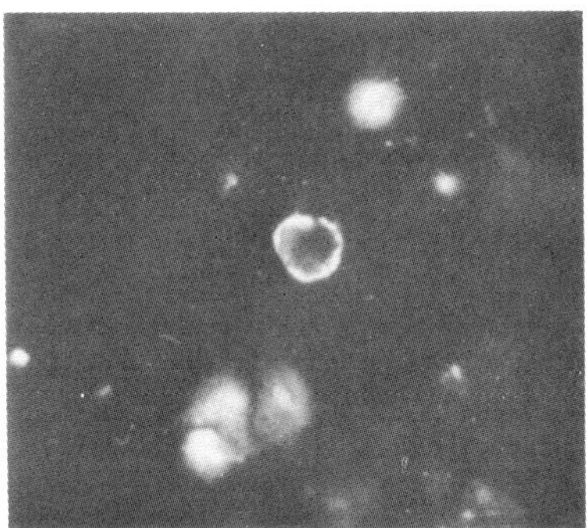

FIG. 11. Fluorescent photomicrograph of cells stained for LCM antigen by indirect immunofluorescence. The culture was infected with LCM virus 48 hr. previously and contained a low proportion of infected cells, one of which shows ring fluorescence. This type of fluorescent staining was completely absent in control, uninfected cultures or in infected cultures exposed to normal mouse serum.

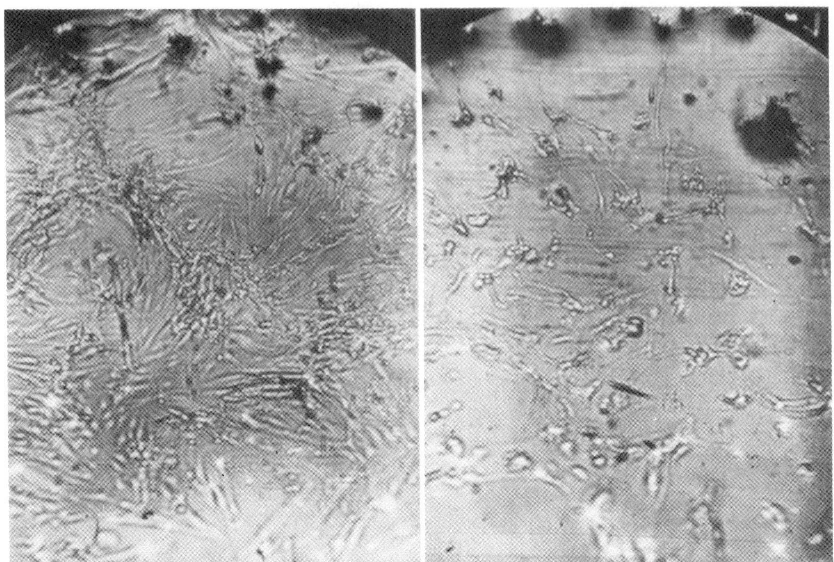

FIG. 12 (left). Cultured monolayer of testis cells from a mouse persistently infected with LCM virus. Photographed 6 days after addition of normal mouse lymphocytes to the culture. Minimal cytopathic effects.

FIG. 13 (right). Cultured monolayer of testis cells from a mouse persistently infected with LCM virus. Photographed 6 days after addition of lymphocytes from a mouse which had suppressed LCM infection 14 days previously. This monolayer has suffered a severe cytopathic response following the addition of LCM immune lymphocytes.

anti-LCM antibody. The cellular immune cytolytic effect is shown in Figures 12 and 13, in which testis cells from a persistently LCM-infected mouse are shown after exposure for 7 days to murine lymphocytes. Lymphocytes were prepared by mincing freshly-excised lymph nodes and gently squeezing and washing the extracted lymphocytes through a fine sieve with balanced salt solution. Lymphocytes from a normal mouse caused only very slight damage, but lymphocytes taken from a mouse 14 days after SC LCM inoculation caused severe destruction of the LCM-infected cells.[11] These findings have been confirmed recently.[62, 70]

It is now clear that LCM virus alters the host cell membrane in such a way that it no longer exactly duplicates the antigenic mosaic recognizable by the host as self. The new pattern can be recognized as foreign, and may be the subject of successful immunologic attack and rejection. The final result of the rejection process determines the status of the animal, *i.e.*, it may die if the rejection is too extensive and severe, be immune if the rejection is successful, or be "tolerant" if the attack fails. Failure of the immune response may be complete, as in some forms of congenital murine LCM, or partial, resulting in "split tolerance," chronic persistent infection, and slow disease. The choice between the alternate pathways of immune conflict or tolerance is probably decided by the degree to which the host's immune organs become rapidly infected with virus during the early stages of infection. Such infection could be expected to paralyze the response of the immune cells against the virus.

At the present time, it seems likely that the acquisition of new virus-induced surface antigens by the animal cell is responsible for a significant proportion of chronic human disease, and possibly some forms of premature aging. Virus-induced autoimmune disease of this type may be more generalized than we have realized. The recently studied examples of slow virus disease, such as Aleutian mink disease, visna, and subacute sclerosing panencephalitis, all have elements of similarity to the LCM model, and collectively cover a very wide spectrum of pathologic effects. Perhaps the best known example of slow virus disease is the sheep encephalopathy known as "scrapie." This transmissible disease is very closely related to the transmissible encephalopathy of mink, and to the human disease called kuru, the virus of which appears to be transmitted by cannibalism. It may be significant that, at the present time, one of the major concepts of the nature of the scrapie agent is that it is a piece of replicating "altered" cell membrane.[50] So far no immune response whatsoever has been detected against the scrapie agent, which seems to be an exceptionally small and resistant form of life. The implications of the recent expansion of knowledge on the ubiquity of animal viruses suggests that there are many other as yet undiscovered subtle virus–host interactions operating in the human population. It is likely that many of these will include virus-induced antigenic alterations of the cell surface, resulting in autoimmune disease and derangement of the cell's function.

Acknowledgment. Tom Cutie, Ruth Buckley, and Helen Harpp gave excellent technical assistance, and Doctor F. Baker performed the creatinine estimations.

References

1. Abelson HT, Smith GH, Hoffman HA, *et al.*: Use of enzyme-labeled antibody for electron microscope localization of lymphocytic choriomeningitis virus antigens in infected cell cultures. J Nat Cancer Inst 42:497–515, 1969
2. Annino JS: Clinical Chemistry. Second edition. Boston, Little, Brown, and Co., 1960
3. Armstrong C: Studies on choriomeningitis and poliomyelitis. Harvey Lect 36:39–65, 1940–41
4. Baker FD, Hotchin J: Slow virus kidney disease of mice. Science 158:502–504, 1967
5. Baratawidjaja RK, Morrissey LP, Labzoffsky NA: Demonstration of vaccinia, lymphocytic choriomeningitis and rabies viruses in the leucocytes of experimentally infected animals. Arch Ges Virusforsch 17:273–279, 1965
6. Barlow JL, Hotchin J: The effect of certain drugs on lymphocytic choriomeningitis infection in mice. NY State Dept Health, Ann Rep Div Lab Res, 1960, pp 22–23
7. Barlow JL: The effect of alkylating agents on lymphocytic choriomeningitis infection in mice. NY State Dept Health, Ann Rep Div Lab Res, 1961, pp 47–48
8. Barlow JL, Hotchin J: Induction of persistent tolerant infection with lymphocytic choriomeningitis virus in adult mice by amethopterin treatment. NY State Dept Health, Ann Rep Div Lab Res, 1962, p 39
9. Benda R, Činátl J: Multiplication of lymphocytic choriomeningitis virus in bottle cell cultures. Experimental data for the preparation of highly infectious fluids. Acta Virol 5:159–164, 1962
10. Benda R, Hronovsky V, Červa L, *et al.*: Demonstration of lymphocytic choriomeningitis virus in cell cultures and mouse brain by the fluorescent antibody technique. Acta Virol 9:347–351, 1965
11. Benson L: Effects of immune mouse lymphocytes on normal and virus infected mouse tissue culture. NY State Dept Health, Ann Rep Div Lab Res, 1962, pp 41–42
12. Benson L, Hotchin J: Antibody formation in persistent tolerant infection with lymphocytic choriomeningitis virus. Nature (London) 222:1045–1047, 1969
13. Brown P: Evolution of lymphocytic choriomeningitis virus infection from neonatal inoculation through development of adult "late onset disease" and glomerulonephritis. Arch Ges Virusforsch 24:220–230, 1968
14. Buck LL, Pfau CJ: Inhibition of lymphocytic choriomeningitis virus replication by actinomycin D and 6-azauridine. Virology 27:698–701, 1969
15. Buckley SM, Casals J: Lassa fever, a new virus disease of man from West Africa. III. Isolation and characterization of the virus. Amer J Trop Med Hyg 19:680–691, 1970
16. Collins DN, Hotchin J: Glomerulonephritis and glomerulosclerosis as a late manifestation of persistent tolerant infection of mice with lymphocytic choriomeningitis virus. NY State Dept Health, Ann Rep Div Lab Res, 1963, pp 100–101
17. Collins DN, Weigand H, Hotchin J: The effects of pretreatment with x-rays on the pathogenesis of lymphocytic choriomeningitis in mice. II. The pathological histology. J Immunol 87:682–687, 1961

18. Dalton AJ, Rowe WP, Smith GH, *et al.*: Morphological and cytochemical studies on lymphocytic choriomeningitis virus. J Virol 2: 1465–1478, 1968
19. East J, Parrott DMV, Seamer J: The ability of mice thymectomized at birth to survive infection with lymphocytic choriomeningitis virus. Virology 22:160–162, 1964
20. Földes P, Szeri I, Bános Z, *et al.*: LCM infection of mice thymectomized in newborn age. Acta Microbiol Hung 11:277–282, 1964
21. Farmer TW, Janeway CA: Infections with the virus of lymphocytic choriomeningitis. Medicine 21:1–63, 1942
22. Furusawa E, Cutting W, Furst A: Inhibitory effect of antiviral compounds on Columbia SK, LCM, vaccinia and adeno type 12 viruses in vitro. Chemotherapia 8:95–105, 1964
23. Germuth FG, Senterfit LB, Pollack AD: Immune complex disease. I. Experimental, acute and chronic glomerulonephritis. Johns Hopkins Med J 120:225–251, 1967
24. Gledhill AW: Protective effect of anti-lymphocytic serum on murine lymphocytic choriomeningitis. Nature (London) 214:178–179, 1967
25. Goldberg SA, Brodie M, Stanley D: Effect of x-ray on experimental encephalitis in mice inoculated with St. Louis strain. Proc Soc Exp Biol Med 32:587–590, 1935
26. Haas VH: Studies on the natural history of the virus of lymphocytic choriomeningitis in mice. Public Health Rep 56:285–292, 1941
27. Haas VH, Stewart SE: Sparing effect of amethopterin and guanazolo in mice infected with the virus of lymphocytic choriomeningitis. Virology 2:511–516, 1956
28. Haas VH, Briggs GM, Stewart, SE: Inapparent lymphocytic choriomeningitis infection in folic acid-deficient mice. Science 126:405–406, 1957
29. Hampers CL, Kolker P, Hager EB: Isolation and characterization of antibodies and other immunologically reactive substances from rejecting renal allografts. J Immunol 99:514–525, 1967
30. Helyer BJ, Howie JB: Spontaneous autoimmune disease in NZB/BL mice. Brit J Haemat 9:119–131, 1963
31. Henson JB, Gorham JR, Takaka Y: Renal glomerular ultrastructure in mink affected by Aleutian disease. Lab Invest 17:123–139, 1967
32. Hirsch MS, Murphy FA: The effect of antilymphocyte serum on lymphocytic choriomeningitis (LCM) virus infection in mice. Fed Proc 26:481, 1967
33. Hirsch MS, Murphy FA, Russe HP, *et al.*: Effects of anti-thymocyte serum on lymphocytic choriomeningitis (LCM) virus infection in mice. Proc Soc Exp Biol Med 125:980–983, 1967
34. Hirsch MS, Murphy FA, Hicklin MD: Immunopathology of lymphocytic choriomeningitis virus infection of newborn mice. Antithymocyte serum effects on glomerulonephritis and wasting disease. J Exp Med 127:757–766, 1968
35. Hotchin J: Some aspects of induced latent infection of mice with the virus of lymphocytic choriomeningitis, Symposium on Latency and Masking in Viral and Rickettsial Infections. Minneapolis, Burgess Publishing Co., 1958, pp 59–65
36. Hotchin JE, Cinits M: Lymphocytic choriomeningitis infection of mice as a model for the study of latent virus infection. Canad J Microbiol 4:149–163, 1958
37. Hotchin JE, Weigand H: Relationship between age at inoculation and outcome of infection of mice with lymphocytic choriomeningitis virus. NY State Dept Health, Ann Rep Div Lab Res, 1959, p 21
38. Hotchin JE: The role of immunological tolerance in neonatal infection of mice with lymphocytic choriomeningitis virus. Quart Rev Pediat 16:97–101, 1961
39. Hotchin J, Weigand H: The effects of pretreatment with x-rays on the pathogenesis of lymphocytic choriomeningitis in mice. I. Host survival, virus multiplication and leukocytosis. J Immunol 87:675–681, 1961
40. Hotchin J, Weigand H: Studies of lymphocytic choriomeningitis in mice. I. The relationship between age at inoculation and outcome of infection. J Immunol 86:392–400, 1961
41. Hotchin J: The biology of lymphocytic choriomeningitis infection: Virus-induced immune disease. Cold Spring Harbor Symp Quant Biol 27:479–499, 1962
42. Hotchin J: The foot pad reaction of mice to lymphocytic choriomeningitis virus. Virology 17:214–215, 1962
43. Hotchin J, Benson LM, Seamer J: Factors affecting the induction of persistent tolerant infection of newborn mice with lymphocytic choriomeningitis. Virology 18:71–78, 1962
44. Hotchin J, Benson L: The pathogenesis of lymphocytic choriomeningitis in mice: The effects of different inoculation routes and the footpad response. J Immunol 91:460–468, 1963
45. Hotchin J, Collins DN: Glomerulonephritis and late onset disease of mice following neonatal virus infection. Nature (London) 203:1357–1359, 1964
46. Hotchin J, Sikora E: Protection against the lethal effect of lymphocytic choriomeningitis virus in mice by neonatal thymectomy. Nature (London) 202:214–215, 1964
47. Hotchin J: Chronic disease following lymphocytic choriomeningitis virus inoculation and possible mechanisms of slow virus pathogenesis, NINDB Monograph No. 2, Slow, Latent and Temperate Virus Infections. Washington, D. C., U. S. Dept. of Health, Education and Welfare, 1965, pp 341–359
48. Hotchin J, Benson L, Sikora E: The detection of neutralizing antibody to lymphocytic choriomeningitis virus in mice. J Immunol 102:1128–1135, 1969
49. Hotchin J: A concept of persistent virus infection. Proc Third Int Symp Medical and Applied Virology: Viruses Affecting Man and Animals, in press, 1970
50. Hunter GD, Millson GC, Gibbons RA: Some new information concerning the stability of the scrapie agent. Biochem J 105:7P, 1967

51. Kajima M, Majde J: LCM virus as a carrier of non-viral cellular components. Naturwissenschaften 57:93–101, 1970

52. Kindig D, Spargo B, Kirsten WH: Glomerular response in Aleutian disease of mink. Lab Invest 16:436–443, 1967

53. Larsen JH: On the induction of immunological tolerance to LCM virus in the adult mouse. XV Scand Congr Path Microbiol, 1967, pp 60–61

54. Larsen JH: Studies on immunological tolerance to LCM virus. 9. Induction of immunological tolerance to the virus in the adult mouse. Acta Path Microbiol Scand 73:106–114, 1968

55. Larsen JH: Development of humoral and cell-mediated immunity to lymphocytic choriomeningitis virus in the mouse. J Immunol 102:941–946, 1969

56. Larsen JH: On the induction of immunological tolerance to a self-reproducing antigen. Immunology (London) 16:15–23, 1969

57. Lehmann-Grube F: Lymphocytic choriomeningitis in the mouse. II. Establishment of carrier colonies. Arch Ges Virusforsch 14:351–357, 1964

58. Lerner EM II, Haas VH: Histopathology of lymphocytic choriomeningitis in mice spared by amethopterin. Proc Soc Exp Biol Med 98:395–399, 1958

59. Levy HB, Haas VH: Alteration of the course of lymphocytic choriomeningitis in mice by certain antimetabolites. Virology 5:401–407, 1958

60. Lillie RD, Armstrong C: Pathology of lymphocytic choriomeningitis in mice. Arch Path 40:141–152, 1945

61. Lundstedt C, Volkert M: Studies on immunological tolerance to LCM virus. 8. Induction of tolerance to the virus in adult mice treated with anti-lymphocytic serum. Acta Path Microbiol Scand 71:471–480, 1967

62. Lundstedt C: Interaction between antigenically different cells. Virus-induced cytotoxicity by immune lymphoid cells in vitro. Acta Path Microbiol Scand 75:139–152, 1969

63. Manaligod JR, Pirani CL, Miyasato F, et al.: The renal changes in NZB-Bl and NZB-NZW Fl hybrid mice. Light and electron microscopic studies. Nephron 4:215–230, 1967

64. Maurer F.: Lymphocytic choriomeningitis. Lab Anim Care 14:415–419, 1964

65. Mellors RC: Autoimmune disease in NZB/BL mice. I. Pathology and pathogenesis of a model system of spontaneous glomerulonephritis. J Exp Med 122:25–40, 1965

66. Mims CA: Immunofluorescence study of the carrier state and mechanism of vertical transmission in lymphocytic choriomeningitis virus infection in mice. J Path Bact 91:395–402, 1966

67. Mims CA, Subrahmanyan TP: Immunofluorescence study of the mechanism of resistance to superinfection in mice carrying the lymphocytic choriomeningitis virus. J Path Bact 91:403–415, 1966

68. Murphy FA, Webb PA, Johnson KM, et al.: Morphological comparison of machupo with lymphocytic choriomeningitis virus: Basis for a new taxonomic group. J Virology 4:535–541, 1969

69. Oldstone MBA, Dixon FJ: Lymphocytic choriomeningitis: Production of antibody by "tolerant" infected mice. Science 158:1193–1195, 1967

70. Oldstone MBA, Habel K, Dixon FJ: The pathogenesis of cellular injury associated with persistent LCM viral infection. Fed Proc 28:429, 1969

71. Parikh GC: Cytological changes by lymphocytic choriomeningitis virus in the human amnion cells. Jap J Microbiol 5:129–132, 1961

72. Pedersen IR, Volkert M: Multiplication of lymphocytic choriomeningitis virus in suspension cultures of Earle's strain L cells. Acta Path Microbiol Scand 67:523–536, 1966

73. Peters JM, Boyd EM: Organ weights and water levels in albino rats following 14 days starvation. Toxicol Appl Pharmacol 7:494–495, 1965

74. Pfau CJ, Pedersen IR, Volkert M: Inability of nucleic acid analogues to inhibit the synthesis of lymphocytic choriomeningitis virus. Acta Path Microbiol Scand 63:181–187, 1965

75. Pollard M, Kajima M, Sharon N: LCM virus-induced immunopathology in congenitally infected gnotobiotic mice, Perspectives in Virology. Volume 6. New York, Academic Press, 1968, pp 193–209

76. Pollard M, Sharon N, Teah BA: Congenital lymphocytic choriomeningitis virus infection in gnotobiotic mice. Proc Soc Exp Biol Med 127:755–761, 1968

77. Porter DD, Larsen AE, Porter HG: The pathogenesis of Aleutian disease of mink. I. In vivo viral replication and the host antibody response to viral antigen. J Exp Med 130:575–593, 1969

78. Recher L, Tanaka T, Sykes JA, et al.: Further studies on the biological relationship of murine leukemia viruses and on kidney lesions of mice with leukemia induced by these viruses, Nat Cancer Inst monograph 22, 1966, pp 459–479

79. Remezov PI, Topleninova KA: Detection of the virus of lymphocytic choriomeningitis by means of the indirect method of fluorescing antibodies. Voprosy Paikhiatrii i Nevropatologii 7:113–120, 1961

80. Rowe WP: Studies on pathogenesis and immunity in lymphocytic choriomeningitis infection of the mouse. Bethesda, Md., Res Rep Naval Med Res Inst 12:167–220, 1954

81. Rowe WP: Protective effect of pre-irradiation on lymphocytic choriomeningitis infection in mice. Proc Soc Exp Biol Med 92:194–198, 1956

82. Rowe WP, Black PH, Levey RH: Protective effect of neonatal thymectomy on mouse LCM infection. Proc Soc Exp Biol Med 114:248–251, 1963

83. Rowe WP, Murphy FA, Bergold GH, et al.: Arenoviruses: Proposed name for a newly defined virus group. J Virol 5:651–652, 1970

84. Sidwell RW, Dixon GJ, Sellers SM, et al.: In vivo antiviral activity of 1,3-bis(2-chloroethyl)-1-nitrosourea. Appl Microbiol 13:579–589, 1965

85. Sikora E: Protective effect of neonatal thymectomy on lymphocytic choriomeningitis virus disease in mice. NY State Dept Health, Ann Rep Div Lab Res, 1963, pp 43–44

86. Spector WS: Handbook of Biological Data. Philadelphia and London, W. B. Saunders Co., 1956

87. Traub E: A filterable virus from white mice. Immunology (London) 29:69, 1935

88. Traub E: A filterable virus recovered from white mice. Science 81:298–299, 1935

89. Traub E: The epidemiology of lymphocytic choriomeningitis in white mice. J Exp Med 64:183–200, 1936

90. Traub E: Factors influencing the persistence of choriomeningitis virus in the blood of mice after clinical recovery. J Exp Med 68:229–250, 1938

91. Traub E: Observations on immunological tolerance and "immunity" in mice infected congenitally with the virus of lymphocytic choriomeningitis (LCM). Arch Ges Virusforsch 10:303–314, 1960

92. Traub E: Studies on the mechanism of immunity in murine LCM. Arch Ges Virusforsch 14:65–86, 1963

93. Traub E, Kesting F: Experiments on heterologous and homologous interference in LCM-infected cultures of murine lymph node cells. Arch Ges Virusforsch 14:55–64, 1963

94. Volkert M, Larsen JH: Studies on immunological tolerance to LCM virus. 5. The induction of tolerance to the virus. Acta Path Microbiol Scand 63:161–171, 1965

95. Volkert M, Larsen JH, Pfau CJ: Studies on immunological tolerance to LCM virus. 4. The question of immunity in adoptively immunized virus carriers. Acta Path Microbiol Scand 61:268–282, 1964

96. Volkert M, Lundstedt C: The provocation of latent lymphocytic choriomeningitis virus infection in mice by treatment with anti-lymphocytic serum. J Exp Med 127:327–339, 1968

97. Wagner RR, Snyder RM: Viral interference induced in mice by acute or persistent infection with the virus of lymphocytic choriomeningitis. Nature (London) 196:393–394, 1962

98. Webb HE, Wight DGD, Wiernik G, et al.: Langat virus encephalitis in mice. II. The effect of irradiation. J Hyg (London) 66:355–364, 1968

99. Weigand H, Hotchin J: Studies of lymphocytic choriomeningitis in mice. II. A comparison of the immune status of newborn and adult mice surviving inoculation. J Immunol 86:401–406, 1961

100. Wilsnack RE, Rowe WP: Immunofluorescent studies of the histopathogenesis of lymphocytic choriomeningitis virus infection. J Exp Med 120:829–841, 1964

Radiation Sensitivity of New Zealand Black Mice and the Development of Autoimmune Disease and Neoplasia

JANE I. MORTON AND BENJAMIN V. SIEGEL

Studies from this laboratory (1–4) have demonstrated hyper-responsiveness of young adult New Zealand Black (NZB) mice to immunization with sheep erythrocytes and have culminated in the speculation that this mouse strain possesses a relative abundance of hematopoietic stem cells. In mice of several strains, survival after acute exposures of up to 1000–1500 R largely depends on the number of stem cells present at the time of irradiation (5–7). With this in mind we have tested our hypothesis of enhanced stem cell numbers by determining the susceptibilities of NZB mice of various ages to acute doses of ionizing radiation.

MATERIALS AND METHODS

Animals

The NZB mice employed represented the 4th–6th generations raised in this laboratory from breeding pairs, generations 57 and 58, obtained originally from W. H. Hall, Otago University Medical School, Dunedin, New Zealand. At the time of x-irradiation, equal numbers of male and female mice were selected for each of the following groups: 1-month-old (27–32 days, which are Coomb's negative), 3-month-old (88–94 days which are also Coombs' negative) and 9-month-old (9–9.5 months, Coombs' positive). In an effort to have a homogeneous 9-month-old group, we selected animals with an intense anti-globulin reaction in the test of Norins and Holmes (8) for Coombs' positivity. Mice were housed 5–6 per cage and maintained on Purina laboratory chow and tap water *ad libitum*, with conventional conditions of husbandry both before and after irradiation.

Additional experiments were performed with 3-week-old (17–23 days) animals weaned one day before irradiation and

Abbreviation: NZB, New Zealand Black.

with nursling 2-week-old (11–14 days) NZB mice. For the latter study, babies were removed from mothers just before irradiation, litters were pooled, and individuals were toe-marked for identification and apportioned into different x-irradiation groups. After irradiation, one baby from each of six treatment groups was returned to each mother. Cages were checked daily during the entire experimental period and deaths were recorded.

Irradiation

Irradiations were performed with an x-ray unit (G.E. Maxi-tron) operated at 300 kV (peak) and 20 mA with added filtration, yielding a half-value layer equivalent to 2.0 mm Cu. Exposure rates were measured with Victoreen ionization chambers inserted in mouse phantoms, and averaged 28–29 R/min. Animals were exposed in individual plastic containers mounted around the periphery of a turntable which was rotated during exposure.

The exposure necessary to kill 50% of the animals (LD_{50}) was calculated by computer using an Oregon State University Radiation Center program based on probit analysis (9) as modified for computer by Aitchison and Brown (10). The LD_{50} values were determined from the maximum likelihood regression of the normal equivalent deviate (N.E.D. = probit minus 5) of the percentage mortality on the natural logarithm of the exposure in roentgens. The maximum likelihood method is an iterative procedure that determines the line of best fit to transformed data by applying weights that decrease toward the extremes of the distribution (11).

RESULTS AND DISCUSSION

Radiation sensitivity increased with age for 1-, 3-, and 9-month-old NZB mice, and dose-related deaths for the 1- and 3-month-old animals showed characteristically steep sigmoidal curves (Fig. 1). The erratic 30-day death response of the 9-month-old animals might reflect a heterogeneous population with regard to autoimmune disease development, in spite of efforts to minimize this by prior selection of animals based on the intensity of their Coombs' reactions. Seven-day survivals for 9-month-old NZB mice were likewise observed to be poor ($LD_{50(7)}$ = 699 R) and irregularly related to intermediate irradiation exposures (Fig. 1). These early deaths could reflect bone marrow injury of animals undergoing chronic hematopoietic stress, although gastrointestinal sensitivity, which is reported (12) to become prominent with age in such strains as C57Bl, may also be responsible. Since deaths of untreated NZB mice in our colony ordinarily do not occur as

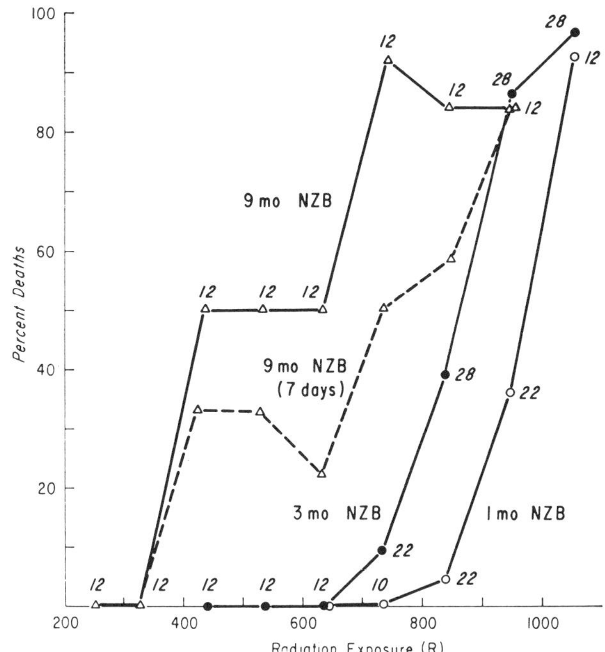

FIG. 1.   Percentage of NZB mice of different ages dying within a period of 30 days after different exposures to x-irradiation. The total number of mice studied at each radiation exposure is recorded beside the corresponding experimental point. Deaths occurring within 7 days after irradiation of 9-month-old mice are also included (- - -) in the figure.

early as 9–11 months, we made no correction for natural mortality in this age group.

Fig. 2 depicts cumulative deaths with time for all mice dying in each of the age groups represented in Fig. 1. Most irradiation deaths among 9-month-old mice occurred between days 5 and 7, and on days 7–12 and 11–13 for 3- and 1-month-old mice respectively. Thus, the incidence of early deaths and high 30-day radiation sensitivity among these mice appeared to be directly related.

In Fig. 3 are plotted $LD_{50(30)}$ values with 95% confidence limits as calculated by computer analysis for these animals and for additional groups of 2- and 3-week-old NZB mice. To more readily visualize the differences with age between the radiation sensitivity of NZB mice and that of a number of nonautoimmune strains, curves derived from data reported by other investigators for C57B1 (13), SAS/4 (14), and CAF1 (15) mice are also presented.

45

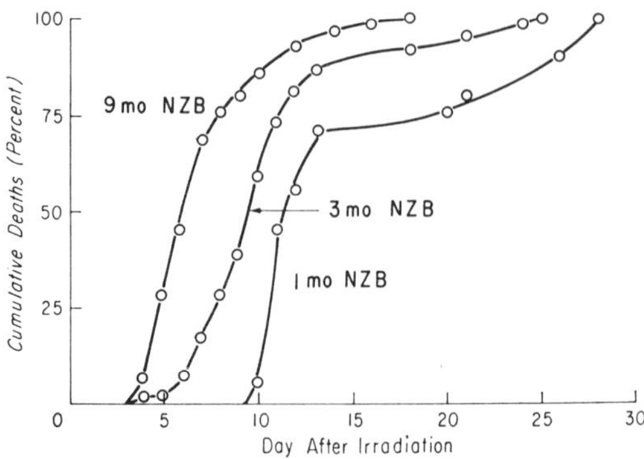

Fig. 2. Pattern of cumulative deaths for all NZB mice in each of the age groups of Fig. 1 which died within 30 days after irradiation.

The most striking characteristic of the NZB response was a peak radiation resistance at 1 month of age, an observation in stark contrast to previous demonstrations (13–15) of minimum or low resistance to irradiation by 30-day-old mice of other strains. The lower resistance of 3-week-old weanling NZB mice (Fig. 3) may, however, correspond to this minimum, which has been attributed (16) to high sensitivity of both gastrointestinal and hematopoietic systems. Our results suggest that by the age of 30 days the NZB mice had a high intestinal resistance to the damaging effects of x-irradiation as well as a superior capacity for hematopoietic recovery. The early appearance of high radiation resistance in NZB mice provides an interesting corollary to the observations of Evans *et al.* (17) and Playfair (18) that suggest an early maturation of the immune system for this mouse strain, and tends to support the concept of a possible relationship between primary immune capacity and the size of the stem cell pool (2).

The radiation $LD_{50(30)}$ of 856 R noted here for 3-month-old NZB mice, although lower than that of the 1-month-old animals, was higher than values previously reported for other mouse strains of similar age, including the highly resistant SJL/J strain (19). We do not yet know whether the further diminished resistance observed for 9-month-old (Fig. 3) as compared to 3-month-old NZB mice was the consequence of a gradual increase in sensitivity with time, or if it represented a precipitous event associated with a particular stage of dis-

46

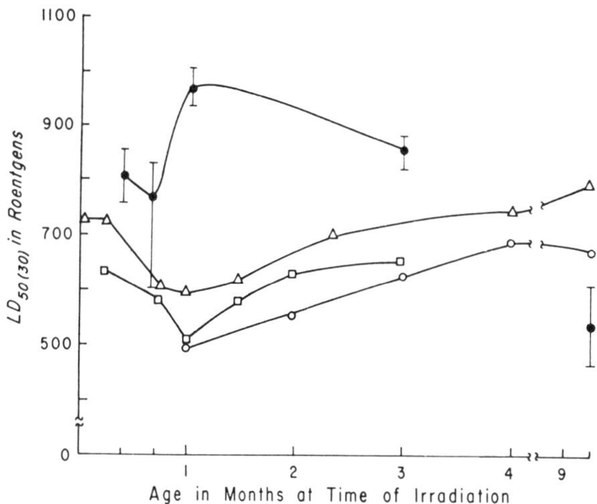

FIG. 3. $LD_{50(30)}$ values for NZB mice (●) of different ages. Upper and lower 95% confidence limits are designated by the vertical bars. Also presented are curves constructed from data reported for three other mouse strains. △, SAS/4 (ref. 14); □, C57B1 (ref. 13); O, CAF₁ (ref.15).

ease development. This depressed capability of Coombs' positive 9-month-old NZB mice to survive irradiation also seemed to parallel the decreased capacity of 9-month-old NZB mice to mount a primary immune response (2–4, 20). Conceivably, both these phenomena might be ascribed to a paucity of stem cells in these anemic animals (2). The high sensitivity of NZB mice of this age to x-irradiation was in marked contrast to the gradual increase in radiation resistance which has been reported for other mice after 1 month of age, where a maximum is reached between 6 and 18 months, with diminished resistance appearing only in advanced old age (13–15). In general, the age-associated changes in radiation resistance observed with NZB mice appeared to represent an acceleration and magnification of those changes which in nonautoimmune strains develop gradually.

The mechanism by which the presence of an enlarged pool of hematopoietic stem cells in young NZB mice might predispose them to the development of autoimmune disease has been discussed previously (2) and envisions an enhanced opportunity for the triggering of autoantibody formation as a consequence of increased availability of potentially responsive target cells. It seems feasible that augmented numbers of stem cells could similarly contribute to the generation of reticular neoplasia observed in many of the old NZB mice (21). In this regard, cytologic studies of the type B neoplasm common to the NZB strain have indicated the involvement of a recticular stem cell capable of lymphocytic, plasmacytic, and histiocytic differentiation (22).

On the basis of a high radiation resistance coupled with immunologic hyper-responsiveness, it could be speculated that the genetic defect responsible for the development of autoantibodies and neoplasia in the NZB strain might involve an early failure to adequately restrict the size of the hematopoietic stem cell compartment. The necessity for such a regulatory mechanism has been defined by previous studies concerned with stem cell repopulation kinetics in the irradiated host (23). Further elucidation of the mechanism controlling stem cell numbers would seem of great importance for the comprehension and management of those disease processes deriving from regulatory dysfunction.

We are grateful to Prof. Donald J. Kimeldorf for supervision and use of the x-ray facility at the Oregon State University Radiation Center, Corvallis, and to Dr. Fred A. Hodge for design and execution of the computer analysis of LD_{50} values, and to both for their critical evaluation of this manuscript. Meir Stampfer and Daniel Suher provided valuable technical assistance.

This work was supported by U.S. Atomic Energy Commission Contract RLO-1927-50 and Public Health Service research grant CA 10089 from the National Cancer Institute.

1. Morton, J. I., C. L. Olson, and B. V. Siegel, *Fed. Proc.*, **26**, 788 (1967).

2. Morton, J. I., and B. V. Siegel, *J. Reticuloendothel. Soc.*, **6**, 78 (1969).

3. Siegel, B. V., R. E. Brooks, and J. I. Morton, *Blood*, **35**, 386 (1970).

4. Morton, J. I., and B. V. Siegel, *Experientia*, **26**, 1008 (1970).

5. Storer, J. B., in "Biology of the Laboratory Mouse," ed. E. L. Green (McGraw-Hill, New York, 1966), p. 427.

6. Doherty, D. G., and L. H. Smith, *Radiat. Res.*, **40**, 85 (1969).

7. Smith, L. H., and H. G. Willard, *Amer. J. Physiol.*, **216**, 493 (1969).

8. Norins, L. C., and M. C. Holmes, *J. Immunol.*, **93**, 891 (1964).

9. Finney, D. J., *Probit Analysis* (Cambridge Univ. Press, London, 1952).

10. Aitchison, J., and J. A. C. Brown, *The Log-normal Distribution* (Cambridge Univ. Press, London, 1957).

11. Nachtwey, D. S., E. J. Ainsworth, and G. F. Leong, *Radiat. Res.*, **31**, 353 (1967).

12. Yuhas, J. M., D. Huang, and J. B. Storer, *Radiat. Res.*, **38**, 501 (1969).

13. Abrams, H. L., *Proc. Soc. Exp. Biol. Med.*, **76**, 729 (1951).

14. Crosfill, M. L., P. J. Lindop, and J. Rotblat, *Nature*, **183**, 1729 (1959).

15. Kohn, H. I., and R. F. Kallman, *Science*, **124**, 1078 (1956).

16. Fred, S. S., S. M. Wilson, and W. W. Smith, in "Gastrointestinal Radiation Injury," ed. M. F. Sullivan (Exerpta Medica Foundation, 1968), p. 413.

17. Evans, M. M., W. G. Williamson, and W. J. Irvine, *Clin. Exp. Immunol.*, **3**, 375 (1968).

18. Playfair, J. H. L., *Immunology*, **15**, 35 (1968).

19. Yuhas, J. M., and J. B. Storer, *Radiat. Res.*, **39**, 608 (1969).

20. Diener, E., *Int. Arch. Allergy*, **30**, 120 (1966).

21. Howie, J. B., and B. J. Helyer, *Advan. Immunol.*, **9**, 215 (1968).

22. Dunn, T. B., and M. K. Deringer, *J. Nat. Cancer Inst.*, **40**, 771 (1968).

23. Gurney, C. W., and W. Fried, *Proc. Nat. Acad. Sci. USA*, **54**, 1148 (1965).

URINARY IMMUNOGLOBULINS IN RHEUMATOID ARTHRITIS AND OTHER CONNECTIVE TISSUE DISEASES

F. D. LINDSTRÖM

INTRODUCTION

Studies on normal human urine have demonstrated free light chains of both types (1, 14) and evidence has been presented by Stevenson (32) and by Gordon, Eisen and Vaughan (12) that urinary light chains are derived predominantly from the anabolic phase in gammaglobulin metabolism. An Fc-like fragment has also been reported to be present in normal urine (2, 35, 36, as well as intact IgG and IgA (14, 34).

In their study of urinary gammaglobulins in patients with rheumatoid arthritis (RA), Gordon et al. (12) found no qualitative difference between normal and RA urines. However, in about half of the number of RA patients the quantity of gammaglobulin excreted was higher than in normals. Cooper and Bluestone (7) quantitated free immunoglobulin light chains in sera, urine and synovial fluids of patients with connective tissue disease and noted increased amounts of free light chains in the synovial fluids and urine of patients with RA. In the current study presented here urinary immunoglobulins in a group of patients with RA and other connective tissue diseases have been quantitated using immunodiffusion in Oudin tubes (25). Also, the homogeneity of urinary immunoglobulin has been studied by electrophoresis. The data obtained indicate increased excretion of IgG and free light chains in patients with rheumatoid arthritis. Also a Bence-Jones-like urinary protein is described in a patient with systemic sclerosis.

MATERIALS AND METHODS

24 hour urine samples were collected from 29 patients and 17 healthy controls. The patient group consisted of 19 patients with RA, 3

"

TABLE 1

Incidence and quantitation of urinary immunoglobulins.

		Incidence of IgG	IgG mg/24 hr	Incidence of free light chains	Free light chains mg/24 hr	Incidence of IgA	IgA mg/24 hr
RA	mean		26.6		29.7		9.8
		19/19		19/19		7/19	
	range		4-83		2-80		5.5-24
Other connective tissue diseases	mean		19.4		34		5.1
		10/10		10/10		4/10	
	range		3-70		6-117		4-9
Controls	mean		7.6		8.2		3
		17/17		12/17		8/17	
	range		2-19	2 N.Q.	3.9-15		1.5-4.6

N.Q. = Not quantitatable

with juveline rheumatoid arthritis (JRA), 2 with systemic lupus erythematosus (SLE), 2 with systemic sclerosis (SS) and a mixed group consisting of 3 patients, representing ankylosing spondylitis, Reiter's disease and dermatomyositis. Only patients who showed negative tests for proteinuria by the Albustix method (Ames Company, Elkhart, Ind.) and who lacked other evidence of significant renal involvement, were included in the study.

The urine was filtered and then dialysed against cold, running tap water for two days, using dialysis tubing (Union Carbide Corp., Chicago, Ill.) with average pore size 24 Å. This membrane retains lysozyme (mol wt 14,000). The dialyzed urine was then lyophilized and the dry material reconstituted in a small volume of saline. The resulting urine-concentrate was used for quantitation using single diffusion in Oudin tubes as previously described (20). Immunoelectrophoresis was done using the method of Scheidegger (28). Agarose-gel-electrophoresis utilized the technique of Laurell (19).

Antisera against light chains were obtained by injecting rabbits with Bence-Jones protein of kappa or lambda type purified by zone electrophoresis on starch-block (17) and chromatography on Sephadex G-200 (Pharmacia Fine Chemicals, Upsala, Sweden), as described elsewhere (22). Antisera to free light chains were prepared by the method of Tan and Epstein (33). These antisera were made group specific (for kappa or lambda type light chain) by absorption with the opposite type light chain (lambda and kappa, respectively), IgG and IgA antisera were obtained from commercial sources (Hyland Laboratories, L.A., Calif.). They were specific for γ- and α-chains respectively, and showed no reactivity for light chains.

Gel filtrations of urine concentrates were performed in a few instances, using Sephadex G-200. The fractions were tested by double diffusion in agar against the antisera mentioned above.

All urine concentrates were studied by the latex fixation test described by Singer and Plotz (30) to see, if results obtained by Bienenstock, Goldstein and Tomasi (5) concerning urinary IgA rheumatoid factor could be confirmed. In association with this eluate fractions from Sephadex G-200 chromatography of urine concentrates were also screened with the latex slide test (RA-test, Hyland Laboratories, L.A., Calif.).

Statistical analysis of excretion data utilized the rank-sum-test (8).

RESULTS

In Table 1 relevant data on urinary immunoglobulin excretion are tabulated.

Patients with JRA, SLE, SS, ankylosing spondylitis, Reiter's disease and dermatomyositis were taken together in one group named »other connective tissue diseases», since their excretion data were similar. One exception to this, however, occurred in one of the two patients with systemic sclerosis (EN), whose immunoglobulin excretion will be described in some detail.

Control group. All normal urines showed some material reacting with IgG antisera, although the amount was significantly less than for the patient group. 12/17 urines showed free light chains,

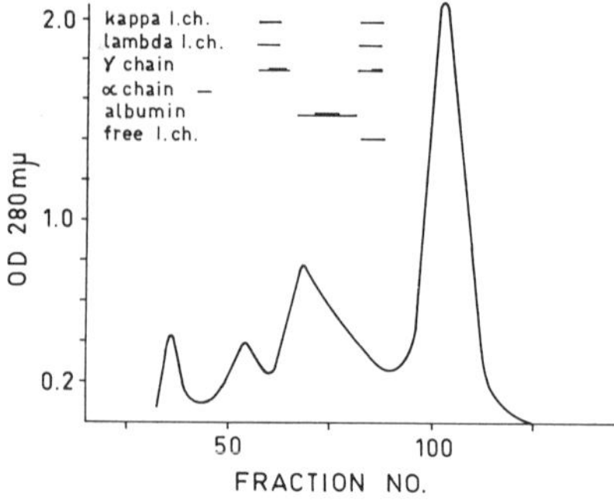

Fig. 1. Representative pattern of gel filtration on Sephadex G-200 of urine concentrate from patient with RA. Fraction volume 8 ml. Result of immunodiffusion of separate fractions against antisera specific for kappa and lambda light chains, γ and α heavy chains, albumin and free light chains are also shown. Fractions were read on a Beckman DU 2 spectrophotometer at 280 mμ.

which were always of kappa type, when appearing in measureable amounts. These data indicate that lambda type light chains were present either in trace amounts (4 instances) or not at all. The quantity excreted was significantly less than in the patient group.

The incidence and level of urinary IgA showed no difference from the patient group.

Rheumatoid arthritis

All RA patients had IgG or fragments thereof in their urine; the amounts excreted were significantly higher than in the control group (p < 0.01).

The free light chain excretion in this group was significantly higher than in the control group (p < 0.01). There was a domination of K type light chains, but most (11/19) had measurable amounts of lambda type light chains. The kappa type domination was no stronger than would be expected from the 2:1 ratio (kappa:lambda) in the immunoglobulin of the peripheral blood (23). When ordinary light chain antisera were used for quantitation, slightly higher excretion data were obtained, since these antisera recognize not only free light chains, but also light chains bound to heavy chains in intact immunoglobulin molecules.

Several urine-concentrates were studied by gel filtration on Sephadex G-200. Fig. 1 shows a representative pattern. The fractions were tested by immunodiffusion in agar. IgA was present in the first peak and was composed predominantly of the secretory (11S) type of immunoglobulin (3). Anti-Fc antiserum detected material with a biphasic distribution, first in the 7S region on the chromatograph and again in the area immediately following the albumin peak. Light chains were also present in a biphasic pattern, first in the 7S peak and again after the albumin peak. Free light chains, however, were present only in the postalbumin region. IgM was not present in any fraction. The last large peak consisted of low molecular weight material including urinary pigments.

All urine concentrates were tested for rheumatoid factor activity using the latex fixation test. In 19 RA patients tested only one showed a positive test, with a titre of 1/10. Efforts to localize this rheumatoid factor activity through gel filtration and screening of eluate fractions with the latex slide test were not successful.

Other connective tissue diseases

The urinary immunoglobulins in the connective tissue disease group showed the same general pattern as had been noted in the RA group, but quantities were generally somewhat lower. One patient with SS, who excreted relatively large amounts of kappa type light chains, was included in this group, and thus affecting the figure for mean free light chain excretion. When IgG and light chain excretion data for this group were considered together with those for the RA group they were still significantly higher than those for the control group (p < 0.01).

The incidence of urinary IgA and quantitative data regarding this immunoglobulin did not differ significantly between the patient group as a whole and the control group.

TABLE 2

Urinary immunoglobulin excretion in patient EN
with systemic sclerosis in mg/24 hr.

	IgG	IgA	Free light chains	
			K	L
Oct. -68	4	0	80	8
Dec. -68	40	6	178	5
June -69	40	0	127	1
Nov. -69	24	0	63	4

Agarose gel electrophoresis of the urine concentrates showed no evidence of increased homogeneity in the gammaglobulin region. The gammaglobulins usually appeared as a heterogenous, smear-like material.

Several 24 hour urine samples from patient EN with systemic sclerosis were studied; quantitative data are tabulated in Table 2. This patient had a striking elevation of K type light chain excretion, while the amount of lambda type light chains was quite small. Agarose gel electrophoresis of the urine concentrate showed a narrow »band» in the γ-region, and immunoelectrophoresis using kappa antiserum showed a precipitin bow with limited electrophoretic dispersion (Fig. 2). The Bence-Jones heat test, however, was negative. Clinical investigation did not show any sign of myeloma (no serum M-component, normal bone-marrow, no lytic lesions in the skeleton), but a polyclonal hypergammaglobulinaemia. However, immunoelectrophoresis showed presence of free kappa type light chains in the patient's serum (33).

DISCUSSION

The findings in this study of increased free light chains in the urine from patients with rheumatoid arthritis and other connective tissue disease confirms results obtained by Gordon, Eisen and Vaughan (13) and Cooper and Bluestone (7). However, the latter authors did not find any free light chains at all in the urine of their control group of ten samples, while in this study the majority of controls (12/

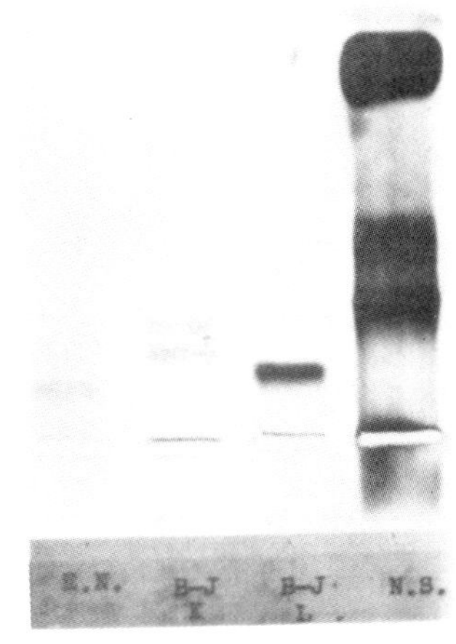

Fig. 2. A. Agarose gel electrophoresis of urine concentrate from patient EN, isolated Bence-Jones protein type kappa and lambda and normal human serum (NS). Anode towards the top.

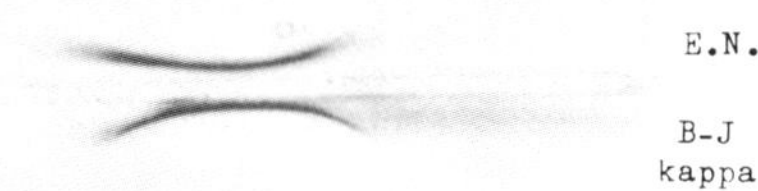

Fig. 2. B. Immunoelectrophoresis of EN urine concentrate and isolated Bence-Jones protein type kappa. Antiserum against kappa type light chains is used. Anode to the left.

17) showed the presence of small amounts free light chains. Free light chains have previously been demonstrated in normal human urine by Berggård and others (1, 14).

Cooper and Bluestone (7) found no free light chains in the urine from 14 patients with systemic sclerosis. Two patients with this disease were studied here, and both showed elevated level of urinary free light chains. Actually one of the patients (EN) showed a monoclonal Bence-Jones-like protein in her urine.

Elevated levels of free light chains in the urine probably reflect increased immunoglobulin synthesis. The study by Gordon and associates (12) and Vaughan, Jacox and Grey (36) has demonstrated that urinary light chains represent an anabolic product in gammaglobulin metabolism, rather than breakdown products from the immunoglobulin molecule. Also, studies by Shapiro, Scharff, Maizel and Uhr (29) indicate that there is synthesis and release of excess light chains by cells from the lymph nodes of hyperimmunized rabbits.

Solomon, Waldman, Fahey and McFarlane (31) showed that free light chains were rapidly catabolized in the healthy kidney, which means that urinary free light chains are only a portion of the free light chains synthesized per day. Studies by Wochner, Strober and Waldman (40) in nephrectomized mice also clearly stress the importance of the kidneys in the metabolic fate of free light chains. In renal insufficiency, the catabolism is diminished and the level of free light chains in serum increases, as does the amount of free light chains excreted in the urine (9). However, none of the patients in this study had any evidence of renal disease; this makes it unlikely that poor renal function contributed to the increased level of urinary light chains.

The gel filtration experiments on urine concentrates from RA patients showed elution patterns very similar to that obtained on urine concentrates from normal human urine (4). This suggests that the relative proportions of intact IgG molecules and Fc-like material are approximately the same in rheumatoid arthritis and normal people. The occurrence in the urine concentrate of low molecular weight material reacting with antisera to IgG might influence the quantitation procedure in the Oudin tubes, since this depends on diffusion of molecules through an agar-antiserum mixture, tending to give falsely high figures for IgG. However, the same source of error applies equally to quantitations on control urine concentrates (for reasons given above), making comparison between IgG excretion data relevant. The increased excretion of IgG + Fc-like fragments in patients with rheumatoid arthritis probably reflects increased immunoglobulin synthesis. It is conceivable that hypergammaglobulinaemia, which was present in most of the RA patients, can cause increased secretion of the intact IgG molecule in the urine, since this molecule is normally present in urine. The demonstration of an Fc-like protein in the urine and plasma of patients with heavy chain disease (10, 24) suggests that Fc synthesis may be part of an anabolic process in the formation of the complete IgG molecule. This is supported by the finding of Berggård and Bennich (2) of Fc in normal plasma. On the other hand urinary Fc-piece may be due to catabolism of IgG. This is supported by the report of Vaughan and associates (36) who demonstrated Fc-like material in urine after parenteral administration of labelled IgG to agammaglobulinaemic patients.

The finding of IgA rheumatoid factor in urine of patients with rheumatoid arthritis (5) could not be confirmed in this study. However, this could be because Bienenstock and coworkers used more concentrated urine specimens (1000 times versus 200 times). Also the group of patients studied by Bienenstock et al. had higher serum latex titres than those reported here.

Studies of the urinary immunoglobulins on electrophoresis showed no evidence of increased homogeneity. Also the presence of both types of light chain (kappa and lambda) with the expected average kappa/lambda ratio of approximately 2:1 (41), is similar to the heterogeneity observed in normal immunoglobulins.

The patient EN with systemic sclerosis, however, was a notable exception to this. She excreted what might be called a Bence-Jones type of protein in her urine. The fact that the Bence-Jones heat test was negative is a result of the low sensitivity of this test (20). This patient had a polyclonal type of hypergammaglobulinaemia, but no serum M-component or other evidence of myeloma or macroglobulinaemia of Waldenström. Though this case may fall into some light chain variant (39) of what has recently been called lanthanic disease (41) or benign monoclonal gammopathy of Waldenström (18, 37), it is conceivable that this monoclonal urinary protein is in some way directly related to systemic sclerosis and the hypergammaglobulinaemic state. It may be that this urinary monoclonal immunoglobulin represents the initial stage of transition from polyclonal to monoclonal type immunoglobulin response. This kind of transition has been documented in Aleutian disease of mink (26), which probably is a viral disease of mustelids, accompanied by marked hypergammaglobulinaemia (15, 16, 38). In these animals a viral infection leads to plasmacytosis with polyclonal hypergammaglobulinaemia, and may evolve into monoclonal paraproteinaemia and Bence-Jones proteinuria (6, 13, 26).

Evidence presented in several recent publications (11, 42, 43) suggests a greater than chance incidence of paraproteinemia in rheumatoid arthritis. It is argued that prolonged antigenic stimulation, for example by rheumatoid arthritis, may be a factor in the evolution of immunoproliferative disorders. It is conceivable that similar pathogenic mechanisms could be operating in systemic sclerosis. The patient EN is being carefully followed in order to detect further evidence of a transition of the kind mentioned above.

ACKNOWLEDGEMENT

The study was supported by grant B70-61P-2917-01 from the Swedish Medical Research Council, Alfred Österlunds Stiftelse, Riksföreningen mot Reumatism and Medicinska Fakulteten, University of Lund, Sweden. I want to thank Dr. Ralph C. Williams, Jr. for reviewing the manuscript. The expert technical assistance of Mrs. Maj Lis Svensson is gratefully acknowledged.

REFERENCES

1. *Berggård I:* On a γ-globulin of low molecular weight in normal human plasma and urine. Clin Chim Acta 6: 413, 1961
2. *Berggård I, Bennich H:* Fc fragment of immunoglobulin G in normal human plasma and urine. Nature (London) 214: 697, 1967
3. *Bienenstock J, Tomasi TB:* Secretory γA in urine. Clin Res, 15: 292, 1967
4. *Bienenstock J:* Urinary Fc and F'c fragments. J Immun 100: 280, 1968
5. *Bienenstock J, Goldstein G, Tomasi TB:* Urinary γA rheumatoid factor. J Lab Clin Med 73: 389, 1969
6. *Buko L, Kenyon AJ:* Aleutian disease gammopathy of mink induced with an ultrafiltrable agent. Nature (London) 216: 69, 1967
7. *Cooper A, Bluestone R:* Free immunoglobulin light chains in connective tissue disease. Ann Rheum Dis 27: 537, 1968
8. *Dixon WJ, Massey FJ:* Introduction to statistical analysis. McGraw-Hill, York Pa 1957
9. *Epstein WV, Gulyassy PF, Tan M, Rae AI:* Effect of renal homotransplantation on the metabolism of the light chains of immunoglobulins. Ann Intern Med 68: 48, 1968
10. *Franklin EL, Lowenstein J, Bigelow B, Meltzer M:* Heavy chain disease — a new disorder of serum γ-globulins. Amer J Med 37: 332, 1964
11. *Goldenberg GJ, Paraskevas F, Israels LG:* The association of rheumatoid arthritis with plasma cell and lymphocytic neoplasms. Arthritis Rheum 12: 569, 1969
12. *Gordon DA, Eisen AZ, Vaughan JH:* Studies in urinary γ-globulins in patients with rheumatoid arthritis. Arthritis Rheum 9: 575, 1966
13. *Gordon DA, Franklin AE, Karstad L:* Viral plasmacytosis (Aleutian disease) of mink resembling human collagen disease. Canad Med Ass J 96: 1245, 1967
14. *Hanson LÅ, Tan EM:* Characterisation of antibodies in human urine. J Clin Invest 44: 703, 1965
15. *Henson JB, Leader RW, Gorham JR:* Hypergammaglobulinemia in mink. Proc Soc Exp Biol Med 107: 919, 1961
16. *Kenyon AJ, Trautwein G, Helmboldt CF:* Characterization of blood serum protein from mink with Aleutian disease. Amer J Vet Res 24: 168, 1963
17. *Kunkel HG:* Zone electrophoresis. In: Methods of biochemical analysis. Interscience Publishers, Inc., New York 1954
18. *Kyle RA, Bayrd ED:* »Benign» monoclonal gammopathy: a potentially malignant condition? Amer J Med 40: 426, 1966
19. *Laurell CB:* Antigen-antibody crossed electrophoresis. Anal Biochem 10: 358, 1965
20. *Lindström FD, Williams RC Jr, Swaim WR, Freier EF:* Urinary light chain excretion in myeloma and other disorders — an evaluation of the Bence-Jones test. J Lab Clin Med 71: 812, 1968
21. *Lindström FD, Williams RC Jr., Theologides A:* Urinary light chain excretion in leukemia and lymphoma. Clin Exp Immun 5: 83, 1969
22. *Lindström FD:* Kappa/lambda light chain ratio in IgG eluted from rheumatoid arthritis synovium. Clin Exp Immun 7: 1, 1970
23. *Mannik M, Kunkel HG:* Two major types of normal 7S γ-globulin. J Exp Med 117: 213, 1963
24. *Osserman EF, Takatsuki K:* Clinical and immunochemical studies of four cases of heavy (Hγ) chain disease. Amer J Med 37: 351, 1964

25. *Oudin J:* Specific precipitation in gels and its application to immunochemical analysis. Meth Med Res 5: 335, 1952

26. *Porter DD, Dixon FJ, Larsen AE:* The development of a myeloma-like condition in mink with Aleutian disease. Blood 25: 736, 1965

27. *Porter DD, Dixon FJ, Larsen AF:* Metabolism and function of gammaglobulin in Aleutian disease in mink. J Exp Med 121: 889, 1965

28. *Scheidegger JJ:* Une micro-méthode de l'immunoélectrophorèses. Int Arch Allerg 7: 103, 1955

29. *Shapiro AL, Scharff MD, Maizel JV Jr, Uhr JW:* Synthesis of excess light chains of gammaglobulin by rabbit lymph node cells. Nature (London) 211: 243, 1966

30. *Singer JM, Plotz CM:* The latex fixation test. I. Application to the serological diagnosis of rheumatoid arthritis. Amer J Med 21: 888, 1956

31. *Solomon A, Waldmann TA, Fahey JL, McFarlane AS:* Metabolism of Bence-Jones proteins. J Clin Invest 43: 103, 1964

32. *Stevensson GT:* Further studies of the gamma-related proteins of normal urine. J Clin Invest 41: 1190, 1962

33. *Tan M, Epstein WC:* A direct immunologic assay of human serum for Bence-Jones proteins (L-chains). J Lab Clin Med 66: 344, 1965

34. *Turner MW, Rowe DS:* Characterization of human antibodies to Salmonella typhi by gel-filtration and antigenic analysis. Immunology 7: 639, 1964

35. *Turner MW, Rowe DS:* A naturally occurring fragment related to the heavy chains of immunoglobulin G in normal human urine. Nature (London) 210: 130, 1966

36. *Vaughan JH, Jacox RF, Grey BA:* Light and heavy chain components of gamma-globulins in urines of normal persons and patients with agammaglobulinemia. J Clin Invest 46: 266, 1967

37. *Waldenström J:* The occurrence of benign, essential monoclonal (M type) nonmacromolecular hyperglobulinemia and its differential diagnosis. IV. Studies in the gammopathies. Acta Med Scand 176: 345, 1964

38. *Williams RC Jr, Russel JD, Kenyon AJ:* Antigammaglobulin factors and immunofluorescent studies in normal mink and mink with Aleutian disease. Amer J Vet Res 27: 1447, 1966

39. *Williams RC Jr, Brunning RC, Wollheim FA:* Light chain disease — an abortive variant of multiple myeloma. Ann Intern Med 65: 471, 1966

40. *Wochner RD, Strober W, Waldmann TA:* The role of the kidney in the catabolism of Bence-Jones proteins and immunoglobulin fragments. J Exp Med 126: 207, 1967

41. *Zawadzki ZA, Edwards GA:* Dysimmunoglobulinemia in the absence of clinical features of multiple myeloma and macroglobulinemia. Amer J Med 42: 67, 1967

42. *Zawadzki ZA, Benedek TG, Ein D, Easton JM:* Rheumatoid arthritis terminating in heavy-chain disease. Ann Intern Med 70: 335, 1969

43. *Zawadzki ZA, Benedek TG:* Rheumatoid arthritis, dysproteinemic arthropathy and paraproteinemia. Arthritis Rheum 12: 555, 1969

Rheumatoid Arthritis in Man
and Immune Complexes

LYSOSOMAL MECHANISMS OF TISSUE INJURY IN ARTHRITIS

GERALD WEISSMANN, M.D.

STUDIES during the past decade have indicated that lysosomes mediate, at least in part, acute and chronic inflammation in joints.[1-4] This association in no way implies that etiologic agents have been identified in human arthritis, except in such discrete entities as crystal-induced or infectious arthritis. Two main points have been appreciated, however. First of all, it is clear that materials present in lysosomes can provoke inflammation, tissue injury and breakdown of connective tissue. Secondly, it is the normal function of lysosomes, as part of the "vacuolar apparatus" described by DeDuve,[5] to extrude enzymes from cells into surrounding tissues.

Since many of these studies have been directed toward an analysis of human rheumatoid arthritis, it is important to consider the features of this disease in which a role can be postulated for lysosomes.[6] The local lesions of rheumatoid arthritis are characterized by the margination of leukocytes and their appearance in synovial fluid; hypertrophy and hyperplasia of synovial lining cells, many of which contain abnormal numbers and configurations of lysosomes; infiltration of the synovium by many lymphocytes, frequently in clusters; the transformation of synovium into granulation tissue, which, as pannus, invades cartilage; and erosion of cartilage, initially of matrix and followed by chondrocyte death and attempts at regeneration.

The primary reason for implicating lysosomes in such changes is that each of the local lesions of human disease can develop in laboratory animals injected with lysates of purified lysosomes.[4] Moreover, analysis of synovia and synovial fluid from patients with rheumatoid arthritis has documented

Supported by grants from the National Institutes of Health (AM-11949), the New York Heart Association and the New York Chapter of the Arthritis Foundation.

considerable increases in activity of many lysosomal enzymes (acid phosphatase, beta-glucuronidase, cathepsin D and lysozyme). Histochemical and ultrastructural studies show that lysosomes of synovial lining cells from patients with rheumatoid arthritis have an abnormal appearance and may be more permeable to substrate.[6] This observation does not necessarily mean that the membranes of ordinary lysosomes are more "fragile," but may reflect formation of new kinds of digestive vacuoles, the membranes of which differ in various reactions from those of resting lysosomes. Finally, agents that disrupt biomembranes (especially those of lysosomes) produce changes in joints morphologically similar to lysosome-induced arthritis and to human disease.[3,4] But to draw firmer conclusions from these indirect observations, it must be shown that lysosomes contain discrete substances capable of mediating the various components of the chronic, local lesions. These substances are listed in Table 1.[7]

Table 1. Hydrolysis of Macromolecules by Lysosomal Hydrolases.*

SUBSTRATE	ENZYME	SOURCE
EXTRACELLULAR STRUCTURES		
Collagen	Collagenase	Leukocytes
Protein polysaccharides	Hyaluronidase	Liver
Protein polysaccharides	Neutral protease	Leukocytes
Protein polysaccharides	Cathepsin D	Liver, cartilage
Hyaluronate, chondroitin sulfate	Hyaluronidase	Liver, bone
Cartilage matrix	Cathepsin D	Cartilage
Elastin	Elastase	Leukocytes
Arterial walls	Elastase	Leukocytes
Basement membranes	Cathepsins D, E	Leukocytes
Erythrocyte membranes	?	Liver
Amyloid	?	Macrophages
CIRCULATING MATERIALS		
C'1	Neutral protease	Leukocytes
C'3, C'5	Neutral protease	Leukocytes
Kininogens, kinins	Neutral protease	Leukocytes
Fibrin	Acid peptidases	Leukocytes
Thyroglobulin	Cathepsins D, E	Spleen
Gamma globulin	Neutral, acid proteases	Beef, human spleen
Endotoxin	?	Liver
Plasminogen	Urokinase	Kidney

*Modified from Weissmann & Dukor,[7] in which primary references are listed.

Lysosomal Mechanisms

Chemotaxis (Attraction of Leukocytes to Local Site)

After the initial demonstration that leukocytes or their lysosomes could generate chemotactic factors from fresh serum, Ward and Hill[8] identified a neutral protease in rabbit leukocyte lysosomes that was capable of generating chemotactic activity by means of a complement component. Indeed, lysates of the granules cleaved complement component C5 into fragments varying in molecular weight from 4000 to 15,000. These authors had previously shown that a neutral protease from heart tissue could generate chemotactic activity from C3. Taubman et al.[9] recently confirmed the generation of chemotactic activity from C5 and demonstrated, furthermore, that neutrophil lysosomes can cleave C3 into large and small fragments.

Hypertrophy and Hyperplasia

When lysates of polymorphonuclear leukocytes are injected into the joints of rabbits, the synovial lining cells undergo hypertrophy, and new mitoses are evident as early as 24 hours after injection. Such changes could be brought about if lysosomal proteases were able to influence gene activity in mammalian cells; in fact, one such mechanism has been documented. After Ryan and Cardin[10] reported that lysates of purified lysosomes induced mitoses in cultured cells, it was found that a neutral protease, present in leukocyte lysosomes, could hydrolyze histones.[11] Indeed, lysates of granulocyte lysosomes were found to act like trypsin in augmenting the template activity of isolated nuclei or chromatin for exogenous RNA-polymerase (perhaps by removing regulatory proteins from DNA).[12] It is possible, therefore, that if lysosomal hydrolases gained access to the cell nuclei, they could act to derepress them by hydrolyzing regulatory proteins. Furthermore, protease-sensitive steps in the translational process have also been identified, and it will be a challenging task to determine whether purified, neutral proteases of human lysosomes can cause similar alterations of transcription or translation.

Lymphocyte Clustering

Many of the lymphocytes that appear as follicular

clusters in the synovium of patients with rheumatoid arthritis, or in animals injected with lysosomal lysates, appear to have "activated" nuclei and an abundant cytoplasm filled with vacuoles. In this respect, they resemble lymphocytes stimulated by phytohemagglutinin or by specific antigen. Stimulated, or transformed, human lymphocytes differ from resting cells in their content of lysosomal enzymes. Hirschhorn et al.[14] found that the content of lysosomal enzymes in the transformed cells was markedly augmented. Such cells, which elaborate various factors capable of injuring cells with which they have come in contact, are therefore also equipped with a complement of lysosomal hydrolases. Indeed, Allison and Mallucci[15] have suggested, and Hirschhorn et al.[16] have documented, that lysosomal hydrolases of resting lymphocytes undergo redistribution within the first two hours of the cells' encounter with phytohemagglutinin. It is at this time that the template capacity for exogenous RNA-polymerase of isolated lymphocyte nuclei is dramatically increased and that the normal trypsin-induced augmentation of RNA synthesis is abolished.[17] Such observations suggest that when lymphocytes become activated by antigen or phytohemagglutinin, they have undergone changes that could result from the pre-emptive action of an endogenous neutral protease, akin to the histonase described in leukocyte lysosomes. This hypothesis was supported by the finding that inhibitors of proteolysis also inhibited lymphocyte stimulation.[18]

Granulation Tissue

Allison et al.[19] suggested that the overgrowth of fibroblasts induced by agents such as silica is due to the release of lysosomal hydrolases. Silica is engulfed by lysosomes, forms membrane-disruptive hydrogen bonds with their inner walls, and therefore kills cells by inducing a kind of "perforation of the cell's digestive tract," to use the terminology of DeDuve. No direct relation between a discrete lysosomal component and fibroplasia has yet been identified, but repeated injections of lysates of leukocyte lysosomes lead to fibroplasia and pannus formation in homologous animals.[4]

Degradation of Cartilage Matrix

Experiments carried out in the laboratories of

Lewis Thomas, in New York City, and Dame Honor B. Fell, in Cambridge, England, first showed that the depletion of cartilage matrix due to breakdown of a large glycoprotein called PP-L[20] can be induced by an excess of vitamin A. The vitamin acts in vivo in rabbits and in vitro in limb-bone organ cultures to liberate a cathepsin from chondrocyte lysosomes (reviewed by Dingle[21]). This enzyme was purified and identified as cathepsin D[22]; antiserums to the purified enzyme were capable of inhibiting cartilage degradation. Cathepsin D has a pH optimum of 3.5; its major role is presumably intracellular. It was therefore of considerable interest to find that lysosomes of leukocytes contained a neutral protease capable of breaking down PP-L,[23] of degrading cartilage matrix[23] and of hydrolyzing histones.[11] ·This neutral protease was found to be concentrated in leukocyte granules, and indeed in one of their subgroups.

Collagenase is required, however, if cartilage is to be completely eroded, since breakdown of glycoproteins can account only for loss of metachromasia or softening. Harris et al.[24] recently reported that rheumatoid synovium and fluid contain a collagenase capable of degrading insoluble collagen at neutral pH. The source of this enzyme is as yet unclear, but it appears to differ from the lysosomal enzyme isolated from leukocytes by Lazarus et al.[25] The lysosomal enzyme, unlike synovial collagenase, is not inhibited by serum and is less active upon collagen in fibrillar form. It appears to arise as a consequence of synovial pannus formation, which I believe is a result of earlier release of lysosomal hydrolases.

Tissue Injury in Rheumatoid Arthritis

A sequence of events consistent with the outline described above is summarized in Figure 1. The primary stimulus to the formation of rheumatoid factor is unknown. Once immune complexes form, they are taken up by phagocytes (not only polymorphonuclears, but lining cells as well), and lysosomal hydrolases are extruded. Direct activation of the complement sequence after the union of rheumatoid factor with altered 7S gamma globulin (IgG) can be inferred from studies of synovial fluid. In joint fluids of patients with rheumatoid arthritis, depletion of specific components of complement (C1, C4,

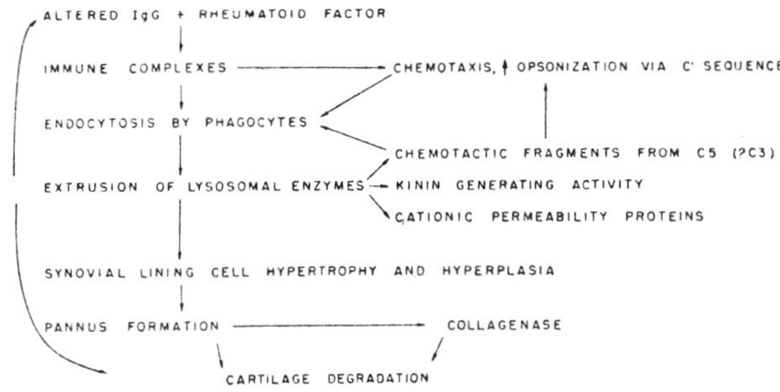

Figure 1. One possible Sequence of Tissue Injury in Rheumatoid Arthritis.

C2 and C3) has been documented, in association with the appearance of C3 convertase and the activation of C5, C6 and C7.[26] But lysosomal enzymes can also generate biologically active materials from C5 and the kinin system; indeed, Hegner[27] demonstrated the presence of kinin-forming and kinin-degrading enzymes in leukocyte lysosomes. Cationic permeability-promoting proteins that act independently of kinins or complement components have also been demonstrated in lymphocyte lysosomes.

After acute injury, pannus formation results from synovial hypertrophy and hyperplasia as well as the cellular immune factors elaborated by transformed lymphocytes. It was previously suggested that the antigen or antigens that give rise to humoral antibody (rheumatoid factor) and cellular immune reactions (lymphocyte clusters) may be native constituents altered by lysosomal enzymes.[3] The recent description by LoSpalluto, Fehr and Ziff[28] of the partial degradation of gamma globulin by lysosomal proteases tends to support such a hypothesis.

Lysosomal Enzyme Extrusion

If lysosomal contents can be held responsible for many of the local lesions of rheumatoid arthritis, how can one account for their release into synovial fluid and surrounding tissues? Lysosomes are abundant in the lining cells of the synovial membrane, many of which are nothing but specialized forms of fixed tissue macrophages. They are also present in cartilage cells. We are therefore presented with a number of possible cellular sources for enzyme release. But perhaps the most readily available sources are polymorphonuclear leukocytes, which crowd the inflamed synovial cavity in rheumatoid arthritis. These cells, filled with engulfed complexes of rheumatoid factor and altered IgG, have been called "R.A. cells," or ragocytes, and constitute a hallmark of the disease. It is therefore reasonable to assume that the engulfment of large particles such as immune complexes leads to extrusion of lysosomal constituents..

Three main hypotheses have been proposed to account for extrusion of hydrolases from cells engaged in the uptake of bulky materials. The first, advanced by Metchnikoff,[29] attributes hydrolase release to death of the phagocyte, with subsequent escape of ferments (cytases) into surrounding tissues. The second, which may be described as "regurgitation during feeding," suggests that phagosomes still open at the external surface of the cell are joined by leukocyte lysosomes at their innermost borders (Fig. 2). Under such circumstances, lysosomal hydrolases could escape from the open end of incompletely fused, secondary lysosomes. Electron microscopical images consistent with this hypothesis have been presented.[30] The third hypothesis has been proposed to account for selective extrusion of lysosomal enzymes by cells or bone rudiments in culture. Dingle[21] suggested that uptake of macromolecules by such tissues results in perturbation of lysosomal membranes, causing them to merge selectively with similarly perturbed portions of the external cell membrane that has been called "reverse endocytosis," which is the exact opposite of events observed during uptake.

We have shown that when mouse peritoneal macrophages or human polymorphonuclear leukocytes take up zymosan or latex particles, they selectively release lysosomal enzymes without extruding cytoplasmic enzymes[31] or suffering cellular injury. Selective extrusion of lysosomal hydrolases could effectively be retarded by agents that raised the intracellular level of cyclic 3',5' adenosine monophosphate (cAMP) — for example, prostaglandin E_1 and theophylline — or by cyclic nucleotides themselves. These studies suggested that the Metchnikoff

hypothesis could not account for hydrolase release
after uptake of inert particles since extrusion of
lysosomal enzymes was not accompanied by death
of the cell or leakage of cytoplasmic enzymes. It is
not possible, however, to decide between the other
two possibilities — that is, "regurgitation" and
"reverse endocytosis" — although the former seems
more likely.

INHIBITION OF ENZYME RELEASE FROM HUMAN POLYMORPHONUCLEAR LEUKOCYTES

To determine whether the ingestion of immune
complexes produced changes similar to those induced by inert particles or, on the other hand, to
those induced by crystals that cause death of the
cell by perforation, we have compared the uptake
by human polymorphonuclear leukocytes of immune
complexes with the uptake of inert zymosan particles and monosodium urate crystals. It has been
suggested that these crystals are taken up by phagocytes, enter secondary lysosomes and cause death of
the cell by virtue of direct membrane perforation
from within the lysosomes.[32]

These studies showed that human polymorphonuclear leukocytes selectively released a portion of
their intracellular lysosomal hydrolases without
leaking cytoplasmic lactate dehydrogenase or losing
viability when they encountered immune complexes
of rheumatoid arthritis with heat-aggregated IgG. In
direct contrast, monosodium urate crystals caused
polymorphonuclear leukocytes to leak lactate dehydrogenase and beta glucuronidase simultaneously;
cell viability was grossly impaired earlier, and to a
greater extent. Therefore, leukocytes are killed
when exposed to membrane-lytic crystals, but they
respond to immune complexes in the same manner
as to inert particles: by releasing lysosomal hydrolases into their surrounding medium.

Previous work by Dorothea Zucker-Franklin[30]
documented the entry into polymorphonuclear leukocytes of immune complexes. Indeed, electron
photomicrographs show that uptake of RF-aIgG proceeds, at least in some cases, by pathways compatible with the "regurgitation-during-feeding" hypothesis, as shown in Figure 2. Since such images were
rarely seen, it could not be inferred that other pathways were excluded as means by which enzymes
are released. Previous work had indicated that

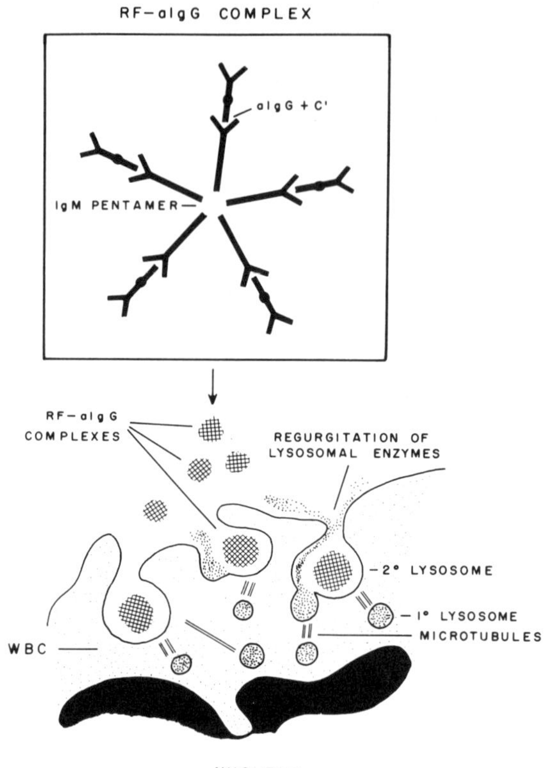

Figure 2. Regurgitation of Lysosomal Hydrolases on Exposure to Immune Complexes Composed of Rheumatoid Factor (IgM Pentamer) and Aggregated IgG (aIgG).

As the complexes enter phagosomes, the latter merge with primary lysosomes to form secondary lysosomes within which digestion takes place. In some circumstances, fusion with lysosomes at the internal border of the phagosome proceeds before the external opening has sealed off completely. Merger of primary lysosomes with phagosomes, or the cell membrane, is thought to depend upon intact microtubules. Extrusion of hydrolases takes place from lysosomes of living cells, since the enzymes do not gain access to the free cytoplasm, and the cell remains viable. Drugs such as colchicine and vinblastine are believed to prevent hydrolase release by interfering with granule flow and merger, a process that is also dependent upon the level of AMP within cells.

polymorphonuclear leukocytes respond to uptake of bacteria or other particles with extrusion of hydrolases, but such experiments had not clearly excluded cell death or damage to the plasma membrane as factors in enzyme release. Similarly, several studies have documented redistribution of acid hydrolases from granular to less easily sedimentable forms after polymorphonuclear leukocytes were exposed to bacteria or RF-aIgG complexes. Unfortunately, these experiments could not distinguish between enzymes that have been released from lysosomes within living cells and those that have come to reside in a population of secondary lysosomes, which are more fragile during homogenization than the lysosomes of resting cells.

cAMP and Enzyme Release

The mechanisms by which cyclic nucleotides, prostaglandin E_1 and theophylline inhibit selective release of lysosomal hydrolases from polymorphonuclear leukocytes exposed to particles or immune complexes are unclear. These agents could block uptake of the particles, retard merger of primary lysosomes with the phagosomes or prevent merger of lysosomes with the plasma membrane. We could detect no gross interference with the initial stages of particle uptake: no inhibition of zymosan-particle uptake was detected, and equal numbers of cells took up visible crystals or stainable complexes. However, these agents may have effects both upon phagocytosis per se and upon the subsequent fate of the phagocytosed material. When heat-aggregated protein (^{125}I-labeled bovine serum albumin) was fed to macrophages in the presence of such agents, uptake was indeed retarded. But if one followed the intracellular degradation of the radiolabeled material once it had been ingested, it was found that high concentrations of cAMP retarded digestion, as did colchicine or incubation at 4°C.[33] Prostaglandin E_1 (which stimulates formation of cAMP in polymorphonuclear leukocytes at the concentrations used in these experiments) and theophylline (which inhibits the phosphodiesterase capable of hydrolyzing cAMP) were synergistic. It is therefore likely that these agents acted to block lysosomal enzyme release by means of increasing intracellular cAMP concentrations. It has been suggested that the intracellular level of cAMP might act to regulate the traffic of lysosomes to the digestive vacuole or to the cell periphery by an effect on microtubules or microfilaments.[31,33]

THERAPEUTIC CONSIDERATIONS

If extrusion of lysosomal hydrolases is central to tissue injury in acute and chronic arthritis, how do the drugs that are thought to be useful in treating joint disease work? Table 2 lists the agents that

Table 2. Effect of Some Drugs on Lysosomal Function.

DIRECT STABILIZATION OF LYSOSOMAL MEMBRANE

Cortisone	Chloroquine
Cortisol	Phenylbutazone
Prednisolone	Acetylsalicylic acid
Betamethasone	Stilbamidines

UPTAKE & CONCENTRATION WITHIN LYSOSOMES

Chloroquine, stilbamidine, gold salts

INHIBITION OF LYSOSOMAL ENZYMES

Gold Salts, Trypan Blue

INHIBITION OF LYSOSOMAL ENZYME RELEASE OR VACUOLE MERGER (OR BOTH)

Colchicine, vinblastine, cAMP, theophylline, prostaglandin E_1

have been shown to affect the function of lysosomes in vivo and in vitro; many of these agents are used in connective-tissue diseases.[2] In general, they may be considered to act either directly upon the lysosome or upon its function in the vacuolar system, but these effects are by no means mutually exclusive. Thus, steroids, which stabilize lysosomal membranes, also retard merger of the phagocytic vacuole with pre-existent lysosomes, and chloroquine, which stabilizes lysosomes in vitro, appears to induce autophagy in living cells by mechanisms that are not well understood.[2] It is of interest that many of the agents that inhibit extrusion of lysosomal hydrolases also have effects upon phagocytosis per se or on leukocyte motility; colchicine is a prime example. The selective effects of colchicine in gouty arthritis are still unexplained by these actions.

DISCUSSION

DR. LEE WITTERS: Do you think that aspirin works on inflammatory states by acetylating the membrane for release of lysosomal enzymes as it does in the platelet and possibly in the mast cell?

DR. WEISSMANN: Whether salicylates can acetylate receptors on the membrane or cytoplasmic structural proteins (microtubles and microfilaments) themselves remains to be determined.

DR. WITTERS: Could informational macromolecules introduced within a mammalian cell by endocytosis possibly reach the nucleus without becoming destroyed by lysosomal enzymes?

DR. WEISSMANN: That is a difficult question, not only to us but to virologists. Some viruses, such as double-stranded RNA reovirus, can escape ribonuclease attack. Chromosomal breaks can be produced in cultured cells incubated with purified deoxyribonuclease, suggesting that large enzymes can gain access to the nucleus. There is also evidence that exogenous peroxidase may enter the inner cisternae of the endoplasmic reticulum, which is coexistent with the outer nuclear membrane. Thus, some data do suggest that macromolecules, by mechanisms that we need not postulate now, can gain entry to the cell, escape destruction and produce nuclear changes.

DR. ALFRED GOLDBERG: In Figure 2 you did not mention any of the inhibitors of lysosomal protease. I wonder whether an agent like amino caproic acid would be useful pharmacologically?

DR. WEISSMANN: A number of lysosomal proteases differ considerably in their spectrum of inhibition by various protease inhibitors. This is a promising area of investigation.

DR. HOWARD H. HIATT: If you visualize extra lysosomal protease activity, for example, as attacking histones and making the DNA more available to the polymerase, what mechanism do you visualize to protect the polymerase from the same enzyme that is attacking the histones?

DR. WEISSMANN: Interestingly enough, when we do the experiments in vitro, we get very little degradation of polymerase at neutral pH, but very much at acid pH (measured with pure DNA as template). The proteases of lysosomes appear relatively specific in many ways — just as limited proteolysis activated in plasma accounts for selective activation of kinins or complement components; the substrate specificity may be extremely important in this regard. Indeed, the postulate of substrate specificity might explain why the enzymes of lysosomes do not degrade themselves. For example, leukocyte lysosomes incubated under sterile conditions for about 24 hours show no decrement in activity at neutral pH, whereas if they are acidified, or if other proteins are added, digestion will proceed rapidly.

DR. CARL HIRSCH: The problem of specificity is a very interesting one. There seems to be a high degree of recognition, even of specific proteins. This is so specific that if one invested this specificity in a different enzyme, one would need as many enzymes as there are protein species. Do you have any evidence for a better model that would also provide recognition under certain conditions of specific proteins?

DR. WEISSMANN: There is evidence for a system that recognizes older, effete proteins in liver autolysis. However, within the waves of autophagy that follow shock, anoxia or glucagon, whole organelles are removed indiscriminately. Within the autophagic vacuoles formed after chloroquine administration, indiscriminate and random removal of organelles and proteins has also been suggested. If the bulk of cellular turnover is due to autophagy, few mechanisms for selectivity of enzyme turnover can be postulated. I do not know how autophagic removal of organelles can possibly provide one with specificity of hydrolysis.

DR. HOWARD LEVIN: Are there systems in which the lysosomes function independently of complement?

DR. WEISSMANN: One of our earlier hypotheses was that complement is taken up by phagocytes together with immune complexes. We thought that subsequently its components might act in very much the way monosodium urate crystals do — that is, to have terminal complement components perforate lysosomes from within. Unfortunately, in our hands and those of Peter Henson (personal communication), who has been studying hydrolase extrusion when polymorphonuclear leukocytes encounter a filter coated with immune complexes, complement enhances, but its absence does not completely impair, hydrolase extrusion. Extrusion is relatively independent of complement; it apparently is the general response of cells to ingestion of particles, whether or not they are immune. Complement components are crucial, of course, in regulating the uptake of materials, in the absence of which no extrusion can occur.

Dr. Goldberg: Is there any direct evidence in this system for an effect of colchicine on the release process? Isn't there an inconsistency in saying that colchicine may be useful in gout by blocking the release of lysosomal enzymes and, at the same time, saying that urate crystals act by causing intracellular lysis?

Dr. Weissmann: I agree completely; that is a paradox. If colchicine worked only by inhibiting the merger of the primary lysosome with the secondary lysosome (a merger that is dependent upon the integrity of microtubules) cholchicine would be an ideal anti-inflammatory agent in all systems. It should therefore be very effective in pseudogout, associated with uptake of calcium pyrophosphate crystals. It is not; therefore, we are studying whether colchicine inhibits hydrogen bonding between crystals and membranes, and our results in this regard are as yet inconclusive.

References

1. Weissmann G, Dingle JT: Release of lysosomal protease by ultraviolet irradiation and inhibition by hydrocortisone. Exp Cell Res 25:207-210, 1961
2. Weissmann G: The effects of steroids and drugs on lysosomes. Lysosomes in Biology and Pathology. Edited by JT Dingle, HB Fell. Amsterdam, North-Holland Publishing Company, 1969, pp 276-298
3. Idem: Lysosomes, autoimmune phenomena, and diseases of connective tissue. Lancet 2:1373-1375, 1964
4. Weissmann G, Spilberg I, Krakauer K: Arthritis induced in rabbits by lysates of granulocyte lysosomes. Arthritis Rheum 12:103-116, 1969
5. DeDuve C, Wattiaux R: Functions of lysosomes. Annu Rev Physiol 28:435-492, 1966
6. Hamerman D: Views on the pathogenesis of rheumatoid arthritis. Med Clin North Am 52:593-605, 1968
7. Weissmann G, Dukor P: The role of lysosomes in immune responses. Adv Immunol 12:283-331, 1970
8. Ward PA, Hill JH: C5 chemotactic fragments produced by an enzyme in lysosomal granules of neutrophils. J Immunol 104:535-543, 1970
9. Taubman SB, Goldschmidt PR, Lepow IH: Effects of lysosomal enzymes from human leukocytes on human complement components. Fed Proc 29:434, 1970
10. Ryan WL, Cardin C: Lysosomal stimulation and inhibition of the growth of cells in tissue culture. Proc Soc Exp Biol Med 126:112-114, 1967
11. Davies P, Krakauer K, Weissmann G: Subcellular distribution of neutral protease and peptidases in rabbit polymorphonuclear leucocytes. Nature (Lond) 228:761-762, 1970
12. Weissmann G, Hirschhorn R, Troll W, et al: A mechanism for widespread gene activation of mammalian cells. J Clin Invest 47:101a-102a, 1968
13. Velez R, Farrell NL, Freedman ML: Selective proteolytic dissociation of rabbit reticulocyte single ribosomes not attached to messenger RNA. Biochim Biophys Acta 228:719-727, 1971

14. Hirschhorn R, Hirschhorn K, Weissmann G: Appearance of hydrolase rich granules in human lymphocytes induced by phytohemagglutinin and antigens. Blood 30:84-102, 1967
15. Allison AC, Mallucci L: Lysosomes in dividing cells, with special reference to lymphocytes. Lancet 2:1371-1373, 1964
16. Hirschhorn R, Brittinger G, Hirschhorn K, et al: Studies on lysosomes. XII. Redistribution of acid hydrolases in human lymphocytes stimulated by phytohemagglutinin. J Cell Biol 37:412-423, 1968
17. Hirschhorn R, Troll W, Brittinger G, et al: Template activity of nuclei from stimulated lymphocytes. Nature (Lond) 222:1247-1250, 1969
18. Hirschhorn R, Grossman J, Troll W, et al: The effect of epsilon amino caproic acid and other inhibitors of proteolysis upon the response of human peripheral blood lymphocytes to phytohemagglutinin. J Clin Invest 50:1206-1217, 1971
19. Allison AC, Harington JS, Birbeck M: An examination of the cytotoxic effects of silica on macrophages. J Exp Med 124:141-154, 1968
20. Pal S, Doganges PT, Schubert M: The separation of new forms of the proteinpolysaccharides of bovine nasal cartilage. J Biol Chem 241:4261-4266, 1966
21. Dingle JT: The extracellular secretion of lysosomal enzymes, Lysosomes in Biology and Pathology, Vol II. Edited by JT Dingle, HB Fell. Amsterdam, North-Holland Publishing Company, 1969, pp 421-436
22. Barret AJ, Dingle JT: Tissue Proteinases. Amsterdam, North-Holland Publishing Company, 1971, pp 109-133
23. Weissmann G, Spilberg I: Breakdown of cartilage proteinpolysaccharide by lysosomes. Arthritis Rheum 11:162-169, 1968
24. Harris ED Jr, Evanson JM, DiBona DR, et al: Collagenase and rheumatoid arthritis. Arthritis Rheum 13:83-94, 1970
25. Lazarus GS, Daniels JR, Brown RS, et al: Degradation of collagen by a human granulocyte collagenolytic system. J Clin Invest 47:2622-2629, 1968
26. Zvaifler N: Further speculation on the pathogenesis of joint inflammation in rheumatoid arthritis. Arthritis Rheum 13:895-901, 1970
27. Hegner D: Isolierung und Enzymbestand von Granula aus polymorphkernigen Leukozyten des peripheren Rinderblutes. Hoppe Seylers Z Physiol Chem 349:544-554, 1968
28. LoSpalluto JJ, Fehr K, Ziff M: Degradation of immunoglobulins by intracellular proteases in the range of neutral pH. J Immunol 105:886-897, 1970
29. Metchnikoff E: Immunity in Infective Diseases (Reprint of 1905 edition). New York, Johnson Reprint Corporation, 1968
30. Zucker-Franklin D, Hirsch JG: Electron microscope studies on the degranulation of rabbit peritoneal leukocytes during phagocytosis. J Exp Med 120:569-576, 1964
31. Weissmann G, Dukor P, Zurier RB: Effect of cyclic AMP on release of lysosomal enzymes from phagocytes. Nature [New Biol] (Lond) 231:131-135, 1971
32. Weissmann G, Zurier RB, Spieler PJ, et al: Mechanisms of lysosomal enzyme release from leukocytes exposed to immune complexes and other particles. J Exp Med 134 (3):149s-165s, Part 2, 1971
33. Weissmann G, Dukor P, Dukor S, et al: Studies of lysosomes, mechanisms of enzyme release from endocytic cells and a model for latency *in vitro*, Immunopathology of Inflammation. Edited by BK Forscher, JC Houck. Amsterdam, Excerpta Medica, 1971, pp 107-117

Immune Complexes in Systemic Lupus Erythematosus and Glomerulonephritis

THE ROLE OF STREPTOCOCCI IN HUMAN GLOMERULONEPHRITIS

By JOHN B. ZABRISKIE

It is now generally accepted that a majority of the various forms of the disease glomerulonephritis with perhaps some direct toxic modifications at the onset are primarily immunologic in nature. The work of a number of investigators (1) has pointed out that this immunologic insult may take two basic forms. The first depends upon the production of antigen–antibody complexes which are subsequently trapped in the glomerular capillary walls or filter. The second mechanism may involve the formation of injurious agents (humoral and/or cellular) capable of reacting with the renal basement membrane tissue of the host. The end result of both forms of immunological intrusion is inflammation of the renal tissue, primarily basement membrane, with of course, help from complement components and leukocytes.

Keeping these two mechanisms firmly in mind, I would like to review some of the evidence for the role, if any, of the streptococcus in the initiation of pathogenetic events leading to these two separate disease-producing mechanisms. In so doing, I will lean heavily on material gained from renal biopsy studies in human glomerulonephritis but will bring in knowledge gained from studies of experimentally induced nephritis. In certain instances knowledge gained from studies of other more well-defined human antigen–antibody complex diseases will be used to illustrate certain points, or at least to serve as a springboard for future work in streptococcal-related glomerulonephritis.

POSTSTREPTOCOCCAL GLOMERULONEPHRITIS

A large body of clinical epidemiological and immunological data has now accumulated to indicate that the pathogenesis of human poststreptococcal glomerulonephritis is mediated via some form of antigen–antibody complexes (presumably streptococcal) with subsequent damage to the renal glomerulus. In support of this hypothesis we have the following evidence: (*a*) as in experimentally induced immune complex glomerulonephritis, granular deposits of complement and bound gamma globulin are present in the glomerular capillary walls and near the renal basement membrane (2–6); (*b*) complement components are diminished in the sera of patients with this acute proliferative disease (7); (*c*) certain type-specific strains of Group A streptococci are associated with outbreaks of acute glomerulonephritis (8); (*d*) antibodies to streptococcal products are present in high titer in the sera of these patients (9);

(*e*) at least three investigators have demonstrated the presence of streptococcal antigen in the glomeruli of these patients (see Table I).

Regarding the first point, there is relatively little argument that in a large majority of the cases of acute proliferative glomerulonephritis, there is a deposition of both human gamma globulin and $\beta_1 C$ material in the glomeruli of patients with acute poststreptococcal glomerulonephritis (see Table I). While the amount of these proteins varied considerably from case to case in these reports, these components were usually seen in association with each other. An

TABLE I

Results of Immunofluorescent Studies in Renal Biopsy Specimens of Patients with Acute Poststreptococcal Glomerulonephritis

| | Tabulated results | | | | |
Antisera to	McCluskey et al.*	Feldman et al.‡	Seegal et al.§	Michael et al.‖	Treser et al.¶
Bound gamma globulin	12/17**	9/9	10/12	12/16	35/35
Bound $\beta_1 C$	12/17	9/9	11/12	13/16	34/35
Fibrinogen or its products	12/17	7/8	NT‡‡	5/10	NT
Albumin	0/17	NT	0/12	0/8	0/35
Streptococcal cellular antigens	0/17	0/9	7/12	3/10	12/35
Streptococcal extracellular antigens	NT	NT	NT	0/5	NT

* Reference 2.
‡ Reference 4.
§ Reference 5; reference 10.
‖ Reference 3.
¶ Treser, G., and Lange, K. Personal communication.
** Numerator refers to the number of positive specimens; denominator refers to the number of biopsies studied.
†† NT = not tested.

examination of the published pictures from these reports also indicates that gamma globulin was rarely, if ever, seen in the mesangial areas, while $\beta_1 C$ was often seen in these cells. When looked for, fibrin was detected in varying amounts in the renal biopsies of these patients and usually not in the same distribution as the bound gamma globulin (2). Indeed, fibrin was most often noted within mesangial cells and in between proliferating endothelial cells and, I emphasize, *not* near the nodular basement membrane deposits of gamma globulin and $\beta_1 C$. This difference in the localization of these products has important implications in the discussion to follow.

Fig. 1 shows these characteristic gamma globulin deposits in the glomeruli of a patient with well-documented acute poststreptococcal glomerulonephritis. These deposits were similar to those seen by other investigators and demonstrate the granular nature of these deposits and their distribution along the basement membrane of the glomerulus. $\beta_1 C$ deposits were almost always associated

with these deposits but the amount of these "fixed" complement components
was usually somewhat less.

With respect to the localization of streptococcal antigens, 7 out of 12 renal
biopsies obtained from patients with acute poststreptococcal glomerulonephritis exhibited positive glomerular staining when fluorescein-labeled antisera
to Type 12 nephritogenic streptococci were layered over these sections. Fig.
2 demonstrates the localization of these antigens and it is clear that the observed immunofluorescent deposits are *not* present in the same region as the
gamma globulin deposits shown previously. Indeed, these deposits were pri-

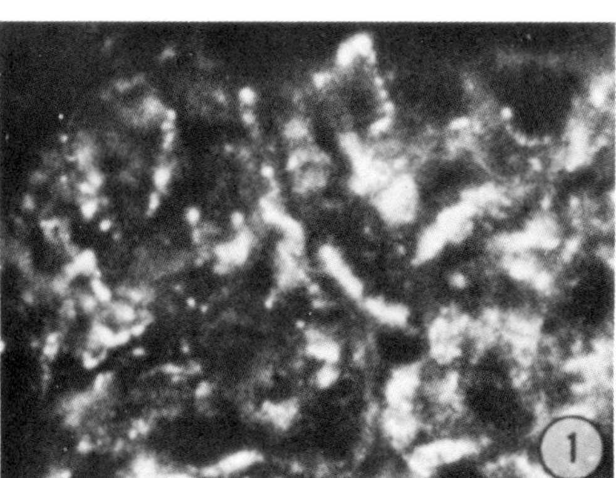 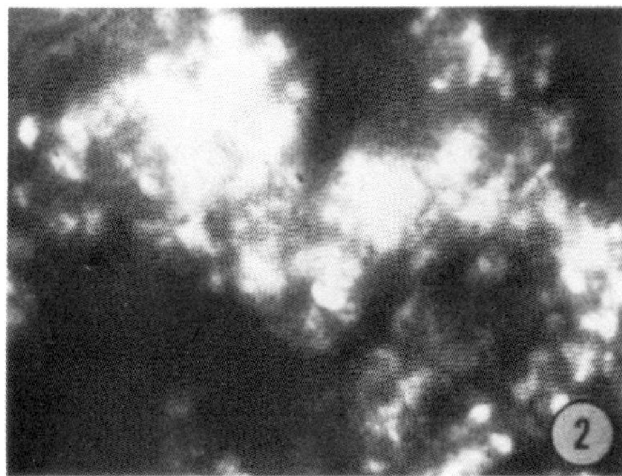

Figs. 1 and 2. Fig. 1 demonstrates deposits of gamma globulin in the glomeruli of a patient
with acute poststreptococcal glomerulonephritis. Note the granular nature of these deposits
along the basement membrane portion of the glomerulus. × 800, approximately. Fig. 2 reveals the presence of diffuse deposits of streptococcal antigen in the glomerulus of a patient
with poststreptococcal glomerulonephritis. These deposits appear to be in the mesangial areas
of the glomerulus and within the cytoplasm of these cells. × 1000, approximately.

marily concentrated in the mesangial cells and in between proliferating endothelial cells of the glomerulus. In many instances these deposits appeared to
be actually within the cytoplasm of the mesangial cells. These deposits are
almost identical to those reported by Michael and his coworkers (3) and were
found in three out of nine patients with acute poststreptococcal glomerulonephritis. Treser et al. (6) also reported a similar distribution in their renal
biopsies.

Since other investigators failed to localize streptococcal antigens in the
renal biopsies of patients with similar gamma globulin deposits, a few comments concerning the streptococcal antisera used in our studies seems appropriate. First, the antisera were prepared by prolonged immunization of rabbits
with heat-killed Type 12 streptococci and only those rabbits demonstrating
high titers to the group-specific carbohydrate and M protein were utilized.

Secondly, the specificity of the reaction was strengthened by the fact that antisera to type-specific streptococcal strains 6, 14, and 49 prepared in the same manner did not give positive staining in these glomeruli. Finally, repeat biopsy specimens of a few of our patients failed to demonstrate these deposits at a later stage in the disease process, suggesting that streptococcal antigenic sites were no longer available for binding to the streptococcal antiserum.

These immunofluorescent studies were confirmed by electron microscopy studies using ferritin-labeled antisera. Andres (10) demonstrated that gamma globulin and β_1C components were present in electron-opaque deposits in the glomeruli of these patients. In addition, ferritin-labeled antisera to streptococcal antigens localized both in electron-opaque deposits in the arteriolar wall as well as in basement membrane-like material between mesangial cells. Of significance was the finding that these electron-opaque deposits, after transport and condensation from the glomerular capillary wall to the basement membrane subepithelial deposit, lost their ability to bind streptococcal antigens but not β_1C or gamma globulin. Andres has suggested this might be due to destruction of the antigen and/or the binding of all available antigenic sites in these deposits by antibody.

If these observations do indeed indicate that streptococcal antigen and antibody are present in the areas of immunologic damage in the glomerulus, how does one explain the failure of other investigators to confirm these results? Concomitantly, why were immunofluorescent deposits of streptococcal antigen found in areas unrelated to the nodular deposits of gamma globulin and β_1C?

The answer to the first question is perhaps related to the time that the initial biopsy was taken, the severity of the disease, and the antisera used. In the case of Michael's studies, positive results were obtained primarily in early cases (within 1st wk). Negative results were more often seen in biopsies that were obtained 2 or more wk after the onset of symptoms. Seegal's cases were examples of severe fulminating glomerulonephritis in which subacute and progressive nephritis was seen in at least two of these patients. In these severe examples of human glomerulonephritis, a second biopsy, while demonstrating an increased deposition of gamma globulin in the glomeruli, no longer exhibited positive staining for streptococcal antigens. Feldman's studies did include a number of early cases but the streptococcal antisera used in these studies were not obtained from hyperimmunized rabbits and were not antisera previously tested by us for their capacity to bind streptococcal antigens in the glomeruli. As Lancefield[1] has recently demonstrated, rabbits differ markedly in their ability to make antibodies to one or another streptococcal cellular structure.

At first glance a satisfactory answer to the second question, namely, the appearance of antigen deposits in areas different from that of the nodular deposits of gamma globulin and complement, appears to be more difficult to achieve. However, evidence from both experimentally induced nephritis and human lupus nephritis supports our hypothesis of the difficulty in demonstrating the presence of the antigen in nodular immunoglobulin deposits. For example, Koffler et al. (11) were able to demonstrate that large deposits of DNA antigen were present in the nodular deposits in glomeruli of lupus erythematosus nephritis patients only after salt elution of the antibody was performed. Similar results were obtained by Edgington et al. (12) after elution of antibody from glomeruli of animals with experimentally induced autologous immune complex disease.

Thus, the inability to detect streptococcal antigens in nodular deposits in the glomeruli of patients with poststreptococcal nephritis may well be dependent on the lack of streptococcal antigenic sites available for binding. Unfortunately, none of the authors noted in Table I carried out elution studies on the renal biopsies of these nephritic patients so that this question still remains unanswered. However, bearing in mind the technical difficulties that might be encountered, this type of elution is feasible and should be carried out in future biopsies.

The fact that streptococcal antigen was present in what appears to be the cytoplasm of mesangial cells and in between proliferating endothelial cells may well be related to the nature of the antigen. Kantor (13) has demonstrated that certain streptococcal proteins such as the M protein have a particular affinity for fibrinogen. Injection of rats or mice resulted in the formation of M protein–fibrinogen complexes which localized in the glomerular capillaries and in between what appear to be epithelial cells of the glomerular tufts (14). A review of the photographs of those authors who studied the localization of fibrin in patients with acute poststreptococcal glomerulonephritis reveals that fibrin was deposited primarily within and around proliferating cells of the glomerulus, a distribution quite similar to that noted for the deposition of streptococcal antigen (2, 4).

The exact nature of the streptococcal antigen is still a matter of dispute. Treser et al., using fluorescein-labeled antisera to purified streptococcal membranes, state that the streptococcal antigen is a part of the membrane structure of the streptococcal cell (15). In contrast, using antisera prepared against the membranes obtained from four different type-specific streptococcal strains, including the Type 12 strain mentioned above, we failed to localize streptococcal membrane antigens in those patients who exhibited positive staining with Type 12 antiserum prepared against whole streptococcal organisms. In addition, absorption studies with T12 cell walls and purified membranes ($<0.01\%$ rhamnose and $<2\%$ muramic acid) revealed that the absorption of immunofluorescent staining was achieved only with streptococcal cell walls.

This ability to abolish the immunofluorescent staining was destroyed by treating the cell wall preparations with either trypsin or hot HCl extraction of these walls.[2]

A number of the points mentioned above are at least open to experimental proof and some suggested avenues of approach are listed below. (*a*) Antibody elution techniques should reveal whether streptococcal or renal antigens are actually present in the nodular deposits seen in positively staining renal glomerular biopsies. (*b*) Previous studies (5) indicated that a fluorescein-labeled streptococcal antigen preparation bound to the fixed gamma globulin deposits in the glomeruli of these patients, suggesting that the fixed antibody contained free antibody molecules specific for streptococcal antigens. However, the streptococcal antigen preparation contained a number of streptococcal antigens, including streptococcal membrane fragments, and these studies should be repeated using more purified fluorescein-labeled antigens. (*c*) The use of immunofluorescence techniques to detect the *early* presence of fibrinogen and/or its products coupled with streptococcal antigen should help to establish the presence or absence of streptococcal-fibrinogen complexes in the glomeruli of these patients. Similarly, a search for extracellular toxins bound to either capillary walls or glomerular structures early in the course of the infection might be of value in establishing the initial renal insult.

In summary, the available evidence still favors a role of streptococcal antigen–antibody complexes in acute poststreptococcal glomerulonephritis. The conflicting results reported in Table I may merely represent differences in the type of antisera used or the time at which the biopsy was taken. Obviously, there is still a need for further work on experimentally induced models of glomerulonephritis, as well as more careful studies with human renal tissue.

PROGRESSIVE GLOMERULONEPHRITIS

Perhaps one good controversy deserves another and in the remaining part of the discussion, I would like to turn to our more recent studies done with Dr. Falk and Dr. Möller in Sweden in patients with progressive glomerulonephritis. While our results are open to at least two different interpretations, they are worthy of consideration.

The rationale behind the study of these patients was the concept that the disease, progressive glomerulonephritis, had many characteristics that differed from those of acute streptococcal "immune complex" nephritis. The continuing clinical nature of the disease, the appearance of both linear and granular deposits in the renal biopsy material, and the presence of mononuclear cells in the histological sections of renal tissue of these patients were all factors that suggested that an altered cellular reactivity to renal tissue, in particular to renal basement membrane antigens, might play an important role in this disease.

In view of the known antigenic cross-reaction between renal glomerular basement membrane antigens and streptococcal membrane antigens (16, 17), the possibility existed that the initiating stimulus for this proposed altered cellular reactivity might be streptococcal in nature. Accordingly, patients with clinical, pathological, and immunofluorescent evidence of progressive glomerulonephritis were studied (18). A control group of nonglomerular renal disease patients served as the controls (see Table II).

The techniques for the isolation of leukocytes from these patients and the general preparation of these cells for migration from capillary tubes were based

TABLE II

Degree of Cellular Inhibition of Leukocytes Obtained from Patients with Progressive Glomerulonephritis as Compared with Nonglomerulonephritic Renal Disease Patients and Normal Controls

Disease states	No. of patients	Degree of inhibition to streptococcal antigens		
		Type 12 membranes	Type 12 cell walls	Type 5 membranes
		%	%	%
Progressive glomerulonephritis*	19	34 (±2)	27 (±3)	22.2 (±2)
Nonglomerular renal disease‡	15	8.1 (±1)	8.1 (±2)	5.1 (±1)
Normal controls	10	8.8 (±2.6)	10.9 (±2.3)	NT§

* Cases with clinical and renal biopsy evidence of glomerular diseases.
‡ Patients with pyelonephritis, polycystic disease, lipoid nephrosis.
§ NT = Not tested.

on techniques employed by Bendixen (19) and modified by Falk et al. (20). These methods may be described briefly as follows: 50 cc of venous blood was obtained from each patient, defibrinated with glass beads, and allowed to sediment with equal volumes of 2% gelatin in glass cylinders. After centrifugation and collection of the white cells, the contaminating red cells were removed via lysis with 0.83% ammonium chloride, pH 7.2. The cells were adjusted to a concentration of 2×10^7 cells/ml and allowed to migrate from capillary tubes into small plastic planchettes containing tissue culture media and the antigens to be tested. 10% *homologous* human serum was added to all media used. The degree of inhibition of migration of these cells in the presence of specific antigen was measured by calculating the ratio of

$$\frac{\text{area of migration with antigen}}{\text{area of migration without antigen}} \times 100$$

and then subtracting the observed value from 100%.

Fig. 3 depicts the type of inhibition of migration observed in patients with glomerulonephritis in the presence of sensitizing antigen. On the left is depicted the degree of migration in the normal control planchette; the planchette on the right shows the inhibition achieved with antigen. The nature of this inhibition reaction deserves some comments. First, this reaction is definitely a cell-to-cell interaction involving both granulocytes and lymphocytes. Removal of all the granulocytes results in loss of the observed cellular reactivity. Secondly, this technique depends on the presence of particulate antigens in the surrounding medium and to date only high concentrations of soluble antigens

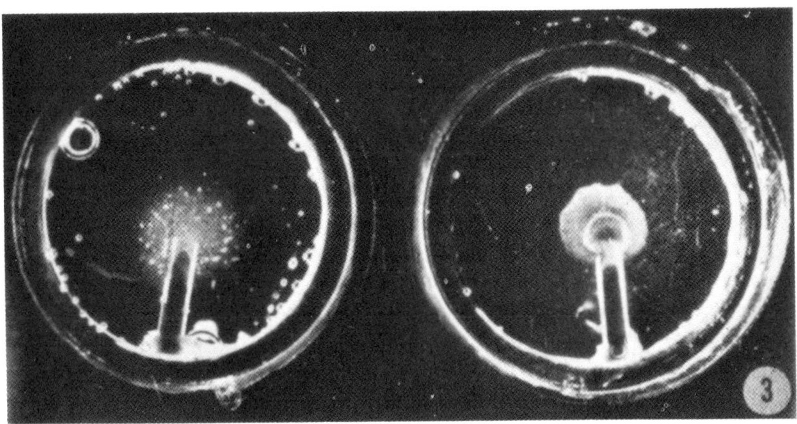

Fig. 3. Migration of human peripheral blood leukocytes in the presence and absence of streptococcal antigens is depicted in this photograph. The planchette on the left contains a migrating fan of cells in the absence of the antigen. The planchette on the right demonstrates inhibition of migration in the presence of streptococcal antigen.

have been effective (21). Thus, in general, the technique is limited to particulate antigens. Preliminary attempts in our laboratory to couple soluble antigen to tanned cells, for example, have been unrewarding.[3]

With these facts in mind, I would now like to present the results of our cellular migration studies in these patients. Table II shows the results obtained with this technique in 19 patients with progressive glomerulonephritis as compared with 13 non-nephritic controls. With respect to the antigens used, both Type 12 and Type 5 streptococcal membranes were used in these studies. These membranes were obtained from Type 12 and Type 5 streptococcal strains, respectively, and contain little or no contaminating cell wall material ($<0.01\%$ rhamnose and $<2\%$ muramic acid). In contrast, the Type 12 streptococcal cell walls contained approximately 20–30% contaminating membrane material. It is clear that the presence of either Type 12 cell walls or membranes resulted in a marked degree of inhibition in patients with progressive glomerulonephritis. Type 5 membranes resulted in a somewhat smaller degree of inhibition than that observed with Type 12 membranes but the results were still four times those observed in control patients. The lack of reactivity to soluble streptococcal substances (i.e. M protein, group-specific carbohydrates, extracellular products) in both groups is not surprising in view of the general lack of reactivity to soluble antigens in this test. In view of the known contamination of Group A streptococcal cell walls by streptococcal membranes (22), we would have to assume that the observed reactivity to Type 12 streptococcal cell walls was due to membrane contamination. This concept is strengthened by the fact that Type 12 membranes contain negligible amounts of streptococcal cell

TABLE III

Effect of Streptococcal Antigens on DNA Synthesis in Lymphocytes from Non-Nephritic and Glomerulonephritic Subjects

Substance tested (0.1 mg)	Non-nephritic patients		Glomerulonephritic patients	
	No.	Mean counts/min (±SE)	No.	Mean count/min (±SE)
Normal media controls	7	88 (±20)	14	66 (±13)
T12 streptococcal membranes	7	832 (±229)	14	2144 (±223)
T12 streptococcal cell wall	7	170 (±96)	14	1079 (±265)
T5 streptococcal membranes	2	759 (±123)	5	1199 (±215)
T5 streptococcal soluble cell wall	6	47 (±5)	2	91 (±6)

walls. Considerably less reactivity was noted in the non-nephritic group to these antigens and actually the degree of reactivity observed in these patients was similar to that observed with normal individuals (approximately 5–10% inhibition). While not shown, the degree of reactivity to tubercle bacilli was similar in all groups, demonstrating that lymphocytes from patients with progressive glomerulonephritis do not respond abnormally to *any* antigenic stimulus.

In order to further explore the above-observed cellular reactivity and to hopefully confirm our results, another parameter of cellular hypersensitivity was employed. The level of DNA synthesis in lymphocytes, as measured by the incorporation of thymidine-^{14}C after exposure to a sensitizing antigen, is another measurement of cellular reactivity to antigenic confrontation. While this reaction measures the response of both antigen-sensitive cells and antibody-producing cells, it is considered a reliable in vitro parameter of cellular reactivity to antigenic stimulation. In addition, this technique has the advantage of longer contact with the antigen (4–5 days vs. 24 hr) and measures lymphocytic reaction to soluble and particulate antigens.

Table III shows the markedly increased DNA synthesis induced in the lymphocytes of patients with chronic glomerulonephritis after cultivation with streptococcal antigens. It is apparent that both streptococcal membranes (T12 and T5), as well as the cell walls from the Type 12 strain, produced 4–10 times the amount of thymidine-^{14}C incorporation in the lymphocytes of nephritic patients as that observed in the lymphocytes of non-nephritic controls. The fact that the non-nephritic patients also responded to the streptococcal antigens is again not surprising, since the general population has had at least minimal exposure to streptococcal infections. However, the reactivity of the lymphocytes of these patients to the streptococcal antigens was always much less than that observed with lymphocytes from patients with progressive glomerulonephritis. While the reactivity to streptococcal cell walls was always less than that observed with membranes in non-nephritic controls, the response of lymphocytes from nephritic patients to streptococcal cell walls was as much or more than that observed with streptococcal membranes. Since altered cellular reactivity to streptococcal membranes (which contain negligible amounts of streptococcal cell walls) was quite pronounced in the lymphocytes of glomerulonephritic patients, these results suggest that the antigenic configuration of the sensitizing antigen (presumably contaminating membrane fragments) was also important for the observed stimulation by the streptococcal walls. Again, soluble streptococcal preparations produced only minimal degrees of lymphocytic stimulation in nephritic and non-nephritic patients. Response to both phytohemagglutinin and purified protein derivative of tubercle bacilli were similar in both groups, suggesting that there was no generalized increased reactivity to any antigen in glomerulonephritic patients.

The fact that streptococcal membranes from both a nephritogenic and a non-nephritogenic strain gave essentially similar results is at first surprising in view of the small number of streptococcal types capable of inducing glomerulonephritis. However, it is conceivable that all streptococcal strains possess "nephritogenic" characteristics and only the ease with which nephritogenic antigens are exposed in vivo separates the nephritogenic and non-nephritogenic strains. The artificial exposure of *both* membranes in this study might explain the similar results obtained with a nephritogenic (T12/126) and a non-nephritogenic (T5) strain. In contrast, the control non-nephritic group failed to respond to any of the streptococcal antigen preparations, indicating the specific nature of the altered state of lymphocytes in glomerulonephritic patients.

How do these results fit in with the generally accepted view concerning either experimentally induced or human progressive glomerulonephritis? Perhaps the most plausible explanation for this observed altered reactivity of leukocytes from these patients would be a primary sensitization to renal basement membrane antigens, either tubular and/or glomerular. The observed reactivity to the streptococcal membranes would be merely a reflection of the known shared antigenicity between the two membranes. This concept would be in keeping with the recent work by Rocklin et al. (23) in which patients with progressive glomerulonephritis, particularly those with proven *linear* immunofluorescent deposits in their glomeruli, had altered cellular reactivity to renal glomerular antigens.

Alternatively, it is conceivable that sensitization to the streptococcal membrane antigens might be the initiating factor in the glomerular damage. Sensitized "killer" cells might result in the damage and release of more glomerular membrane antigens. The presence of cells sensitized to renal antigen coupled with intercurrent streptococcal infections could be responsible for the progressive nature of the disease.

While these hypotheses are attractive and could explain a number of the clinical and pathological features of progressive glomerulonephritis, it must be admitted that the above-mentioned results do not completely mesh with findings obtained in either experimentally induced glomerulonephritis or in the study of human pathological material. For example, the presence of granular deposits in many cases of progressive glomerulonephritis, coupled with the work of Edgington et al. with experimentally induced autologous immune complex disease (24), would suggest that complexes also play an important role in progressive glomerulonephritis. In addition, eluted anti-glomerular membrane antibody found in patients with Goodpasture's disease causes disease in normal monkeys in the absence of cellular sensitivity (25).

Obviously we are again left with many unanswered questions with regard to progressive glomerulonephritis as well. The histological and immunological data available at present would suggest that damage to renal tissue may occur in a number of different ways. Perhaps in the case of progressive glomerulonephritis, both cellular and humoral mechanisms are at work, either concomitantly or at different stages of the disease process.

With the number of in vitro techniques now available, one should be able to begin to clear up some of these difficult points. For example, are sensitized cells from glomerulonephritis patients specifically cytotoxic for renal cell monolayers? Are there differences in the destructive ability of these cells, depending on the immunofluorescent pattern observed in the renal biopsy specimen? Finally, what role does antibody eluted from these renal specimens play in conjunction with sensitized cells with respect to cytotoxicity for renal cell monolayers?

A closer correlation between the nature and deposition of glomerular antibodies and the cellular reactivity to human glomerular membranes and streptococcal membranes in acute and progressive glomerulonephritis, as well as more precise characterization of these antibodies with respect to the antigens involved, will be needed to clearly separate these mechanisms.

BIBLIOGRAPHY

1. McCluskey, R. T. 1970. *Reviewed in* Evidence for immunologic mechanisms in several forms of human glomerular diseases. *Bull. N.Y. Acad. Med.* **46:**769.
2. McCluskey, R. S., P. Vassali, G. Gallo, and D. S. Baldwin. 1966. An immunofluorescent study of pathogenic mechanisms in glomerular diseases. *N. Engl. J. Med.* **274:**695.
3. Michael, A. F., Jr., K. M. Drummond, R. A. Good, and R. L. Vernier. 1966. Acute post streptococcal glomerulonephritis: immune deposit disease. *J. Clin. Invest.* **45:**237.
4. Feldman, J. O., M. R. Mardiney, and S. E. Shuler. 1966. Immunology and morphology of acute post streptococcal glomerulonephritis. *Lab. Invest.* **15:**283.
5. Seegal, B. C., G. A. Andres, K. C. Hsu, and J. B. Zabriskie. 1965. Studies on the pathogenesis of acute and progressive glomerulonephritis in man by immunofluorescein and immunoferritin techniques. *Fed. Proc.* **24**(Pt. I)**:**100.
6. Treser, G., M. Semar, M. McVicar, M. Franklin, A. Ty, I. Sagel, and K. Lange. 1969. Antigenic streptococcal components in acute glomerulonephritis. *Science (Washington)*. **163:**676.
7. Fischel, E. E. 1957. Immune reactions in glomerulonephritis. *J. Chronic. Dis.* **5:**34.
8. Rammelkamp, C. H., Jr. 1957. Microbiologic aspects of glomerulonephritis. *J. Chronic. Dis.* **5:**28.
9. Rammelkamp, C. H., Jr. 1954. Acute hemorrhagic glomerulonephritis. *In* Streptococcal Infections. M. McCarty, editor. Columbia University Press, New York. Chap. 14.
10. Andres, G. A., L. Accinni, K. C. Hsu, and J. B. Zabriskie. 1966. Electron microscopic studies of human glomerulonephritis with ferritin-conjugated antibody. *J. Exp. Med.* **123:**399.
11. Koffler, D., P. H. Shur, and H. G. Kunkel. 1967. Immunological studies concerning the nephritis of systemic lupus erythematosus. *J. Exp. Med.* **126:**607.
12. Edgington, T. S., R. J. Glassock, and F. J. Dixon. 1967. Autologous immune complex pathogenesis of experimental allergic glomerulonephritis. *Science (Washington)*. **155:**1432.
13. Kantor, F. S. 1965. Fibrinogen precipitation by streptococcal M protein. I. Identity of reactants and stoichiometry of the reaction. *J. Exp. Med.* **121:**849.
14. Kantor, F. S. 1965. Fibrinogen precipitation by streptococcal M protein. II. Renal lesions induced by intravenous injection of M protein into mice and rats. *J. Exp. Med.* **121:**861.
15. Treser, G., M. Semar, A. Ty, I. Sagel, M. A. Franklin, and K. Lange. 1970. Partial characterization of antigenic streptococcal plasma membrane components in acute glomerulonephritis. *J. Clin. Invest.* **49:**762.
16. Markowitz, A. S., and C. F. Lange, Jr. 1964. Streptococcal related glomerulonephritis. I. Isolation, immunochemistry and comparative chemistry of soluble fractions from type 12 nephritogenic streptococci and human glomeruli. *J. Immunol.* **94:**565.

17. Holm, S. E. 1967. Precipitinogens in beta hemolytic streptococci and some related human kidney antigens. *Acta Pathol. Microbiol. Scand.* **70:**79.

18. Zabriskie, J. B., R. Lewshenia, G. Möller, B. Wehle, and R. E. Falk. 1970. Lymphocytic responses to streptococcal antigens in glomerulonephritis patients. *Science (Washington).* **168:**1105.

19. Bendixen, G. 1968. Organ-specific inhibition of the *in vitro* migration of leukocytes in human glomerulonephritis. *Acta Med. Scand.* **184:**99.

20. Falk, R. E., L. Collste, and G. Möller. 1969. *In vitro* correlates of transplantation immunity: the release of substances by immune lymphocytes confronted with specific antigens. *Surgery.* **66:**51.

21. Rosenberg, S. A., and J. R. David. 1970. Inhibition of leucocyte migration: an evaluation of this *in vitro* assay of delayed hypersensitivity in man to a soluble antigen. *J. Immunol.* **105:**1447.

22. Zabriskie, J. B., and E. H. Freimer. 1966. An immunological relationship between Group A streptococcus and mammalian muscle. *J. Exp. Med.* **124:**661.

23. Rocklin, R. E., E. J. Lewis, and R. David. 1970. *In vitro* evidence for cellular hypersensitivity to glomerular basement membrane antigens in human glomerulonephritis. *N. Engl. J. Med.* **283:**497.

24. Edgington, T. S., R. J. Glassock, and F. J. Dixon. 1968. Autologous immune complex nephritis induced with renal tubular antigen. *J. Exp. Med.* **127:**555.

25. Lerner, R. A., R. J. Glassock, and F. J. Dixon. 1967. The role of anti-glomerular basement membrane antibody in the pathogenesis of human glomerulonephritis. *J. Exp. Med.* **126:**989.

Procainamide-Induced Lupus Erythematosus

Clinical and Laboratory Observations

STEPHEN E. BLOMGREN, M.D.
JOHN J. CONDEMI, M.D.
JOHN H. VAUGHAN, M.D.

A number of drugs have been implicated in the activation of an illness which resembles idiopathic systemic lupus erythematosus (SLE). These are listed in Table I. The implication is most convincing for hydralazine and procainamide and somewhat less so, but still strong, for isoniazid, diphenylhydantoin, mephenytoin and tridione. Most of the other drugs, however, have been reported in association with lupus erythematosus only sporadically, and in many cases they may have been used to treat symptoms which could have been in fact the earliest manifestations of SLE. Implicit in all such case reports is the speculation that the drug itself is an active participant in eliciting what appears to be an autoreactive immunologic process.

We describe the clinical and laboratory manifestations of the procainamide-induced disease as seen in Rochester, New York, over a four year period. Some of the characteristics of a complex between procainamide and DNA are described, and its possible role in the lupus syndrome is discussed. The types and quantities of antibodies to nucleohistone and deoxyribonucleic acid (DNA) in patients with the syndrome are noted and compared with similar antibodies in patients with idiopathic SLE.

MATERIAL

Over the last four years we encountered fifty-nine patients with clinical and/or serologic evidence of auto-allergic disease associated with routine therapy with procainamide. Of these, forty-four were symptomatic, and the following description will be limited to these. The series of patients reported earlier by Bodman et al. [15] and Vaughan et al. [16] are included in our series of forty-four patients.

Serum from normal persons and from patients with idiopathic SLE in various stages of activity was obtained for comparison with serum from these patients.

METHODS

Immunologic Evaluations. Assays of antinuclear antibody were made using human peripheral blood leukocytes as substrate. By this technic, 2 per cent of undiluted normal serum specimens give positive results [17]. The latex nucleoprotein agglutination test (Hyland) utilizes latex particles coated with nuclear materials. The lupus erythematosus cell test used was the rotary bead method [18]. Rheumatoid factor (anti-IgG) was detected using latex particles coated with human gamma globulin [19]. Coombs' tests were performed using antiserums that detect gamma globulin and/or complement on red cells. Total serum hemolytic complement ($C'H_{50}$) was determined in most cases by a method previously described [20]. When fresh serum was not available, $C'3$ (B_{1c}—B_{1a}) was determined by radial immunodiffusion (Hyland).

DNA-Procainamide Complex. Native calf thymus deoxyribonucleic acid (DNA) was obtained from the Worthington Biochemical Corporation. In designated experiments, heat denaturation was carried out by heating solutions of DNA to 100°C for ten minutes, followed by rapid cooling in an ice bath. Solutions of DNA (1 mg/ml) and ^{14}C-procainamide (1 mg/ml, specific activity 0.15 μc/mg), in pH 7.8 phosphate-buffered saline solution were radiated in the presence of methylene blue (National Aniline Division), protoporphyrin IX (Calbiochem), or riboflavin (Nutritional Biochemical) at 20 to 320 μg/ml. Radiation was with visible light from 150 watt Westinghouse Flood lamps at an intensity of 5,000 foot-candles, carried out at constant temperature, usually 20°C, for periods up to six hours. Mixtures were stirred magnetically. Photo-oxidation was indicated by darkening of all solutions containing photodynamic dye and procainamide. After photo-oxidation, DNA was separated from unbound procainamide by Sephadex® G-200 filtration, dialysis or repeated ethanol precipitation from 1 M sodium chloride. DNA was quantitated by a diphenylamine reaction [21]. Fractions of the isolated DNA were then counted by liquid scintillation to determine the amount of drug bound. This was expressed as a molar ratio relative to guanine, based on a guanine content of 26 per cent. Control preparations of DNA were photo-oxidized in the absence of procainamide.

TABLE I   Drugs Implicated in Induction of the Lupus Syndrome

Procainamide [1]	Ethosuximide [8]
Hydralazine [2]	Penicillin [9]
Isoniazid [3]	Phenylbutazone [10]
Sulfonamides [4]	Tetracycline [11]
Diphenylhydantoin [5]	Streptomycin [12]
Mephenytoin [6]	p-Aminosalicylic acid [13]
Trimethadione [7]	Griseofulvin [14]

Immunization of Rabbits. DNA procainamide complexes, as well as control preparations lacking procainamide, were used to immunize 6-pound New Zealand white rabbits by the method of Plescia et al. [22]. This technic relies upon stabilization of DNA by methylated bovine serum albumin (MBSA) and the use of Freund's complete adjuvant. In order to demonstrate any enhanced immunogenicity of DNA-procainamide complexes, variations were also carried out in which MBSA or adjuvant or both were not used. Antibody was assayed by complement fixation [23].

Antibody to Procainamide. The presence of procainamide attached to DNA was studied using rabbit antibody raised to procainamide diazotized to bovine serum albumin [24]. Specificity was demonstrated by immunodiffusion and complement fixation with procainamide diazotized to equine gamma globulin.

Globulin Precipitation Method for Detection of Antibody. A modification of the Farr [25] technic of ammonium sulfate precipitation of globulins was used to demonstrate antibody to native and denatured DNA and nucleohistone. Heat-denatured DNA was sonicated to reduce nonspecific precipitation in the last step to be described. Nucleohistone (Worthington) was solubilized by sonication in distilled water prior to use. Denatured and native DNA, and nucleohistone, were then passively labeled with ^{3}H-actinomycin D [26]. Unreacted label was removed by extensive dialysis, and the labeled antigens were diluted to 20 μg/ml in phosphate buffered saline solution, pH 7.4. One half milliliter of antigen solution was mixed with 0.1 ml of heat-decomplemented serum and 0.4 ml of buffer. The mixture was incubated one hour at 37°C and eighteen hours at 4°C. Globulins were then precipitated with an equal volume of saturated ammonium sulfate. This brings down antibodies, including so-called non-precipitating antibodies, with the labeled antigen attached. The precipitate was washed with half-saturated ammonium sulfate, the wash discarded, and the precipitate dissolved and counted by liquid scintillation. The precipitated counts can be expressed as a percentage of the total antigen counts added. The more antibody present, the more counts will be precipitated.

RESULTS

The Clinical Syndrome. General statistics: There were twenty-six men, with a mean age of sixty-three years, and eighteen women, with a mean age of sixty-one years. Two patients were Negro. The average duration of therapy before symptoms developed was twelve months, with a range from one month to eight years. The mean dose of procainamide at the time symptoms developed was 1.6 gm/day, with a range from 0.75 to 3.75 gm.

Signs and symptoms: The type and frequency of signs and symptoms in these forty-four patients are listed in Table II. The most common complaint was arthralgias. These were commonly symmetrical and polyarticular, affecting in order of frequency the fingers and hands, shoulders, wrists, elbows and, to a lesser extent, the knees and ankles. They were sometimes migratory. There were three cases of unilateral temporomandibular arthralgia. In eight cases there was heat, redness, swelling and tenderness of at least one joint sufficient to use the term arthritis. The most bitter complaints concerned myalgias. These were diffuse and proximal as well as distal. The patients described stiffness and aching. Although morning

TABLE II Signs and Symptoms in Forty-Four Cases of the Procainamide-Induced Lupus Syndrome

Signs and Symptoms	No. of Cases
Rheumatic symptoms	
Arthralgia	34
Arthritis	8
Myalgia	21
Pleuropulmonic involvement	23
Fever	20
Weight loss	10
Hepatomegaly	9
Lymphadenopathy	4
Abdominal pain	4
Pericarditis	6
Splenomegaly	2
Raynaud's syndrome	2
Rash	2
Central nervous system symptoms	1
History of drug reaction	10

stiffness and stiffness after inactivity were notable, aching often was most severe at the end of the day. In several cases stiffness and aching were most marked in the left arm and shoulder, and this had raised the question of postmyocardial infarction shoulder-hand syndrome.

Pleuropulmonic involvement was usually manifested by pleuritic pain and effusion. There was one case of hemoptysis. Often effusions were accompanied by infiltrates at the base of one or both lungs. The infiltrates were sometimes striking and difficult to distinguish from pulmonary emboli. Figure 1 is the chest film of a sixty year old woman (Case 1) who had been taking procainamide for a year and a half before presenting with fever, polyarthralgias, pleuritic chest pain and cough. She had been treated for arthralgias for several months with prednisone. There were bilateral effusions, with infiltrates at the bases of both lungs. Friction rubs were audible bilaterally. Phlebograms and lung scan were unrevealing. The findings and symptoms subsided in two weeks after the admin-

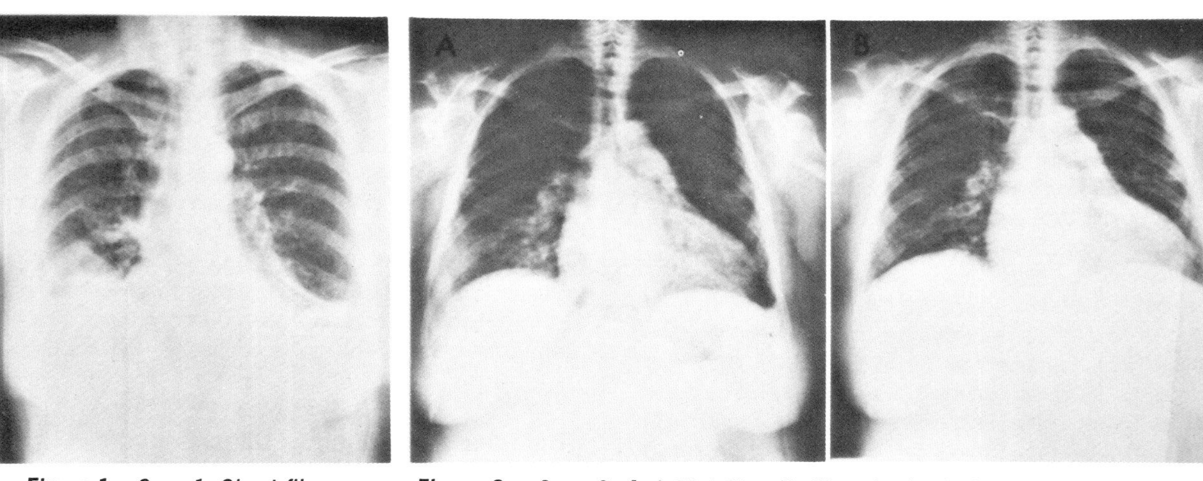

Figure 1. Case 1. Chest film.

Figure 2. Case 2. **A,** initial film. **B,** film obtained eight days later (four days after procainamide therapy was discontinued).

istration of procainamide was stopped. Figure 2A is the initial chest film of a forty-six year old woman (Case 2) with undiagnosed heart disease manifested by biventricular failure and ventricular irritability. She had been receiving procainamide for one year when she presented with cough and pleuritic pain. There were bilateral effusions, an infiltrate in the lower lobe of the right lung and a pleural density laterally on the right. Eight days later, four days after the administration of procainamide was stopped, these findings had virtually cleared (Figure 2B), and she was asymptomatic. Figure 3A is the chest fiim obtained on admission in a fifty-five year old man who presented with a five week history of cough, dyspnea, anorexia, 25 pound weight loss, arthralgias, myalgias and epistaxis. A pleural friction rub was present on the right. There were bilateral effusions, greater on the right, and an infiltrate along the right lower lateral chest wall. The presence of pulmonary embolism and bronchogenic carcinoma had been considered seriously in this case. However the patient had thrombocytopenia, and biopsy was not performed. The effusions cleared rapidly after the administration of procainamide was stopped, but the dense infiltrate persisted for several months (Figure 3B). Eleven months later (Figure 3C) the density had disappeared, but a few markings remain. Although this patient and the previous two may indeed have had pulmonary emboli, the rapid improvement in these and other cases after administration of the drug was stopped suggests that these effusions and infiltrates were part of the drug reaction.

Fever was present in about half the cases. In some it was spiking, with temperatures reaching as high as 40°C. In others it was low grade and remittent. Weight loss and anorexia may be striking when present. One of the earliest patients encountered lost 70 pounds over one year before the diagnosis was made.

The patients with pericarditis had typical rubs and pain. Electrocardiographic changes were minimal to mild.

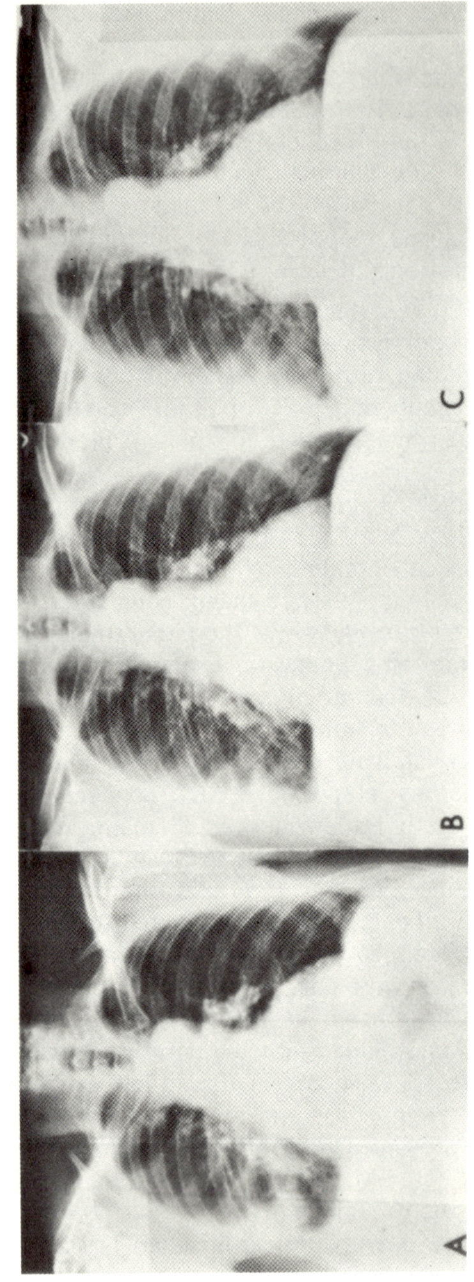

Figure 3. Case 3. **A**, initial film. **B**, film obtained three months later. **C**, film obtained eleven months later.

There were only two instances of skin rash. In both cases the rash was macular and erythematous. Ten patients gave a past history of drug reactions, usually to penicillin, quinidine or sulfonamides.

Laboratory findings: The laboratory data in the forty-four symptomatic cases are summarized in Table III. Antinuclear antibody was present in all. Titers frequently went out beyond 1:1000. Of thirty-nine patients tested for lupus erythematosus cells, thirty were positive. The morphology of the lupus erythematosus cells formed by these patients was indistinguishable from that seen in idiopathic SLE. A nucleoprotein-latex test* was positive in only twenty-five of the forty-four patients. About one third of the group had "rheumatoid factor" (anti-IgG), generally in a titer near 1:320. In seven of thirty patients tested, the Coombs test was positive using a reagent that detects complement on the red cells. In three of these seven IgG globulin was also detectable on their red cells. None of these patients had overt hemolytic anemia. The four instances of anemia were mild, with hematocrit levels ranging from 31 to 33 per cent. Two patients had thrombocytopenia. Only one instance of a leukopenia of under 3,000/cu mm was encountered; this was transient. There were no biologic false-positive tests for syphilis. No cases of renal impairment could be related to procainamide. No patient has had a low total serum complement or C'3.

---

* "LE test," Hyland Laboratories.

TABLE III   Laboratory Findings in Forty-Four Symptomatic Cases of Procainamide-Induced Lupus Erythematosus

Study	No.	Study	No.
ANA	44	Anemia	4
Lupus erythematosus cells	30/39	Thrombopenia	2
		White blood cells < 3,000/cu mm	1
Anti NP (Latex)	25	VDRL	0
Anti IgG (Latex)	14	Abnormal renal function	0
Coombs		Low serum C'	0
Gamma	3/30		
C'	7/30		

Follow-up studies: It was characteristic of the lupus-like reaction that once administration of the drug was stopped, the patient became asymptomatic in days. In patients with more severe reactions resolution was slower, however, and modest doses of prednisone were used to hasten their recovery. Of our earliest fourteen patients, seven required steroid therapy for from one month to three years. Two of the fourteen have continued to receive prednisone in low dosage two and three years, respectively, after treatment with procainamide was stopped. Another patient continued to take prednisone until his death at home of an undiagnosed abdominal catastrophe two years after the administration of procainamide was stopped. The only other death, occurring fifteen months after cessation of procainamide therapy, was due to myocardial infarction in a patient who did not require steroid treatment.

In all fourteen of these early patients symptoms subsided, lupus erythematosus cells or agglutinated nucleoprotein-latex particles no longer formed and the complement or IgG globulin on the red cells, present in some patients, disappeared. Of five who had anti-IgG activity, the low titer persisted in one. All fourteen still had antinuclear antibody after two years, or near the time of death, but their titers had fallen by about one order of magnitude (Figure 4).

Studies on DNA-Procainamide Complexes. The symptoms, signs and laboratory abnormalities described in these cases are clearly related to procainamide administration. Their defervescence was temporally related to cessation of procainamide treatment. Because of these observations and the occurrence of antibodies with specificity for nuclear materials, we sought a complex between procainamide and DNA which might serve as a model for studying the mechanism of the drug-induced syndrome.

Complex with single-stranded DNA: Methylene blue, riboflavin and protoporphyrin IX will mediate the binding of procainamide to denatured (single-stranded) DNA in the presence of visible light. The

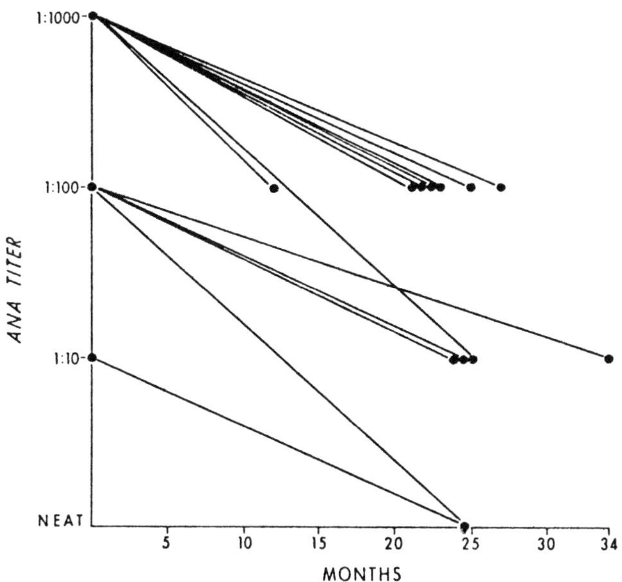

Figure 4. Fall in antinuclear antibody with time.

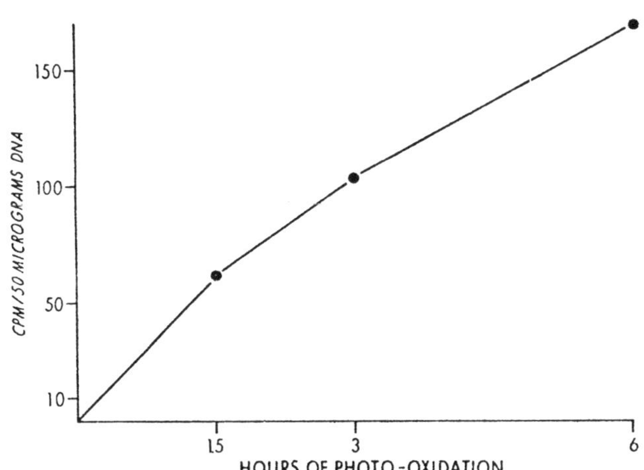

Figure 5. Binding of procainamide as a function of duration of photo-oxidation.

extent of binding depends on the duration of photo-oxidation (Figure 5). In this experiment a mixture of single-stranded DNA (1 mg/ml), procainamide (1 mg/ml) and riboflavin (40 mg/ml) was radiated with 5,000 foot-candles at 20°C with constant mixing. Aliquots were withdrawn at one and a half, three and six hours, the DNA was separated from unbound drugs, and 50 μg samples were counted. The amount of drug bound, as indicated by the rising number of counts in the DNA with time, increased with duration of photo-oxidation.

The extent of drug binding is also a function of the concentration of the photodynamic agent present. Figure 6 is a typical study of the effect of the concentration of riboflavin on the extent of the photodynamic reaction. The amount of drug bound increased with riboflavin concentration up to the limits of solubility of the photodynamic molecule. The same was true for protoporphyrin IX.

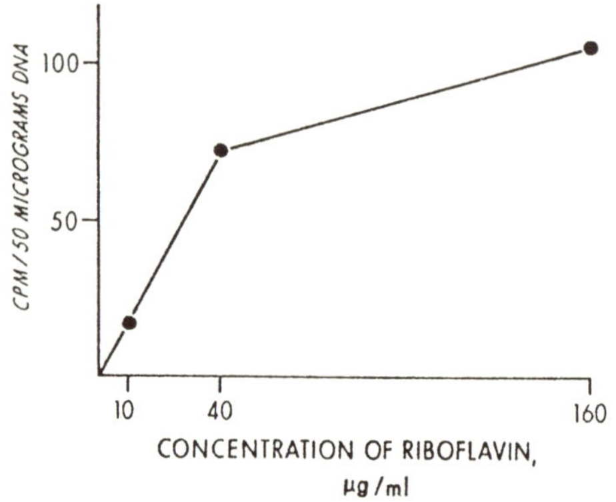

Figure 6. *Effect of riboflavin concentration upon extent of binding of procainamide.*

A different indicator of drug binding was the acquisition of new antigenic specificity. In rabbits immunized with drug-DNA complex an antibody developed which recognized a drug-related antigenic change on DNA. Figure 7 shows the quantitative complement fixation curves of a 1:200 dilution of antiserum from a rabbit immunized with photo-oxidized DNA-procainamide complex (poDNA-P). The reactivity of this serum (R 22) with poDNA-P is shown in the uppermost of the curves. Some cross reactivity existed, as expected, with DNA photo-oxidized in the absence of drug (poDNA), as well as with unaltered DNA. The greater reactivity with poDNA-P provides direct evidence that the drug-DNA complex possesses structural changes that are immunologically recognizable, but it should be noted that the complex induced the production of antibodies reactive with uncomplexed as well as complexed DNA.

The presence of procainamide on the DNA was further confirmed by complement fixation reactions with antibody to procainamide, to be described later.

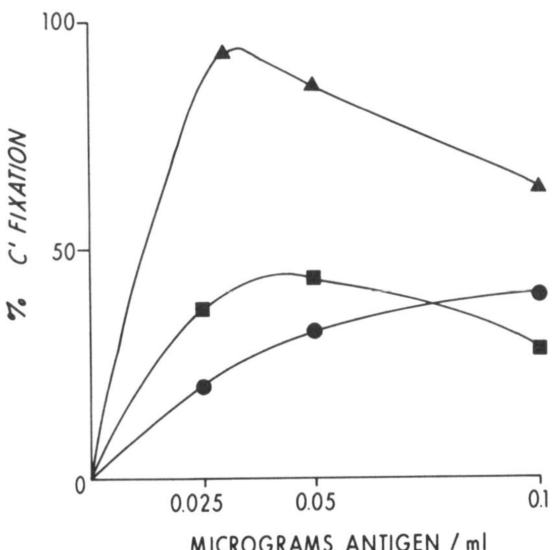

Figure 7. Complement fixation curves of rabbit immunized with photo-oxidized DNA-procainamide complex (poDNA-P); ●—● = unaltered DNA; ■—■ = DNA photo-oxidized in the absence of procainamide (poDNA); ▲—▲ = poDNA-P. Serum is R 22, 1:200.

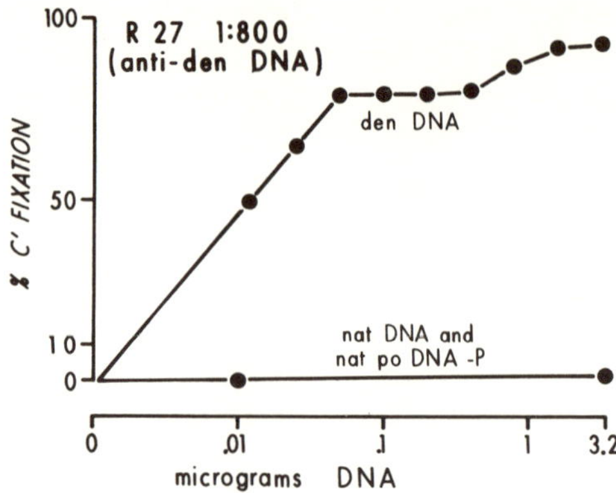

Figure 8. Reactivity of antibody to denatured DNA with denatured DNA (den DNA), native DNA (nat DNA), and renatured photo-oxidized DNA-procainamide complex (nat po DNA-P).

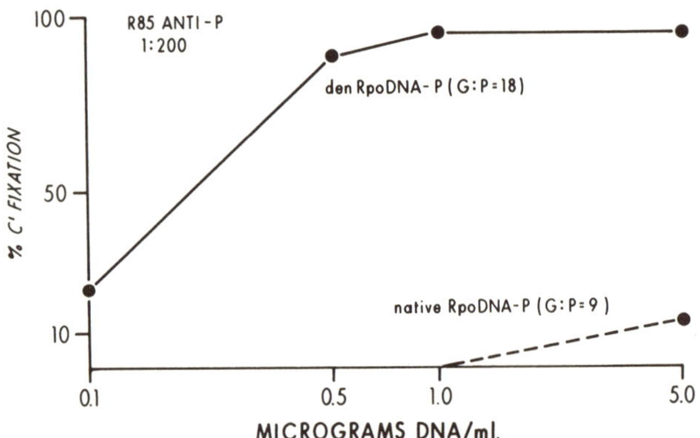

Figure 9. Accessibility of procainamide on DNA. G:P is ratio of guanine bases to procainamide. den R po DNA-P is denatured riboflavin photo-oxidized DNA-procainamide complex.

Complex with double-stranded DNA: When the photo-oxidation studies were repeated using native, double-stranded DNA no significant binding of drug to the native DNA molecule could at first be demonstrated. These early studies were carried out at the low temperatures that were effective in inducing binding with heat denatured DNA (13° to 22°C).

However, when photo-oxidation was carried out at 70°C, at which temperature the native molecule is to some extent uncoiled, binding of the drug to the DNA was as impressive as with single-stranded DNA. Subsequent slow cooling allowed preservation of native, double helix configurations with remarkably little evidence of denaturation. In one preparation made with riboflavin, 1 drug molecule was bound per 3 guanine bases.

An immunologic method was used to assess how much denaturation may have remained in the slowly cooled, double-stranded DNA complex. A rabbit antiserum (R 27) specific for single-stranded DNA (anti-den DNA) was used for this. Figure 8 shows the complement fixation curves of this serum when tested with single-stranded (den) DNA, double stranded (nat) DNA and the drug-DNA complex (nat poDNA-P). Any reactivity of this serum with a presumably "native" DNA would signify denaturation, that is, immunologically reactive areas of single-strandedness. The expected complement-fixing reactivity of the serum with denatured DNA is evident, but the serum showed no reactivity with a standard native DNA or with the slowly cooled ("re-natured") drug-DNA complex. By reference to the concentrations examined, it can be deduced that the native DNA and the drug-DNA complex used had less than 1 per cent of immunologically reactive, single-strandedness in them.

When the nat poDNA-P complex was exposed to antiprocainamide antibodies, again no significant reaction occurred (Figure 9). The serum used (R 85) was from a rabbit immunized with bovine serum albumin to which procainamide had been diazotized. The antibody in R 85 reacted in precipitation and complement fixation with procainamide attached to another carrier (horse gamma globulin) and thus had haptenic specificity for procainamide. Figure 9 shows complement fixation curves obtained with this serum with complexes made with native and denatured preparations of DNA. The complexes with denatured DNA (den R poDNA-P), which in this instance contained only 1 procainamide molecule per 18 guanines, reacted well with the antiprocainamide serum. The complex with native DNA (native R poDNA-P), to which twice as much procainamide was attached, gave only a marginal degree of complement fixation at a very high concentration. This suggests that the procainamide bound to the double-stranded ("native") DNA is buried in the core of the double helix and is inaccessible to the antibody present in the R 85 rabbit antiserum.

Studies of the immunogenicity of the complexes: We attempted to determine whether the DNA-drug complexes we made could be useful in providing a model for the mechanism of the induction of the lupus syndrome by drugs. These efforts can be summarized briefly. After immunizing 134 rabbits, utilizing varying schedules and doses, with and without adjuvant, and with and without methylated BSA stabilization [22], we were unable to demonstrate that procainamide complexed to native or denatured calf thymus DNA is superior to that complexed to unaltered calf thymus DNA as an immunogen in rabbits. In experiments not described here, the complexes we made were not demonstrably resistant to deoxyribonuclease. And lastly, the complexes were not more reactive with serum from patients with procainamide-induced lupus erythematosus when studied in precipitin reactions or complement fixation than was DNA itself.

A study of the antinuclear antibodies in procainamide-induced lupus: precipitation of radiolabeled antigen: The technic of ammonium sulfate precipitation was used to demonstrate antibody to heat-denatured or native DNA, and to nucleohistone in serum from normal subjects, patients with idiopathic lupus erythematosus, and patients with procainamide-induced lupus erythematosus. Figure 10 shows the results when native DNA labeled with ^{3}H-actinomycin D was used. Each point represents the percentage of added antigen that an individual serum bound, so as to make it precipitable by ammonium sulfate. Only the patients with idiopathic lupus erythematosus had significantly more than normal precipitability, and

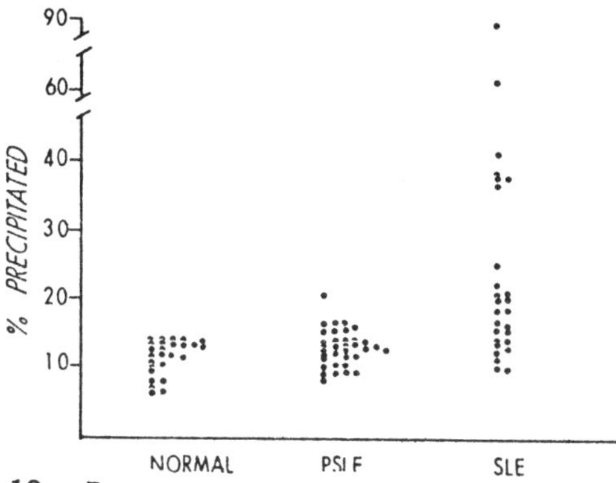

Figure 10. Reactivity of serum with native DNA in globulin precipitation technic.

thus presumably more detectable antibody to native DNA by this procedure. The mean percentage for twenty-seven serum samples from patients with idiopathic lupus erythematosus was 26 per cent. In twenty-seven samples of normal serum it averaged 12 per cent, and in thirty-five samples from patients with procainamide-induced lupus erythematosus it averaged 13 per cent. There was no significant difference between the precipitability of the serum of patients with procainamide-induced lupus erythematosus and that of the normal subjects.

Reactivity with heat-denatured DNA labeled with ^{3}H-actinomycin D gave a different picture (Figure 11). Nineteen specimens of normal serum gave a mean level of 11 per cent, thirty-two specimens from patients with procainamide-induced lupus erythematosus averaged 22 per cent, and twelve specimens from patients with idiopathic lupus erythematosus averaged 23 per cent. The mean levels for serum from patients with procainamide-induced and idiopathic lupus erythematosus were significantly different from normal (P $<$0.05) but not from each other.

All these values for per cent of antigen precipitated can be increased by adding less antigen to the system, as would be expected if the binding by the serum were due to a fixed quantity of binding

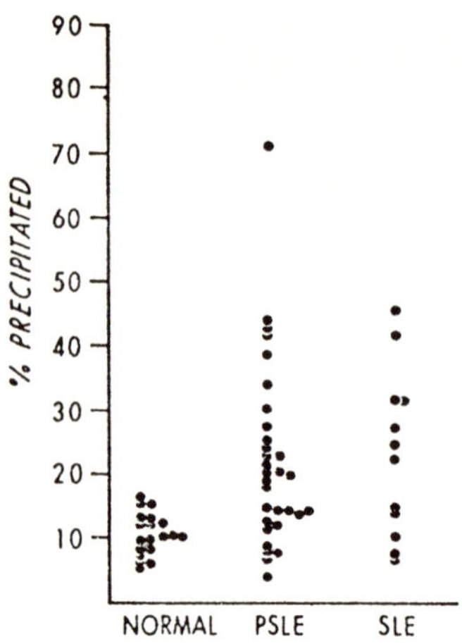

Figure 11.   Reactivity of serum with sonicated denatured DNA in globulin precipitation technic.

globulin. The results shown in the figures are based on the addition of 10 μg of antigen to 0.1 ml of serum. At 3 or 1 μg added, the serum gave a higher percentage precipitated. However, precipitation in normal serum increased also, and no advantage was gained in demonstrating differences.

Because serum from patients with procainamide-induced lupus erythematosus can form lupus erythematosus cells in vitro, it seemed reasonable to expect that antinucleohistone antibody would be present [27]. Twenty-six normal serum samples gave a mean level of 8 per cent precipitation of the 10 μg of nucleohistone added to 0.1 ml of serum (Figure 12). Thirty-four patients with procainamide-induced lupus erythematosus showed a significantly greater per cent of counts precipitated, with a mean of 12 per cent. Twenty-seven serum specimens from patients with idiopathic lupus erythematosus gave a mean of 16 per cent, but a median which was near that for procainamide-induced lupus erythematosus. The serum from patients with procainamide-induced and idiopathic lupus erythematosus was not significantly different from each other, but both were significantly higher than normal (P $<$0.05).
Complement fixing antibody to denatured DNA:

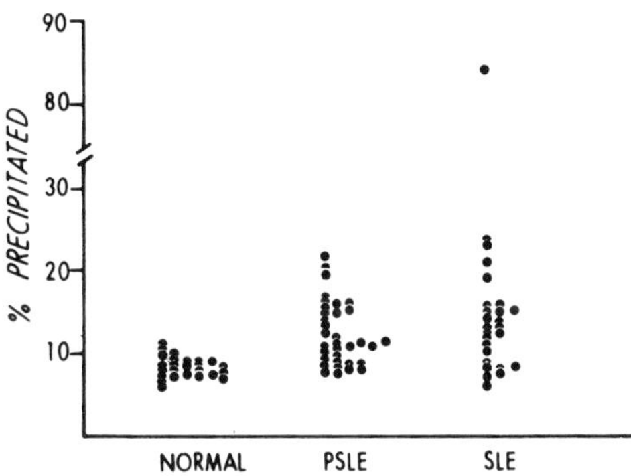

Figure 12. Reactivity of serum with sonicated nucleo-histone in globulin precipitation technic.

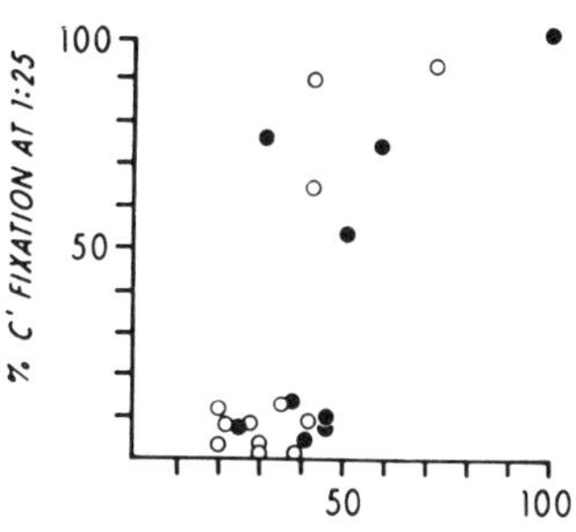

Figure 13. Fixation of complement with denatured DNA at dilution of 1:25 of selected serum which gave high values in globulin precipitation technic. ○ = procainamide-induced lupus. ● = idiopathic lupus.

Serum from patients with procainamide-induced and idiopathic lupus erythematosus giving the highest percentages of precipitation of denatured DNA in the globulin precipitation technic was surveyed for complement-fixing ability against denatured DNA (Figure 13). Serum samples were assayed at a dilution of 1:25 against a single concentration of DNA (0.025 μg/ml). Four of nine serum specimens from patients with idiopathic lupus erythematosus fixed complement under these conditions. The serum giving 100 per cent both for complement fixation and for antigen precipitation was drawn from a patient with intensely active idiopathic lupus erythematosus. The other serum specimens from patients with idiopathic lupus erythematosus were drawn from patients with varying degrees of clinical activity. The serum from patients with procainamide-induced lupus erythematosus was drawn near the time of maximal symptoms. Three of these serum samples fixed complement well at a serum dilution of 1:25, one also at 1:100. The hemolytic complement activities determined in all three serum specimens at the times they were drawn were normal, as has been true of all patients with this syndrome in our experience. All three of the patients with procainamide-induced lupus erythematosus were men in their fifties or sixties, making it less likely that they might actually have had idiopathic lupus erythematosus.

COMMENTS

Drug-induced illness closely resembling lupus erythematosus continues to attract the interest and attention of investigators of autoallergic diseases, particularly since understanding of the mechanism of the drug-induced state might help to elucidate the pathogenesis of idiopathic lupus.

There is no doubt that the administration of procainamide in conventional doses was the proximate cause of the syndrome in the afflicted here described. In a prospective study [28] we demonstrated that in about approximately 50 per cent of persons antinuclear antibody developed after treatment with procainamide for up to six months. We have interpreted [28] this high incidence as making it unlikely that the drug simply unveils a latent predisposition to idiopathic lupus erythematosus, as Alarcon-Segovia suggested might be the case with hydralazine [29], since the estimated frequency of idiopathic lupus erythematosus in the general population is only 1 in 8,000 [30] to 1 in 25,000 [31].

Although the similarity of the drug-induced reaction to idiopathic lupus erythematosus is striking, there are certain differences which ultimately may be important in understanding the pathogenesis of both drug-induced and idiopathic lupus erythematosus. Some of these similarities and differences have recently been reviewed [32], but those brought out by the present series deserve re-emphasis. The preponderance of males in this series is in striking contrast to the preponderance of females in idiopathic lupus erythematosus. Negroes are underrepresented, only two of our patients being black. The pulmonary parenchyma is involved much more often in procainamide-induced lupus erythematosus. Persistence of roentgenographic changes and impaired pulmonary function have been reported [33]. Pulmonary involvement apparently is less common in other drug-induced lupus reactions, however, and one may suspect that the older age or underlying heart disease in the procainamide-induced cases may contribute to this difference. Of particular interest is the rarity or absence of renal damage in procainamide-induced lupus erythematosus.

Our studies suggest that several autoantibodies can appear in procainamide-induced lupus erythematosus. These include antibodies to single-stranded DNA, nucleohistone, red cell membranes and IgG. If these antibodies arise in response to autologous molecules which in some way are altered by procainamide, then a general reactivity of procainamide with several types of macromolecules and/or membranes should be considered.

The appearance of these autoantibodies suggests that a distinct immunologic process has been set in motion. The persistence of slowly falling titers of antinuclear antibody for years after administration of the drug has been stopped indicates that a significant alteration in tolerance to self has occurred and that antinuclear antibody continues to be made as a result. A similar persistence of antinuclear antibody after cessation of drug administration was noted in patients studied prospectively [28].

The means by which procainamide leads to lupus-like symptoms and serologic abnormalities is still unknown. It is possible that the drug activates latent viral infection. Arthralgias, myalgias, serositis, pulmonary infiltrates and systemic symptoms occur in a variety of viral illnesses, and their presence in drug-induced lupus syndromes should at least raise this possibility. Procainamide may elicit autoantibodies by causing the release of immunogenic forms or amounts of host antigens, latent viral antigens, or virus-altered host macromolecular or membrane antigens, but no specific evidence exists for any of these possibilities.

Our efforts have been concerned with the possibility that procainamide may combine with nuclear macromolecules or other potential autoantigens to render them more highly immunogenic. Sela and Arnon [34] have demonstrated that nonimmunogenic macromolecules, such as gelatin, can be made immunogenic by enrichment with aromatic substituents such as tyrosyl, tryptophanyl or phenylalanyl groups. Procainamide, which is similar in size and structure to these substituents, could conceivably convert DNA from its notably poor immunogenic form to a more potent immunogen. The means of coupling of the procainamide to the DNA might be crucial. Simple addition of procainamide to DNA fails to produce observable change in the mixture, although Tan [35] has reported interesting effects when hydralazine is simply mixed with soluble nucleohistone. Some form of general reaction of procainamide with many macromolecules or membranes must be postulated because of the occurrence of antibodies not only to single-stranded DNA but also to nucleohistone, red cells and IgG. Our choice of photo-oxidation as a means of complexing procainamide to DNA was based on the observations of Van Vunakis et al. [36] that any molecule with an unsubstituted amino group could be bound to denatured DNA under the relatively gentle conditions of photo-oxidation, using methylene blue as the photodynamic agent. Our further modification in the use of protoporphyrin IX or riboflavin in place of methylene blue was based on the established photodynamic qualities of these natural substances and the fact that they are part of our normal biologic constitution. The drug-DNA complexes we have described herein have not proved to have enhanced immunogenicity in rabbits, nor have we detected antibody specifically directed to them in the serum of patients with the drug-induced disease. Nevertheless, we believe the type of compound formed continues to be highly interesting and to provide an important model for our thinking about the origin of the disease.

Three findings of prime interest have emerged from our studies. Patients with procainamide-induced lupus erythematosus do not have renal involvement; antibody to native DNA is not present in their serum; and antibody to denatured DNA is present in most serum but fixes complement in low titer in only a few.

The absence of antibody to native DNA in procainamide-induced lupus erythematosus has been reported by Koffler et al. using a hemagglutination technic [37], and the globulin precipitation studies reported here confirm this. Although antibody to denatured DNA is present, this appears to be less specific for lupus erythematosus than does antibody to native DNA [37]. Moreover, in the few instances of active lupus erythematosus or malignant disease in which circulating DNA has been demonstrated, it appears to be in the native form [38,39]. The DNA which has been demonstrated in kidney deposits in lupus nephritis is also native [40], although a recent report has demonstrated that single-stranded DNA can be present [41]. These observations, together with the lack of lowered serum complement in procainamide-induced lupus erythematosus, make it attractive to postulate that the apparent absence of renal disease in this condition may be due to lack of antibody to native DNA and perhaps to lack of circulating native DNA. Tojo and Friou [42] have reported that the occurrence of lupus nephritis is correlated with the complement-fixing ability of antinuclear antibodies. If denatured DNA in complex with complement-fixing antibody to denatured DNA contributes at all to nephritis in lupus erythematosus, then the weak to absent complement-fixing ability of this antibody might also be an important factor in the absence of renal disease in procainamide-induced lupus erythematosus.

REFERENCES

1. Ladd AT: Procainamide-induced lupus erythematosus. New Eng J Med 267: 1957, 1962.
2. Dustan HP, Taylor RD, Corcoran AC, et al.: Rheumatic and febrile syndrome during prolonged hydralazine treatment. JAMA 154: 23, 1954.
3. Auquier L, Meyer A, Seligman M, et al.: Maladie lupique (L.E.E.) au cours d'un traitement par l'isoniazide. Bull Soc Med Hop Paris 118: 371, 1967.
4. Hoffman BJ: Sensitivity to sulfadiazine resembling acute disseminated lupus erythematosus. Arch Derm (Chicago) 51: 190, 1945.
5. Jacobs JC: Systemic lupus erythematosus in childhood. Pediatrics 32: 257, 1963.
6. Benton JW, Tynes B, Register HB Jr, et al.: Systemic lupus erythematosus occurring during anti-convulsant drug therapy. JAMA 180: 115, 1962.
7. Willske K, Shalit IE, Willkens RF, et al.: Findings suggestive of systemic lupus erythematosus in subjects on chronic anticonvulsant therapy. Arthritis Rheum 8: 260, 1965.
8. Livingston S, Rodriquez H, Greene CA, et al.: Systemic lupus erythematosus. Occurrence in association with ethosuximide therapy. JAMA 204: 731, 1968.
9. Gold S: Role of sulphonamides and penicillin in the pathogenesis of systemic lupus erythematosus. Lancet 1: 268, 1951.
10. Ogryzlo MA: The LE (lupus erythematosus) cell reaction. Canad Med Ass J 75: 980, 1956.
11. Domz CA, McNamara DH, Holzapfel HF: Tetracycline provocation in lupus erythematosus. Ann Intern Med 50: 1217, 1959.
12. Popkhristov P, Kapnitov S: (Streptomycin: a factor responsible for provocation and exacerbation of lupus erythematosus: clinical observations). Surv Med (Sofia) 10: 81, 1959.
13. Zingale SB, Minzer L, Rosenberg B, et al.: Drug-induced lupus-like syndrome. Arch Intern Med (Chicago) 112: 63, 1963.

14. Alexander S: Lupus erythematosus in two patients after griseofulvin treatment of trichophyton rubrum infection. Brit J Derm 74: 72, 1962.

15. Bodman SF, Hoffman MJ, Condemi JJ: The procainamide-induced lupus syndrome (abstract). Arthritis Rheum 10: 269, 1967.

16. Vaughan JH, Bodman SF, Condemi JJ: Drug-induced systemic lupus erythematosus. Proceedings of the IVth Panama Congress on Rheumatology, Mexico City, 1967, Amsterdam, Excerpta Medica Foundation, International Congress Series No. 165, 1969, p 91.

17. Condemi JJ, Barnett EV, Atwater EC, et al.: Significance of antinuclear factors in rheumatoid arthritis. Arthritis Rheum 8: 1080, 1965.

18. Dubois EL: Lupus Erythematosus. A Review of the Current Status of Discoid and Systemic Lupus Erythematosus and Their Variants, New York, McGraw-Hill Book Co., 1966, p 302.

19. Singer JM, Plotz CM: The latex fixation test. I. Application to the serologic diagnosis of rheumatoid arthritis. Amer J Med 21: 888, 1956.

20. Cass RM, Mongan ES, Jacox RF, et al.: Immunoglobulins G, A and M in systemic lupus erythematosus. Relationship to serum complement titer, latex titer, antinuclear antibody, and manifestations of clinical disease. Ann Intern Med 60: 749, 1968.

21. Giles KW, Myers A: An improved diphenylamine method for the estimation of deoxyribonucleic acid. Nature (London) 206: 93, 1965.

22. Plescia OJ, Braun W, Palczuk NC: Production of antibodies to denatured deoxyribonucleic acid (DNA). Proc Nat Acad Sci USA 52: 279, 1964.

23. Wasserman E, Levine L: Quantitative microcomplement fixation and its use in the study of antigenic structure by specific antigen-antibody inhibition. J Immun 87: 290, 1961.

24. Russell AS, Ziff M: Natural antibodies to procaine amide. Clin Exp Immun 3: 901, 1968.

25. Farr RS: A quantitative immunochemical measure of the primary interaction between I*BSA and antibody. J Infect Dis 103: 239, 1958.

26. Carr RI, Koffler D, Agnello V, et al.: Studies on DNA antibodies using DNA labeled with actinomycin D (^{3}H) sulfate. Clin Exp Immun 4: 527, 1969.

27. Holman H, Deicher HR: The reaction of the lupus erythematosus (LE) cell factor with deoxyribonucleoprotein of the cell nucleus. J Clin Invest 38: 2059, 1959.

28. Blomgren SE, Condemi JJ, Bignall MC, et al.: Antinuclear antibody induced by procainamide. A prospective study. New Eng J Med 281: 64, 1969.

29. Alarcon-Segovia D, Wakim KG, Worthington JW, et al.: Clinical and experimental studies on the hydralazine syndrome and its relationship to systemic lupus erythematosus. Medicine (Balt) 46: 1, 1967.

30. Leonhardt T: Family studies in systemic lupus erythematosus. Acta Med Scand 176 (supp 416): 1, 1964.
31. Siegel M, Lee SL, Widelock D, et al.: The epidemiology of systemic lupus erythematosus. Preliminary results in New York City. J Chron Dis 15: 131, 1962.
32. Condemi JJ, Blomgren SE, Vaughan JH: The procainamide-induced lupus syndrome. Bull Rheum Dis 20: 604, 1970.
33. Byrd RB, Schanzer B: Pulmonary sequelae in procainamide-induced lupus-like syndrome. Dis Chest 55: 170, 1969.
34. Sela M, Arnon R: Studies on the chemical basis of the antigenicity of proteins. Biochem J 75: 91, 1960.
35. Tan EM: The influence of hydralazine on nuclear antigen-antibody reactions (abstract). Arthritis Rheum 11: 515, 1968.
36. Van Vunakis H, Seaman E, Kahan L, et al.: Formation of an adduct with tris (hydroxymethyl) aminomethane during the photo-oxidation of deoxyribonucleic acid and guanine derivatives. Biochemistry (Wash) 5: 3986, 1966.
37. Koffler D, Carr RI, Agnello V, et al.: Antibodies to polynucleotides: distribution in human serums. Science 166: 1648, 1969.
38. Tan EM, Schur PH, Carr RI, et al.: Deoxyribonucleic acid (DNA) and antibodies to DNA in the serum of patients with systemic lupus erythematosus. J Clin Invest 45: 1732, 1966.
39. Hughes GRV, Cohen SA, Lightfoot RW Jr, et al.: The occurrence of DNA in biological fluids (abstract). Arthritis Rheum 13: 324, 1970.
40. Koffler D, Schur PH, Kunkel HG: Immunologic studies concerning the nephritis of systemic lupus erythematosus. J Exp Med 126: 607, 1967.
41. Andres GA, Accinni L, Beiser SM, et al.: Localization of fluorescein-labeled antinucleoside antibodies in glomeruli of patients with active systemic lupus erythematosus nephritis. J Clin Invest 49: 2106, 1970.
42. Tojo T, Friou GJ: Lupus nephritis. Varying complement-fixing properties of immunoglobulin G antibodies to antigens of cell nuclei. Science 161: 904, 1968.

Localization of Fluorescein-Labeled Antinucleoside Antibodies in Glomeruli of Patients with Active Systemic Lupus Erythematosus Nephritis

G. A. ANDRES, L. ACCINNI, S. M. BEISER, C. L. CHRISTIAN, G. A. CINOTTI
B. F. ERLANGER, K. C. HSU, and B. C. SEEGAL

INTRODUCTION

Patients with systemic lupus erythematosus (SLE) may develop proliferative and membranous glomerulonephritis with deposits of foreign material along glomerular basement membranes (1–3). The presence of immunoglobulins and complement has been demonstrated in glomerular lesions by immunofluorescence techniques (4–7), and antinuclear antibodies have been found in eluates from the glomeruli (8–11). Fluorescein-labeled, highly purified antibody to DNA obtained from the serum of a lupus patient has localized in the glomeruli of two patients with SLE nephritis. Antibodies reacting with DNA, nucleoprotein, or neuclei were eluted from the glomeruli. These studies support the hypothesis that human lupus nephritis is provoked by circulating antigen-antibody complexes containing DNA and antibody to DNA (11).

This report describes the results of the studies of renal tissues from 13 SLE patients: nine with active glomerulonephritis, two with chronic glomerulonephritis,

113

and two without glomerulonephritis. The presence of
immunoglobulins, complement, and denatured DNA in
these tissues was determined by the immunofluorescence
technique. Antibodies specific for the pyrimidine bases
of DNA, thymine and cytosine, were used in searching
for denatured DNA (12–14). Unlike the DNA-reactive
antibodies in sera of some patients with SLE, the antibodies specific for the pyrimidines do not react with
native DNA (13–15).

MATERIALS AND METHODS

Patient Material

Patients with SLE. 13 female patients, 18–47 yr old, had
shown symptoms associated with SLE for 3 months to
15 yr. The more pertinent clinical, laboratory, and pathologic
findings in these patients are summarized in Table I, where
it is seen that eight patients were under the care of Dr.
Andres in the Renal Unit at the II Clinica Medica, University of Rome, and that four were from the Columbia
Presbyterian Medical Center (CPMC), where Dr. Christian
had charge of them. We are indebted to Dr. D. Davids of
St. Luke's Hospital for making available the tissue and the
clinical and laboratory findings of patient BW.

Patients with nephropathies other than SLE nephritis.
Renal tissues from 53 patients with various nephropathies
summarized in Table III were selected for testing with
fluorescein-labeled antibodies specific for thymine and cytosine, as well as with labeled antibodies to immunoglobulins
and to complement. They were chosen to serve as controls
because in most instances the amount of immunoglobulins
and complement and the pattern of distribution in GCW
resembled those found in active SLE nephritis. The age
range was comparable with the lupus patients. One-third
of the patients were women. This group of 53 patients,
from whom biopsy or autopsy specimens were obtained,
included 39 cared for at the Rome Clinic by Dr. Andres,
4 at the CPMC under the care of Dr. Christian, and 10
with renal allografts from Dr. T. E. Starzl, Colorado University Medical Center, Denver, Colo., or Dr. K. A. Porter,
St. Mary's Hospital, London. Clinical, laboratory, and light
and electron microscopic data have been used for the
diagnosis, and most of the findings have been reported
elsewhere (16–20).

Tissue processing

Renal biopsies were obtained with a Silverman needle
with Franklin modification under local anesthesia or by
"open biopsy." The tissues were divided into three parts;
one part was fixed in formalin or Bouin's solution for light
microscopy, the second was treated with osmium tetroxide
in preparation for embedding in Araldite for electron
microscopy, and the third part was quick-frozen in a bath
of dry ice and alcohol and was sectioned in a cryostat at
4μ thickness for immunofluorescent study.

Antisera: preparation and control

The following antisera were purchased, supplied by courtesy of various investigators, or prepared in our laboratories: anti-IgM, Hyland Div., Travenol Labs, Inc., Costa Mesa, Cal.; anti-IgA, Dr. R. D. Rosen (21); anti-lambda, Dr. E. R. Osserman (22); anti-kappa, Dr. E. R. Osserman (22); anti-β1C, Hyland Laboratories and Farbwerke Hoechst; anti-fibrinogen, Dr. F. Gorstein[1]; Anti-IgG, prepared in our laboratories or by Dr. A. J. L. Strauss (23); anti-BSA, prepared in our laboratories; anti-C'1q, Doctors J. H. Morse and C. L. Christian (24); and anti-T and anti-C, prepared by Doctors Beiser and Erlanger (12–13).

All antisera were tested by immunoelectrophoresis to establish their potency and specificity. Globulins were separated from the above antisera by sodium sulfate precipitation and were labeled with fluorescein using a technique already reported (25). Before any new fluorescein-conjugated antibody was used, its optimal dilution was determined by testing on a series of sections of tissue known to contain the specific antigen.

The preparation of the antisera reactive with thymine and cytosine has been described (12–13). Conjugates of bovine serum albumin (BSA) with 5-methyluridine (T) and with cytidine (C) were prepared, and rabbits were injected in the foot pads with the conjugates in complete Freund's adjuvant (26). Antibody for BSA, when present, was removed by absorption, and the antisera reacted only with homologous nucleoside-BSA conjugates and with denatured DNA. There was no crossing with heterologous nucleoside-BSA conjugates (15). The tests used were quantitative complement fixation (27) and quantitative precipitin reactions (28). Controls for the fluorescein staining experiments were prepared by absorbing aliquots of the fluorescein-labeled antisera with T, C, or with denatured DNA. Three successive absorptions were performed with T and C using 5 μg N antigen each time per 0.5 ml of serum and with denatured DNA using 40 μg of denatured human DNA each time per milliliter of serum. DNA was denatured by placing a solution (800 μg/ml) containing 1% formaldehyde in a boiling water bath for 10 min, followed by chilling quickly in an ice bath. After each antigen addition, the mixture was placed in a 37°C water bath for 1 hr and then was refrigerated overnight. After centrifugation, the procedure was repeated. The supernatant fluids after the third addition of antigen had been diluted less than 20%.

Staining of tissues

Staining of sections with the fluorescein-labeled globulins was carried out according to a technique already described (25). In an attempt to sharpen the staining with anti-T and anti-C, in six instances (EC [second biopsy], MTN [postmortem biopsy], VC, ID, LS, and DW), additional sections were first treated with 0.02 M citrate buffer, pH 3.2, for 15–30 min, or with 0.2 M NaCl for 1–2 hr at room tempera-

---

[1]Gorstein, F., and E. Puszkin. Immuno-electronmicroscopic appearance of fibrin. Data in preparation.

ture (11). They were then washed with phosphate buffer at pH 7.2 before staining with Fl-anti-T and with Fl-anti-C. Some sections were also eluted with physiological saline for the same interval of time. Unlabeled antibody was applied first to some tissue sections in order to test for blocking of the subsequent reaction with the labeled antibody.

RESULTS

Histologic studies (Table I). (*a*) In the tissues obtained on initial renal biopsies from the first nine patients (CM, EC, MTN, VC, AC, LS, ID, DW, and BW), glomerular lesions characteristic of, or compatible with, those seen in patients with diagnosis of active SLE nephritis, were found by light and electron microscopy (1–3). Patients AC, MTN, EC, LS, DW, and BW had a variety of proliferative and membranous changes, the pattern and the severity of which varied from glomerulus to glomerulus. Patients VC and ID had a diffuse membranous glomerulonephritis of moderate severity with slight evidence of proliferation. Patient CM had a severe acute proliferative and membranous glomerulonephritis with polymorphonuclear leukocytes and hematoxylin bodies. In all these patients, the electron microscopic studies showed the presence of aggregates of foreign electron-opaque material between proliferating cells and on both sides of the glomerular basement membrane. In the second and third biopsy of patient EC and in the second biopsy of patient MTN, the glomerular changes appeared less severe than when first seen. By electron microscopy there were fewer electron-opaque foreign depositis seen within the GCW of the second and third biopsies than were found in the first biopsy. In patient EC, lesions of "membranous transformation" (29) began to be evident in the third biopsy. In patients CC and PP, lesions of severe chronic nephritis, with diffuse glomerulovascular sclerosis, were seen, whereas the light and electron microscopic studies of tissues obtained from patients SA and PC showed only normal renal structures.

(*b*) All the renal tissues obtained from the third group of patients with glomerular diseases other than SLE glomerulonephritis have been examined by light and electron microscopy. All of theme were studied with the immunofluorescence technique, and some were also studied with the immunoferritin technique. The histologic and immunologic findings have been reported elsewhere (16–20).

TABLE I

Summary of Clinical and Laboratory Data for 13 SLE Patients

Patient	Age	Prior to biopsy/autopsy		At biopsy/autopsy and after biopsy					Histologic, clinical evaluation, course
		Duration symptoms	Course of disease, treatment	LE cells	Anti-nu.Ab	BUN	Creatinine clearance	Urinary findings	
	yr					*mg/100 ml*	*ml/min*		
CM, Rome Clinic 9/65	19	10 mo	Rash of face, chest, migratory arthralgia, fever, proteinuria, pleural effusion. R_x antibiotics, insufficient steroids. On admission also myo- and pericarditis.	pos	pos	100	40	protein 6–8 g casts rbc	Severe membranous, proliferative nephritis with hematoxylin bodies and wire loops. No improvement with immunosuppressive treatment. Left hospital in extremus.
EC, Rome Clinic 6/67	40	6 yr	Initially migratory arthralgia, fever. R_x salicylates. $5\frac{1}{2}$ yr postsurgery, proteinuria, edema. Admission diagnosis, glomerulonephritis, nephrotic syndrome.	neg	neg	15	89	protein 10–16 g casts rbc	Severe proliferative and membranous GN with wire loops. EM shows subendothelial and subepithelial deposits, also present between mesangial cells. R_x 60 mg prednisone/day.
9/67			Readmitted for biopsy.	neg					EM shows some slight improvement of renal lesion.
3/68			Readmitted, in fairly good condition.	pos	pos	15	94	protein 3 g	Steroids decreased, azathioprine started. 4/68 biopsy: decreased proliferative changes, persist deposits. Clinical condition improving.
2/70			Readmitted for observation. Good condition on prednisone 30 mg, azathioprine 50 mg/day.	neg	neg	25	—	protein 2–3 g	
MTN, Rome Clinic 7/67	23	3 yr	Migratory arthralgia, fever, edema, proteinuria. R_x antibiotics. 1 yr pericardial effusion, LE+, proteinuria, casts.	pos	pos	60	52	protein 10–15 g macroscopic blood	Severe membranous, proliferative GN with hematoxylin bodies and wire loops. R_x steroids and azathioprine. Remarkable clinical improvement.
11/67			Puncture to remove a persistent pericardial effusion during which patient died.						Needle biopsy taken. PM showed a decrease in amounts of deposits in GCW.

TABLE I—(*Continued*)

| Patient | Age | Prior to biopsy/autopsy | | At biopsy/autopsy and after biopsy | | | | | Histologic, clinical evaluation, course |
		Duration symptoms	Course of disease, treatment	LE cells	Anti-nu.Ab	BUN	Creatinine clearance	Urinary findings	
	yr					mg/100 ml	ml/min		
VC, Rome Clinic 12/67	18	14 mo	Migratory arthritis, fever, muscle pain, proteinuria, hematuria, edema, pleural effusion. R_x antibiotics.	pos	pos	90	45	protein 10–12 g	Membranous GN with wire loop changes, mesangial cell proliferation. EM subepithelial and subendothelial deposits. Improvement on azathioprine and prednisone. Condition remains satisfactory.
AC, Rome Clinic 2/68	29	13 mo	Migratory arthralgia. 8 months later edema, hematuria. Diagnosed GN, R_x antibiotics. After development of peritoneal, pericardial, pleural effusion.	neg	pos	80	90	protein 8–10 g	Severe proliferative GN, hematoxylin bodies, wire loops. R_x azathioprine and prednisone. After 5 months improved.
9/69			Readmitted for biopsy. Edema and effusion gone, condition good.	neg	neg	35	—	protein 2–4 g	Proliferative and membranous changes decreased. R_x prednisone and azathioprine continued.
2/70			Readmitted for routine check up. Condition remains satisfactory.	neg	neg	30	95	protein 1–3 g	
LS, CPMC 7/60	25	1 yr	Joint pains, fever, lymph nodes tender, enlarged. Murmurs, in systole, diastole. Proteinuria, hematuria.	pos	pos	45	—	protein 4 g casts rbc	Biopsy 10/68. Severe diffuse, proliferative and membranous nephritis with wire loops. Prednisone, azathioprine started.
ID, CPMC '59	47	10 yr	Original diagnosis mild rheumatoid arthritis. 1/66 developed nephrotic syndrome. LE cells neg. 2/66 renal biopsy showed membranous nephritis. LE cells positive. Final admission 4/69 for cerebral thrombosis, renal failure.	pos	pos	117	—	protein 4–6 g	4/69 autopsy. Membranous nephritis. Thickened GBM resembling wire loops.

118

TABLE 1—(*Continued*)

| Patient | Age | Prior to biopsy/autopsy | | At biopsy/autopsy and after biopsy | | | | | Histologic, clinical evaluation, course |
		Duration symptoms	Course of disease, treatment	LE cells	Anti-nu.Ab	BUN	Creatinine clearance	Urinary findings	
	yr					*mg/100 ml*	*ml/min*		
DW, CPMC	31	15 yr	1945 skin rash. 2 similar episodes in next 9 yr. 1954, polyarthritis, rash. 1956, LE cells neg. 1957, muscle biopsy, vasculitis, episcleritis, '60, arthralgias, pneum. pneumonia. On 2nd admission, viridans sepsis, latex 1:2000, LE cells pos. Pleurisy, gastric washings pos. for AFB. 1963 fever, adenopathy, proteinuria +++ BUN 30. 1968, BUN 162. 5/69 admitted with azotemia BUN 100, started on hemodialysis.	pos	pos	100	—	protein 4–6 g	10/69 renal transplant. Own kidney, most glomeruli with sclerosis. In others, active inflammatory lesions with diffuse subepithelial and subendothelial deposits.
BW, St. Luke's 10/69	41	3 mo	Skin rash, fatigue, loss of appetite and weight. Multiple enlarged lymph nodes. Hypergamma-globulinemia. Improved on prednisone.	pos	pos	85	—	protein 3–4 g	10/69 renal biopsy. Light micros. variable glomerular damage. EM shows sub-endothelial and mesangial deposits.
CC, Rome Clinic 2/5/70	18	3 yr	Fever, arthralgia, rash, purpura. After 3 months pleural and pericardial effusions, glomerulonephritis. LE cells+; Anti-nu.Abs+; proteinuria, 8–10 g; casts, rbc, BUN 70 mg/100 ml. R$_x$ antibiotics, steroids azathioprine with only short intervals, for 2 yr. At admission hypertension and renal failure.	pos	pos	120	15	protein 10 g casts rbc	Severe chronic glomerulonephritis with diffuse sclerosis.

TABLE 1—(*Continued*)

Patient	Age	Prior to biopsy/autopsy		At biopsy/autopsy and after biopsy					Histologic, clinical evaluation, course
		Duration symptoms	Course of disease, treatment	LE cells	Anti-nu.Ab	BUN	Creatinine clearance	Urinary findings	
	yr					*mg/100 ml*	*ml/min*		
PP, CPMC 7/60	22	3 mo	Rash, fever, poliarthralgia. LE cells positive. Pleural effusion, proteinuria, hematuria, maintained on prednisone. 9/67, renal insufficiency, LE cells negative. 10/68, final admission.	neg	neg	195	—	protein 4.3 g	10/68 autopsy. Hypercellularity. Thickened basement membranes, extensive glomerulocapsular adhesions, fibrin deposits. Architecture of glomeruli lost due to severe, diffuse sclerosis.
SA, Rome Clinic 6/13/67	29	3 mo	Rash (face, chest), migratory arthritis, fever, pleural effusion. Salicylates.	pos	pos	15	110	normal	Normal kidney, both by light and EM. Steroids and azathioprine.
5/10/68			Readmitted for routine check up.	neg	neg	20	95	normal	Purpura. Skin vasculitis. Steroids and azathioprine.
3/2/69			Readmitted for 3 months, pregnancy. Spontaneous abortion.	neg	neg	18	116	normal	Satisfactory condition. Rash, face. Steroids and azathioprine.
2/28/70			Readmitted for observation.	neg	neg	20	100	normal	Muscle pain migratory arthralgia. Steroids and azathioprine.
PC, Rome Clinic 8/5/67	25	1 yr	Original diagnosis mild migratory arthritis. 4/67 developed skin rash, muscle pain, pleural and pericardial effusions.	pos	neg	20	98	normal	Normal kidney both by light and EM. Steroids and azathioprine.
5/3/68			Readmitted for routine check up.	neg	neg	15	—	normal	Muscle pain. Satisfactory condition.

Immunofluorescence studies. (*a*) The results of studies in which frozen sections of kidney from 13 SLE patients were tested with Fl-Abs specific for IgG, IgM, IgA, kappa and lambda light chains, βlC, C'lq, fibrinogen, T, C, and BSA are summarized in Table II. Only a few sections containing glomeruli were obtained from the biopsy of patient CM, and they were only tested with Fl-anti-T, Fl-anti-βlC and Fl-anti-fibrinogen. Antibodies to IgG, IgM, βlC, and C'lq were localized in a granular pattern in the GCW of biopsy specimens from eight patients listed in the table. Labeled anti-IgA antibody did not yield significant reaction with any of the tissues studied. Light chain globulin fractions were present in variable degrees in GCW of patients EC, MTN, AC, LS, and ID. Anti-fibrinogen was mainly localized in the glomeruli of patients CM, EC, and ID. The fluorescent staining obtained with anti-T and anti-C in patients CM, EC, MTN, VC, AC, LS, ID, and DW was distributed in GCW in a granular manner (Figs. 1, 2, 5, 9, and 12) similar to that obtained with antibodies to immunoglobulins (Figs. 3 and 7) and complement (Figs. 4 and 8) and similar to the irregular distribution of the deposits of foreign material in GCW, as seen by electron microscopy. Renal tissues from patient BW did not bind the anti-T and anti-C sera. Anti-BSA was employed as control since BSA was part of the conjugate used for the preparation of antibodies against nucleosides, and it was not significantly bound except in one instance (LS).

Prior incubation of renal sections from this group of patients with unlabeled anti-T or anti-C blocked the subsequent staining with the respective Fl-Abs. The staining capacity of the labeled antibodies was removed or greatly reduced by absorption with the homologous antigen, T (Fig. 13) or C (Fig. 10), or with denatured DNA (Figs. 11 and 14), whereas it was not affected by cross-absorption, i.e., labeled anti-T with C or anti-C with T.

The renal tissues of two SLE patients (CC and PP) with chronic nephritis, characterized by diffuse glomerular sclerosis, did not bind significant amounts of Fl-Abs to immunoglobulins, complement, T, and C. The same findings were obtained in two SLE patients (SA and PC) without glomerulonephritis.

(*b*) Tests for the localization of Fl-anti-T and Fl-anti-C were made also in tissues from 53 biopsies and one

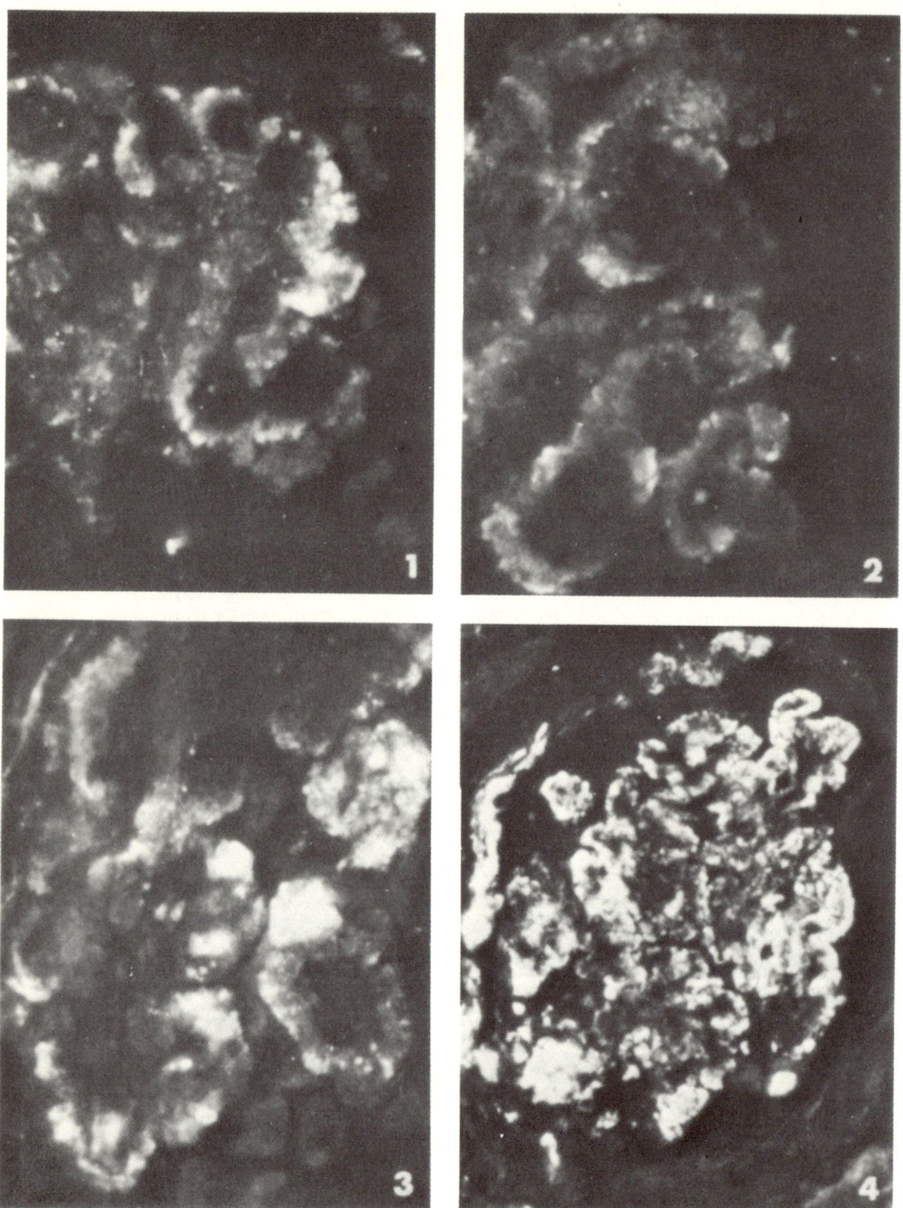

Figs. 1–14 are photomicrographs which show the results of staining with different fluorescein-labeled (Fl-) antibodies on sections of renal tissues of three SLE patients with active glomerulonephritis.

FIGURE 1   Patient MTN. Fl-anti-T localized in a granular manner in GCW. × 350.
FIGURE 2   Same patient. Fl-anti-C similarly localized in GCW. × 350.
FIGURE 3   Same patient. Granular localization in GCW of Fl-anti-IgM. × 450.
FIGURE 4   Same patient. Localization of Fl-anti-C'1q in a glomerulus and in a part of Bowman's capsule. × 300.

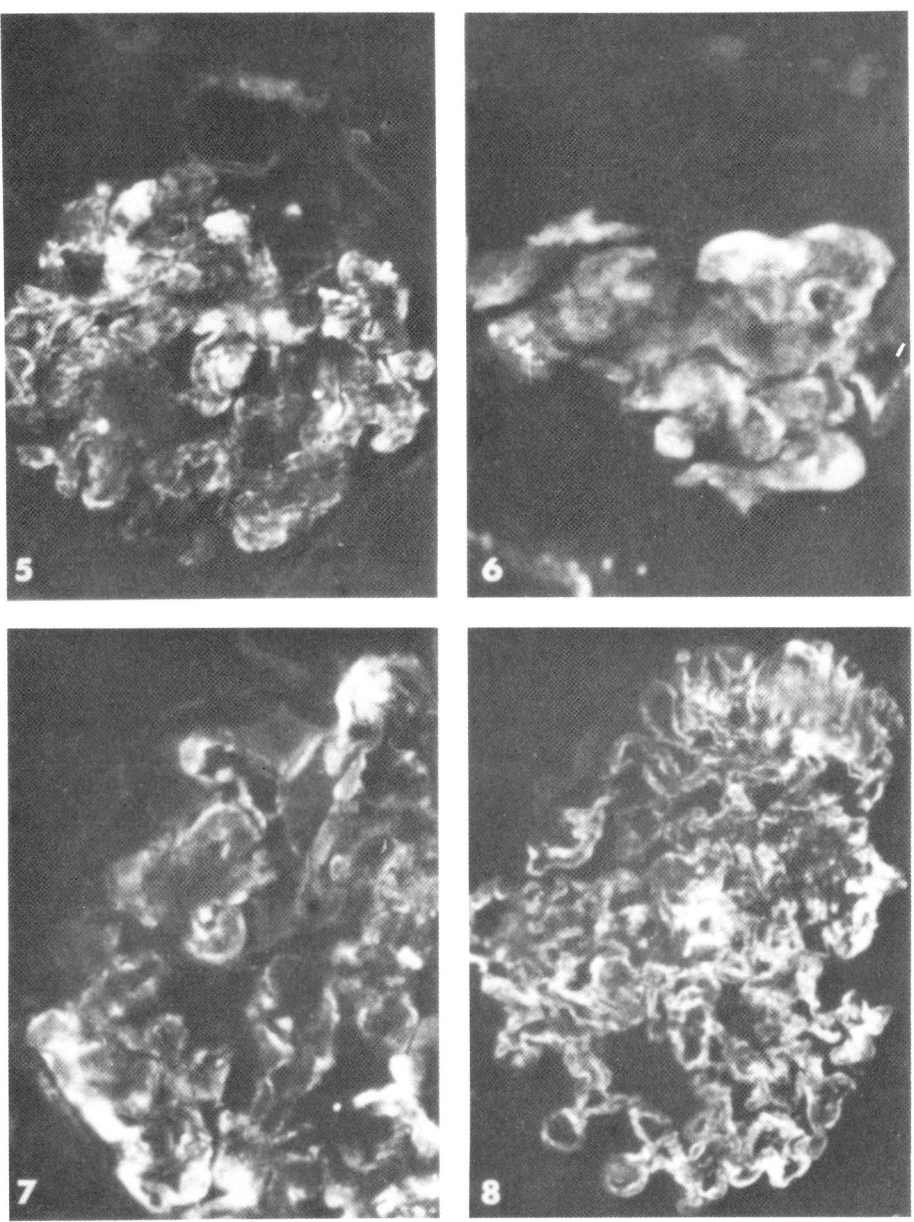

FIGURE 5   Patient LS. Localization in GCW of Fl-anti-T. × 300.
FIGURE 6   Same patient. Localization in a glomerulus of Fl-anti-C. × 300.
FIGURE 7   Same patient. Fl-anti-IgM localized in GCW. × 350.
FIGURE 8   Same patient. Fl-anti-C'1q localized similarly in GCW. × 350.

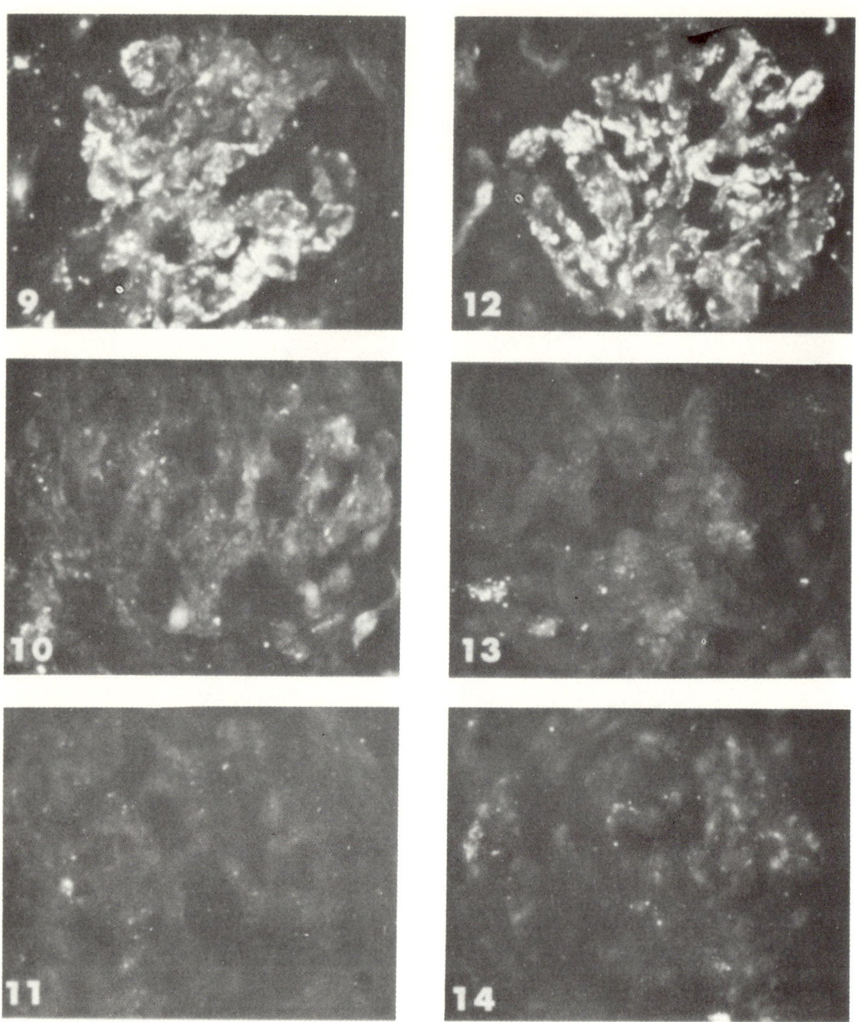

FIGURE 9 Patient ID. Granular localization of Fl-anti-C in GCW. × 100.

FIGURE 10 Same patient. Treated with Fl-anti-C absorbed with C. The staining capacity of this fluorescence is almost completely removed. × 100.

FIGURE 11 Same patient. Treated with Fl-anti-C absorbed with denatured DNA. No fluorescence is seen. × 100.

FIGURE 12 Same patient. Granular localization in GCW of Fl-anti-T. × 100.

FIGURE 13 Same patient. The staining capacity of Fl-anti-T is completely abolished by absorption with T. × 100.

FIGURE 14 Same patient. Treated with Fl-anti-T absorbed with denatured DNA. Very little fluorescence can be seen. × 100.

TABLE II

*Localization of Fl-Antibodies to Immunoglobulins, Complement, and Nucleosides
in Glomeruli of Renal Tissues from 13 SLE Patients*

Patient and date of biopsy	Antisera to										
	IgG	IgM	IgA	Lam	Kap	C'1q	βIC	Fngn	T	C	BSA
CM 10/65	−	−	−	−	−	−	+	++	+++	−	−
EC 6/67	++	++++	−	−	−	++++	+	++	+++	+++	±
9/67	+++	++	−	−	−	++++	++	0/+	++++	++++	0
4/68	++	0	−	++	−	++	+	0/++	++	+	±
MTN 7/67	++++	+++	0	+	++/+++	++++	++	+	+++	+++	±
11/67 (PM)	++	+++	−	−	−	++++	+	±	++	++	0
VC 2/68	++++	±	±	±	0	++++	+++	0	++	±	0
AC 3/68	++++	+	0	+/+++	++/+++	++++	+++	+	++	++	0
9/69	++++	++++	−	−	−	−	++++	−	+++	++	−
LS 10/68	++	+++	−	+++	+++	++++	++++	+	+++	+++	+
ID* 4/69	++++	+++	0/+	+++	±/+	±/+	+++	++	+++	++/+++	0
DW 10/69	+++	+++	−	−	−	−	±/+	±	+/+++	++/+++	0
BW 10/69	+++	+++	−	−	−	−	++++	−	0	0	0
CC 4/70	±	±	−	−	−	±	±	0	0	0	0
PP* 10/68	0	0	0	0	0	0	0	0	0	0	0
SA 7/67	0	0	−	−	−	0	0	0	0	0	0
PC 11/67	0	0	−	−	−	0	0	0	0	0	0

* Autopsy specimen.

Abbreviations: Fl-, fluorescein-labeled; SLE, systemic lupus erythematosus; lam, lambda light chain; kap, kappa light chain; Fngn, fibrinogen; PM, postmortem; T, 5-methyluridine-BSA; C, cytidine-BSA; −, test not done or no glomeruli in sections; 0, negative; ±, minimal in amount; +, slight in amount; ++, moderate in amount; +++, marked in amount; ++++, very marked in amount and extent.

autopsy of patients with glomerular diseases other than SLE nephritis (Table III). All the tests for nucleosides were negative except for one tissue obtained at autopsy from a patient with idiopathic membranous nephropathy, in which both LE cell and antinuclear antibody tests were negative. In this case, a one plus binding of anti-T and anti-C in the GCW was detected after elution with citrate buffer. The 53 renal tissues also were examined with antibodies to immunoglobulins, complement, fibrinogen, and BSA. There were numerous positive stainings of GCW similar in distribution and intensity to those seen in the nine SLE patients with active glomerulonephritis. This suggested that binding of anti-T and anti-C was specific for active lupus nephritis, whereas the other antibodies investigated were bound frequently by tissues obtained from patients with other nephropathies.

DISCUSSION

During the last 12 yr, a number of studies have contributed to a better understanding of immunological disorders characteristic of SLE in man. Several circulating antibodies reactive with native or altered nuclear antigens have been described (30–33). One potential antigen, DNA, has been found in the sera of patients with active SLE nephritis (34). Immunoglobulins and complement are localized in GCW (4–6) with a granular distribution resembling the pathology produced by circulating antigen-antibody complexes (35). Antinuclear antibodies are also concentrated in the glomerular lesions together with the antigen, DNA. The presence of DNA was demonstrated by means of anti-DNA antibody isolated from the serum of a patient with SLE. These last findings give strong support to the hypothesis that SLE nephritis in man is provoked by renal deposition of circulating antigen-antibody complexes formed by DNA, specific antinuclear antibodies, and complement (11).

The purpose of this paper is to report the localization in glomerular lesions of human SLE nephritis of fluorescein-conjugated antibodies of defined specificity. These antibodies are specific for pyrimidine bases of DNA, and react with denatured, but not with native, DNA. The specificity of localization was demonstrated by blocking experiments and also by the removal of the localizing activity by absorption with the homologous nucleoside-protein conjugate. The results reported in human SLE

TABLE III

Results of Tests for the Binding of Fl-Anti-T and Fl-Anti-C in Glomeruli of Kidneys from 53 Patients with Glomerular Diseases other than SLE GN

Disease	Number of cases	LE test and anti-nu.Ab	Number of binding A-T/A-C	Presence of immunoglobulins and complement
Acute poststreptococcal GN	12	both neg	0	Varying amounts of immunoglobulins and C' were bound in glomeruli.
Idiopathic membranous nephropathy	11	both neg	1	All had large amounts of immunoglobulins and C' in glomeruli. One had +binding with anti-T and anti-C.
Chronic nephritis	9	—	0	Small amounts of immunoglobulins and C' in glomeruli.
Renal allografts	10	—	0	Some with large amounts of immunoglobulins and C' in GCW. All contained some immunoglobulins.
Diabetic nephropathy	2	—	0	(Tissue from one obtained at autopsy). One had C' in GCW. The second was negative.
Pyelonephritis	3		0	None or little immunoglobulins and C' in glomeruli.
Polyarteritis	1	both neg	—	Severe renal disease with immunoglobulins and C' in glomeruli and vessels.
Goodpasture's disease	2	—	0	Marked localization of immunoglobulins and C', linear distribution in GCW.
Renal vein thrombosis with neph. syn.	2	both neg.	0	Marked localization of immunoglobulins and C'. Granular distribution in glomeruli.
Familial GN	1	—	0	Moderate amount of immunoglobulins and C'.

Abbreviations: GN, glomerulonephritis; C', complement.

nephritis are similar to those found in a study of lupus-like nephritis of NZB/NZW F1 mice (36).

The data obtained suggest the presence of denatured DNA in the foreign material forming granular deposits in the GCW (1-3) of eight SLE patients with active glomerulonephritis. Only one patient with active glomerulonephritis failed to localize the Fl-Abs to T and C. Failure of staining in two SLE patients with diffuse glomerular sclerosis and in two SLE patients with normal glomerular structures may be explained by the lack of reactive antigen in these areas. It is difficult to evaluate the role of denatured DNA in the pathogenesis of the disease. The presence in the same areas of immunoglobulins and of complement could be the result of accumulation of immune complexes formed by denatured DNA, antibodies to nucleosides, and complement, implying the presence of circulating denatured DNA, possibly as a result of a viral infection (38). Antibodies to denatured DNA have been described in SLE serum (27); and recently, in a study of a large series of SLE sera with the complement fixation text, Seligmann and Arana have shown that antibodies to denatured DNA are found more frequently than those to native DNA (37).

Another possible interpretation of the observations is that native DNA subsequent to deposition in GCW becomes denatured to a degree that permits interactions with anti-T and anti-C. In membranous nephropathies, morphologic appearances and immunologic reactivity of material contained in the foreign deposits may undergo changes during the course of the disease. This was also observed in the third biopsy of patient EC, since glomerular lesions of membranous transformation (29) appeared, and the intensity of staining for immunoglobulins and for T and C were markedly decreased. The determination of the specificity of antibodies eluted from the glomeruli of patients with SLE nephritis may present further evidence in elucidating the role of denatured DNA in the pathogenesis of the disease.

ACKNOWLEDGMENTS

This study was supported in part by the Consiglio Nazionale delle Richerche (CNR), Italy, National Institute of Health Grants HE03929, AM13200, AI04527, AI06860, and contract NONR 4259(11) with the Office of Naval Research.

REFERENCES

1. Farquhar, M. G., R. L. Vernier, and R. A. Good. 1957. An electron microscope study of the glomerulus in nephrosis, glomerulonephritis, and lupus erythematosus. *J. Exp. Med.* **106**: 649.

2. Faith, G. C., and B. F. Trump. 1966. The glomerular capillary wall in human kidney disease: acute glomerulonephritis, systemic lupus erythematosus, and preeclampsia eclampsia. Comparative electron microscopic observations and a review. *Lab. Invest.* **15**: 1682.

3. Comerford, F. R., and A. S. Cohen. 1967. The nephropathy of systemic lupus erythematosus. An assessment by clinical, light and electron microscopic criteria. *Medicine (Baltimore)*. **46**: 425.

4. Vazquez, J. J., and F. J. Dixon. 1957. Immunohistochemical study of lesions in rheumatic fever, systemic lupus erythematosus, and rheumatoid arthritis. *Lab. Invest.* **6**: 205.

5. Freedman, P., and A. S. Markowitz. 1962. Gamma globulin and complement in the diseased kidney. *J. Clin. Invest.* **41**: 328.

6. Paronetto, F., and D. Koffler. 1965. Immunofluorescent localization of immunoglobulins, complement, and fibrinogen in human diseases. I. Systemic lupus erythematosus. *J. Clin. Invest.* **44**: 1657.

7. Freedman, P., and A. S. Markowitz. 1962. Isolation of antibody-like gamma globulin from lupus glomeruli. *Brit. Med. J.* **1**: 1175.

8. Graf, M., and D. Koffler. 1966. Elution of glomerular-bound antibody in systemic lupus erythematosus. *Fed. Proc.* **25**: 659.

9. Krishnan, C., and M. H. Kaplan. 1966. Antinuclear activity in acid eluates of glomeruli from lupus nephritis kidneys. *Fed. Proc.* **25**: 309.

10. Krishnan, C., and M. H. Kaplan. 1967. Immunopathologic studies of systemic lupus reythematosus. II. Antinuclear reaction of γ-globulin eluted from homogenates and isolated glomeruli of kidneys from patients with lupus nephritis. *J. Clin. Invest.* **46**: 569.

11. Koffler, D., P. H. Schur, and H. G. Kunkel. 1967. Immunological studies concerning the nephritis of systemic lupus erythematosus. *J. Exp. Med.* **126**: 607.

12. Butler, V. P., Jr., S. M. Beiser, B. F. Erlanger, S. W. Tanenbaum, S. Cohen, and A. Bendich. 1962. Purine-specific antibodies which react with deoxyribonucleic acid (DNA). *Proc. Nat. Acad. Sci. U. S. A.* **48**: 1597.

13. Erlanger, B. F., and S. M. Beiser. 1964. Antibodies specific for ribonucleosides and ribonucleotides and their reaction with DNA. *Proc. Nat. Acad. Sci. U. S. A.* **52**: 68.

14. Klein, W. J., Jr., S. M. Beiser, and B. F. Erlanger. 1967. Nuclear fluorescence employing antinucleoside immunoglobulins. *J. Exp. Med.* **125**: 61.

15. Garro, A. J., B. F. Erlanger, and S. M. Beiser. 1968. Specificity in the reaction between anti-pyrimidine nucleoside antibodies and DNA. *In* Nucleic Acids in Im-

munology. O. J. Plescia and W. Braun, editors. Springer-Verlag New York Inc., New York. 47.

16. Accinni, L., G. Badalamenti, G. A. Cinotti, G. DeMaio, A. Fabbrini, K. C. Hsu, P. Natali, G. Saguì, B. C. Seegal, and L. Saguì. 1967. Studio morfologico e immunologico dei glomeruli renali nella sindrome nefrosica idiopatica. *Rass. Fisiopatol. Clin. Ter.* **39**: 545.

17. Porter, K. A., G. A. Andres, M. W. Calder, J. B. Dossetor, K. C. Hsu, J. M. Rendall, B. C. Seegal, and T. E. Starzl. 1968. Human renal transplants. II. Immunofluorescent and immunoferritin studies. *Lab. Invest.* **18**: 159.

18. Meltzer, J. I., M. Tannenbaum, B. C. Seegal, and S. C. Sommers. Immunopathologic study of 4 consecutive patients with renal vein thrombosis and the nephrotic syndrome. Proceedings of the 4th International Congress of Nephrology, Stockholm, Sweden, June 1969. 251.

19. Andres, G. A., L. Accinni, K. C. Hsu, and B. C. Seegal. 1970. The role of glomerular basal lamina in renal disease. *In* Chemistry and Molecular Biology of the Intercellular Matrix. E. A. Balazs, editor. Academic Press, Inc., New York. **1**: 575.

20. Andres, G. A., L. Accinni, K. C. Hsu, I. Penn, K. A. Porter, J. M. Rendall, B. C. Seegal, and T. E. Starzl. 1970. Human renal transplants. III. Immunopathologic studies. *Lab. Invest.* **22**: 588.

21. Rossen, R. D., C. Morgan, K. C. Hsu, W. T. Butler, and H. M. Rose. 1968. Localization of 11 S external secretory IgA by immunofluorescence in tissues lining the oral and respiratory passages in man. *J. Immunol.* **100**: 706.

22. Tischendorf, F. W., and E. F. Osserman. 1969. Two antigenic subtypes of human lambda immunoglobulin chains. *J. Immunol.* **102**: 172.

23. Strauss, A. J. L., P. G. Kemp, Jr., W. E. Vannier, and H. C. Goodman. 1964. Purification of human serum γ-globulin for immunologic studies. γ-globulin fragmentation after sulfate precipitation and prolonged dialysis. *J. Immunol.* **93**: 24.

24. Morse, J. H., and C. L. Christian. 1964. Immunological studies of the 11 S protein component of the human complement system. *J. Exp. Med.* **119**: 195.

25. Strauss, A. J. L., B. C. Seegal, K. C. Hsu, P. M. Burkholder, W. L. Nastuk, and K. E. Osserman. 1960. Immunofluorescence demonstration of a muscle binding, complement-fixing serum globulin fraction in myasthenia gravis. *Proc. Soc. Exp. Biol. Med.* **105**: 184.

26. Leskowitz, S., and B. H. Waksman. 1960. Studies in immunization. I. The effect of the route of injection of bovine serum albumin in Freund adjuvant on production of circulating antibody and delayed hypersensitivity. *J. Immunol.* **84**: 58.

27. Stollar, D., and L. Levine. 1961. Antibodies to denatured desoxyribonucleic acid in a lupus erythematosus serum. *J. Immunol.* **87**: 477.

28. Kabat, E. A. 1967. Experimental Immunochemistry. Charles C Thomas, Publisher, Springfield, Ill. 3rd edition.

29. Ehrenreich, T., and J. Churg. 1968. Pathology of membranous nephropathy. Pathology Annual. S. C. Sommers, editor. Appleton-Century, New York. **3:** 145.

30. Ceppellini, R., E. Polli, and F. Celada. 1957. A DNA-reacting factor in serum of a patient with lupus erythematosus diffusus. *Proc. Soc. Exp. Biol. Med.* **96:** 572.

31. Robbins, W. C., H. R. Holman, H. Deicher, and H. G. Kunkel. 1957. Complement fixation with cell nuclei and DNA in lupus erythematosus. *Proc. Soc. Exp. Biol. Med.* **96:** 575.

32. Seligmann, M., and F. Milgrom. 1957. Mise en évidence par la fixation du complément, de la réaction entre l'acid désoxyribonucléique et le sérum de malades atteints de lupus érythémateux dissemine. *C. R. Hebd. Séances Acad. Sci. Paris.* **245:** 1472.

33. Miescher, P., and R. Strässle. 1957. New serological methods for the detection of the L.E. factor. *Vox Sang.* **2:** 283.

34. Tan, E. M., P. H. Schur, R. I. Carr, and H. G. Kunkel. 1966. Deoxyribonucleic acid (DNA) and antibodies to DNA in the serum of patients with systemic lupus erythematosus. *J. Clin. Invest.* **45:** 1732.

35. Dixon, F. J. 1963. The role of antigen-antibody complexes in disease. *Harvey Lect. Ser.* **58.** 21.

36. Seegal, B. C., L. Accinni, G. A. Andres, S. M. Beiser, C. L. Christian, B. F. Erlanger, and K. C. Hsu. 1969. Immunologic studies of autoimmune disease in NZB/NZW F1 mice. I. Binding of fluorescein-labeled anti-nucleoside antibodies in lesions of lupus-like nephritis. *J. Exp. Med.* **130:** 203.

37. Seligmann, M., and R. Arana. 1968. The various types of DNA antibodies in lupus sera. *In* Nucleic Acids in Immunology. O. J. Plescia and W. Braun, editors. Springer-Verlag New York Inc., New York. 98.

38. Tonietti, G., M. B. A. Oldstone, and F. J. Dixon. 1970. The effect of induced chronic viral infections on the immunologic diseases of New Zealand mice. *J. Exp. Med.* **132:** 89.

The Pathogenic Significance
of Immune Complexes in other Diseases

THE INFLUENCE OF INFECTION ON TITRES OF ANTI-GLOBULIN ANTIBODIES

MARION WALLER, R. J. DUMA, E. D. FARLEY, Jr
AND JANE ATKINSON

INTRODUCTION

A growing body of information is defining the characteristics of the anti-Fab antibodies known as serum agglutinators (Osterland, Harboe & Kunkel, 1963; Natvig, 1966a and b; Waller, 1967; Waller, Curry & Richard, 1968). These anti-globulin antibodies are found in most human sera and are stable in titre in normal individuals for up to 5 years (Waller & & Blaylock, 1966). The specificity of these antibodies is determined by the modification of the Fab fragment characteristic of the particular proteolytic enzyme used for hydrolysis. Different proteolytic enzymes split IgG globulin molecules at different sites; and antibodies against these sites are named according to the enzymes used for hydrolysis (Waller, Curry & Mallory, 1968; Waller, Richard & Mallory, 1969), e.g., trypsin agglutinators, papain agglutinators, and pepsin agglutinators.

Speculation as to the biological significance of this group of anti-globulin antibodies has been expressed by two basic postulates: (1) regulation of the catabolism of IgG globulins, including possibly the elimination of antigen–antibody complexes; and (2) an auxiliary immune mechanism, whereby these antibodies help to restore the physiologic potential of specific immune antibodies.

This study is an outgrowth of the observation that under rare circumstances very high titres of serum agglutinators are demonstrable in human sera, and these titres are found associated with severe and protracted infection.

Sera used in study

Sera from patients with chronic infections were obtained from the Chest Clinic of the Medical College of Virginia Hospitals. Sera from patients with septicaemia were obtained 1–2 days after the first positive blood culture, and a repeat sample was obtained 3–4 weeks later. In some instances, the blood sample was obtained more than 2 weeks after the report of positive blood cultures, and in these instances only a single blood sample was tested. Samples were also obtained from normal individuals and patients with diseases characterized by hypergammaglobulinaemia.

Tests for serum agglutinators

Anti-Rh serum Ri (Ripley) was used, this having been utilized for almost all of the studies on human serum agglutinators (Harboe, Rau & Aho, 1965; Natvig, 1966a; Natvig, 1966b; Osterland, Harboe & Kunkel, 1963; Williams & Kunkel, 1963; Williams & Lawrence, 1966). The IgG fraction of this serum was isolated by methods previously described (Waller, 1967).

Selection of enzymes to be used for hydrolysis of anti-Rh serum Ripley

Hydrolysis of anti-Rh serum Ripley has been studied previously, immunochemically and serologically with nine different proteolytic enzymes (Osterland *et al.*, 1963; Kormeier, Ing & Mandy, 1968; Waller *et al.*, 1969; Waller & Curry, 1970). The results indicated that serum agglutinator titres vary in normal individuals. Bromelin and elastase agglutinators are usually demonstrable in high titre ($>1:160$) while pepsin agglutinator titres are low ($<1:40$). Agglutinator titres for papain, ficin, subtilisin, plasmin, trypsin and chymotrypsin rarely exceed $1:160$ in normal individuals. Ficin agglutinators cross-react with papain agglutinators and plasmin agglutinators cross-react with trypsin agglutinators. Therefore, papain, subtilisin, chymotrypsin and trypsin were used in this study.

Tests for rheumatoid factor

The SHC (sensitized human cell) test (Waller *et al.*, 1961) using Ri anti-Rh antibody and Group O Rh positive erythrocytes from a single individual were used to quantitate rheumatoid factor.

Serum electrophoresis

Serum electrophoresis was performed on paper strips using the Spinco Model R Paper Electrophoresis System.

CASE REPORTS

The following are case reports of two patients with very high titres of serum agglutinators.

J.W. This 49-year-old male lumber worker was admitted to the Medical College of Virginia Hospitals on 21 September 1969 with fever, diarrhoea, dehydration, weakness and dyspnoea of recent onset. Pertinent physical findings included a puncture wound of the right foot, cellulitis of the right calf and a urethral stricture. β haemolytic streptococcal (Group A) septicaemia (six blood cultures), enterobacterial urinary tract infection, and acute renal failure were present. He was treated with human tetanus antitoxin, penicillin G, kanamycin, and 4 weeks of arterial dialysis. His hospital course was complicated by a consumptive coagulopathy requiring heparin, aortic and mitral valve endocarditis, purpura gangrenosa of the feet, bilateral sterile pyarthrosis of the knees treated with corticosteroids, and possible allergy to penicillin.

The patient's protracted course and unusual elevation of immunoglobulins led to speculation that an underlying 'connective tissue' disease process was present; however, skeletal muscle, skin and testicular biopsies were not remarkable. A synovial biopsy revealed acute inflammation while rectal and scalene lymph node tissue demonstrated chronic inflammation. Amyloid stains were negative.

A weight loss of 54 lb occurred during the first 10 weeks of hospitalization, and he required 14 units of whole blood. 8 months following admission all toes had autoamputated. At present the patient is alive, gaining weight and is able to walk.

This patient's serum showed very high titres of serum agglutinators and this patient was the propositus for this study of the influence of infection on the serum agglutinators.

W. Y. This 15-year-old school boy was admitted to the Medical College of Virginia Hospitals on 1 February 1970 with fever, chills and painful knees of 3 days' duration. 17 days before, he sustained abrasions of both knees from a fall from his bicycle. 1 week later he had rhinorrhoea, sore throat and felt warm for 3 days. There was no history of repeated infections or bruising tendency. He appeared well-nourished but acutely ill with an elevated temperature. Several small cervical lymph nodes were palpable, and the throat was infected. The skin of both knees was abraded and inflamed. The knee joints were tender, swollen and hot.

Multiple blood cultures grew *Staph. aureus* and β haemolytic streptococci. Joint fluid was grossly bloody but sterile. Christmas disease or haemophilia B was diagnosed and treated over a 4 day period with 12 units of frozen plasma. Human tetanus antitoxin was given on admission. Penicillin G and nafcillin were administered for 38 days.

After 1 week he received two units of whole blood because of a falling haematocrit. On day 18, the left antitibial compartment was incised and drained of 200 ml of sterile pus. During the 5th week, because of painful swelling of the left knee, repeated arthrocentesis were performed and 100–150 ml of sterile pus was evacuated. Thirteen additional units of plasma were given at this time.

The right thigh gradually increased in size. Serial X-rays showed progressive periosteal new bone formation and myositis ossificans. This was thought to represent subperiosteal and muscle haematomas. By the 5th week the patient's weight fell from 121 to 97 lb.

2 months after admission his temperature gradually returned to normal. The knee effusions disappeared, but the right thigh remained enlarged.

RESULTS

Changes in serum agglutinator titres and electrophoretic patterns of patient J.W. following recovery from a severe and protracted illness

Fig. 1 shows the results of the serum electrophoretic patterns of a series of serum samples from patient *J.W.* over an 8-month period. This patient suffered severe, near-fatal streptococcal (Group A) septicaemia as described in Materials and Methods. The high levels of immunoglobulins present in October, 1969, were gradually reduced, and the pattern obtained in May, 1970, approaches that of normal serum. At no time during the period of study did the patient's serum show positive tests for rheumatoid factor (SHC test). Serum agglutinator titres in October, 1969, were the highest ever observed in our laboratory; and unlike titres observed in normal sera, all of the agglutinators were present in high titre. Agglutinator titres began to fall as the patient recuperated.

Two outstanding characteristics of the illness of patient *J.W.* were massive hypergammaglobulinaemia and septicaemia. In order to elucidate the circumstances or initiating factors leading to the very high titres of serum agglutinators, two groups of patients were selected for study. In the first group were patients with hypergammaglobulinaemia unassociated with microbial infection and in the second group were patients with infections of various types.

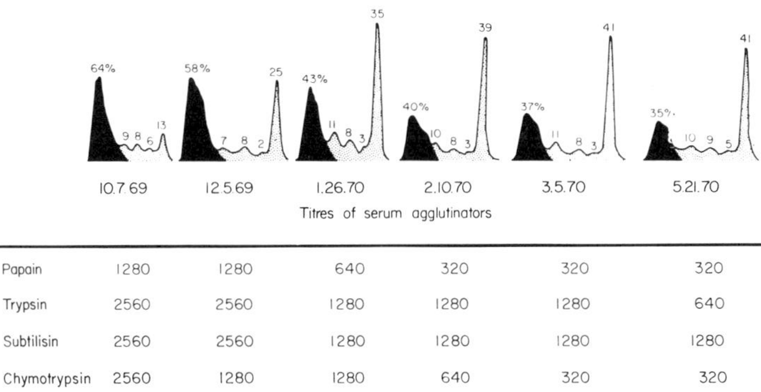

	10.7.69	12.5.69	1.26.70	2.10.70	3.5.70	5.21.70
Papain	1280	1280	640	320	320	320
Trypsin	2560	2560	1280	1280	1280	640
Subtilisin	2560	2560	1280	1280	1280	1280
Chymotrypsin	2560	1280	1280	640	320	320

FIG. 1. Electrophoretic patterns and titres of serum agglutinators in consecutive serum samples of patient *J.W.*

Table 1 shows the results of testing the sera of selected groups of patients with diseases characterized by hypergammaglobulinaemia. Only patients with rheumatoid arthritis and one of the patients with lupus erythematosus showed positive tests for rheumatoid factor. The patients with rheumatoid arthritis were selected for their high titres of rheumatoid factor as well as for their hypergammaglobulinaemia. Although the patients with sarcoidosis show a higher incidence of elevated agglutinator titres than patients with the other diseases represented, the titres are not in excess of what may be observed in normal individuals. Whether or not this degree of activity is significant would require a much larger study of sarcoid patients and their matched controls.

As had been noted before (Waller, 1968), individuals differ in their agglutinator titres. Some patients will only show elevated titres of trypsin agglutinator (patient No. 1, purpura) while others will only show elevated titres of chymotrypsin agglutinator (patient No. 4, lupus erythematosus). In normal individuals, elevated titres of all the agglutinators have not been observed, and apparently this is also true for most patients. A group of normals were included as controls, and as can be seen with No. 1, occasionally elevations of some agglutinators are observed. Normal individuals have never shown titres in excess of 1:320,

Table 1. Serum agglutinator titres and rheumatoid factor titres in patients with hypergammaglobulinaemia

Patient No.	SHC*	Agglutinator titres (>1:80)			
		Papain	Subtilisin	Trypsin	Chymotrypsin
Rheumatoid ai thritis†					
1	1280	0	160	160	0
2	1280	0	160	0	0
3	1280	0	160	160	0
4	5120	0	160	0	0
5–8‡	640	0	0	0	0
9–19	1280	0	0	0	0
20–24	2560	0	0	0	0
Purpura					
1	0	0	0	160	0
2–12	0	0	0	0	0
Sarcoidosis					
1	0	320	160	160	320
2	0	160	160	0	160
3	0	160	0	0	160
4	0	0	160	0	160
5	0	0	0	0	160
6	0	0	0	0	160
7–12	0	0	0	0	0
Myeloma					
1	0	0	160	0	160
2–12	0	0	0	0	0
Lupus erythematosus					
1	40	0	0	0	0
2	0	160	0	0	0
3	0	0	320	160	0
4	0	0	0	0	320
5–13	0	0	0	0	0
Controls (normals)					
1	0	320	0	160	320
2–12	0	0	0	0	0

* SHC—sensitized human cell test.

† Rheumatoid arthritis—Unusual degree of uniformity is due to selection of patients with titres of 1:640 or above.

‡ Sera from individuals with the same serologic results are combined (e.g., 5–8 represents patients 5, 6, 7, and 8).

with this group of agglutinators, and the majority have titres <1:40. The bromelin and elastase agglutinators were purposely excluded from this study because normal individuals almost always have these agglutinators, and marked elevations in titre are not uncommon.

Table 2 shows the results of agglutinator titres in patients with a variety of infections and apparently unrelated diverse conditions. Patients with septicaemia were purposely selected

TABLE 2. Serum agglutinator titres and rheumatoid factor titres in patients with acute and chronic infections

Patient No.	SHC	Agglutinator titres (> 1 : 80)			
		Papain	Subtilisin	Trypsin	Chymotrypsin
Septicaemia					
1 (*S. aureus*)	0	0	160	160	0
2 (*S. aureus*)	0	320	320	320	320
		320*	320	320	640
3 (*S. aureus*)	0	160	320	640	640
		0†	0	0	160
4 (Strep. Group A)	0	640	640	320	160
		10,240	10,240	10,240	5120
5 (Klebsiella)	0	0	0	0	0
	0	0	0	0	160
6 (Bacteroides)	0	0	0	0	0
7–9 (*E. coli*)	0	0	0	0	0
10–11 (Klebsiella)	0	0	0	0	0
12 (Klebsiella, Candida)	0	0	0	0	0
13 (Salmonella)	0	0	0	0	0
14 (Serratia)	0	0	0	0	0
Resolving pneumonia					
1	0	320	640	160	160
2	0	320	320	160	320
3	0	640	160	0	640
4	0	0	160	0	320
5–10	0	0	0	0	0
Bronchiectasis					
1	0	160	0	0	0
2–8	0	0	0	0	0
Diverse diseases					
Diabetes, gangrene,	0	0	640	640	640
renal disease, retinopathy,					
CNS syphilis	0	0	640	640	1280
Hepatitis (drug induced)	80	0	0	160	0
Tuberculosis	0	0	0	0	320
Herpes zoster meningitis	0	0	0	0	0
Metastatic carcinoma	0	0	0	0	0
Leukaemia	0	0	0	0	0
Glomerulonephritis	0	0	0	0	0
Psoriatic arthritis	0	0	0	0	0

* Second blood sample obtained 7 days after first sample. Patient died 6 weeks after admission to hospital.
† Blood sample obtained 4 months after discharge from hospital.

because patient *J.W.* had six consecutive positive blood cultures for Group A β haemolytic streptococci.

It is noted that patients whose blood grew gram positive organisms generally had high titres whereas those with gram negative organisms did not show positive titres. However, because concern was expressed that perhaps blood was tested before some patients had an opportunity to respond to septicaemia, whenever possible a second blood sample was tested 2–3 weeks later. Patient No. 2 (septicaemia) was tested 1 week after admission but approximately 6 weeks after onset of illness. His second blood sample was obtained 1 week after the first. This patient was a diabetic for many years. He died of septicaemia and subacute bacterial endocarditis with multiple lung abscesses. Patient No. 3 (septicaemia) was tested 1 week after admission. She had multiple admissions for hypercalcaemia, arteriosclerotic heart disease, multiple infections, renal disease and empyema; and in addition, she had been treated with alkeran because of a monoclonal spike on serum electrophoresis. However, it was doubtful that she had myeloma, since bone pain, osteoporosis, Bence-Jones protein-uria and plasmacytosis were absent. Also, her elevated agglutinator titres were not characteristic of the usually low response that we have observed in patients with multiple myeloma. A serum sample obtained from her 4 months later showed a marked drop in agglutinator titres. Patient No. 4, *W. Y.*, whose illness is presented in Case Reports, showed the highest titres of serum agglutinators that we have seen. His blood was tested soon after it was reported that blood cultures were growing Group A β haemolytic streptococci and *Staph. aureus*. Another sample could not be obtained until 3 months later, and by then a marked elevation in agglutinator titres had occurred. During this time, the patient's γ-globulin level had doubled (Table 2).

In order to evaluate the influence of chronicity of infection, patients with bronchiectasis and resolving pneumonia were studied. In these patients there was no correlation between γ-globulin levels and titres of serum agglutinators.

Among patients with diverse diseases, only one showed elevated agglutinator titres. This patient had diabetes mellitus, gangrene of the leg requiring amputation, tertiary syphilis, polyclonal gammopathy, and anaemia. Her serologic reactions were of interest because except for papain all agglutinators were elevated. A second blood sample obtained 6 weeks later showed almost the same serologic findings. Only one patient included in the group of diverse diseases showed a positive test for rheumatoid factor.

Penicillin sensitivity and titres of serum agglutinators

Most patients with infection were treated with a penicillin derivative. Two patients (*J.W.* and *W.Y.*—see Case Reports) showed symptoms (unexplained rise in temperature and/or articular effusion) that were attributed to penicillin sensitivity. One received treatment with corticosteroids. However, blood obtained from two other patients with classical penicillin sensitivity but without septicaemia did not contain elevated agglutinator titres.

The effect of changes in rheumatoid factor titres on agglutinator titres

It was apparent that changes in agglutinator titres had no effect on titres of rheumatoid factor and *vice versa*. One patient's rheumatoid factor titre was 1:640 in 1967 (SHC test). In 1970, she was admitted to the hospital with a profuse nose bleed, and a re-evaluation of her rheumatoid factor titre showed an increase to over 1:200,000. Her serum immuno-globulins also had increased spectacularly, especially her IgM which was 3000 mg%. A 1967 study of her serum agglutinators showed that papain, subtilisin, trypsin and chymotrypsin agglutinators were all <1:40, and in 1970 they did not show a rise.

Another patient was studied whose serum had even more of a rise in rheumatoid factor (1,000,000), and once again the titre of the agglutinators remained low with no rise.

DISCUSSION

Although much research has been done on anti-globulin antibodies, we do not know the factors involved in eliciting these responses. Rheumatoid factors have been described in most of the diseases afflicting man and even in normal individuals (Waller, 1969). One of the most interesting tests for demonstrating rheumatoid factors is the sensitized human cell test. This test uses an Rh positive erythrocyte coated with the anti-Rh antibody Ripley. This same anti-Rh serum was the reagent used to demonstrate the first pepsin agglutinator (Osterland *et al.*, 1963). Rheumatoid factors are anti-Fc antibodies and agglutinators are anti-Fab antibodies. However, rheumatoid factors will bind to the Fc piece of IgG globulin whether or not it has been fragmented from the Fab piece, while the anti-Fab antibodies will only bind to the Fab fragment following hydrolysis, presumably because the sites on the Fab fragment are hidden in the intact molecules (Goodman, 1961; Franklin, 1961; Osterland *et al.*, 1963). Another difference between these two groups of antibodies is that anti-Fc antibodies are almost always IgM globulins while anti-Fab antibodies are almost always IgG globulins.

From the present studies we have learned another difference between these antibodies. The most important initiating factor for the appearance of anti-Fc antibodies is the disease rheumatoid arthritis, but this disease does not provoke the appearance of anti-Fab antibodies in excess of that found in normals. Although anti-Fc antibodies have been described in infection (Williams & Kunkel, 1962; Cathcart *et al.*, 1961), they are not present most of the time or in very high titre. However, anti-Fab antibodies reach their highest level following severe and protracted infection. Apparently, the condition which best favours the appearance of high titres of agglutinators is septicaemia due to gram positive cocci.

Many investigators have been intensely interested in elucidating the pathogenetic significance of both of these anti-globulin antibodies. One suggestion has been that they regulate γ-globulin catabolism. However, we have no evidence at this time to suggest that this is the case. The titre of serum agglutinators is not altered when a patient's level of γ-globulin falls to 1/4 or 1/5 of its former value, as in treated myeloma. On the other hand, the level of γ-globulin can increase four-fold, as in some patients with rheumatoid arthritis, and the level of agglutinators is unaffected. To us, it seems more likely that their role may be that of an auxiliary immune mechanism.

For years, we have noted the stability of titre of anti-Fab antibodies in normal individuals but we cannot explain the interesting pattern of titres in normal sera. We were unable to confirm an increased incidence of rheumatoid factors in sarcoidosis using the sensitized human cell test.

Benign monoclonal gammopathy has interested many clinicians. For one reason, immunosuppressive therapy would be withheld if they were sure they were dealing with a benign and possibly remitting condition. Patient No. 3 (Table 2, septicaemia) was studied because her electrophoretic pattern showed a monoclonal spike; yet she did not fulfil other criteria for the diagnosis of multiple myeloma. When we studied her, she was recuperating from staphylococcal septicaemia. On the basis of elevated agglutinator titres we believe that this patient did not have malignant disease. However, we noted that her titre of agglutinators fell more rapidly than those of others previously studied. In the future, test for serum agglutinators may help in evaluating this type of patient.

ACKNOWLEDGMENTS

The authors are grateful for the invaluable technical assistance of Mrs Nellie Curry and Mrs Jean Mallory. This study was supported in part by Public Health Service Research Grant Am 04549 from the National Institutes of Health. This is publication No. 37 from the Charles W. Thomas Arthritis Fund.

REFERENCES

CATHCART, E.S., WILLIAMS, R.C., JR., ROSS, H. & CALKINS, E. (1961) The relationship of the latex fixation test to the clinical and serological manifestations of leprosy. *Amer. J. Med.* **31**, 758.

FRANKLIN, E.C. (1961) Interaction of rheumatoid factor and gamma globulin. *Proceedings of 10th International Congress of Rheumatology, Roma, Torino, Minerva Medica,* **2**, 804.

GOODMAN, J.W. (1961) Reaction of rheumatoid sera with fragments of papain-digested rabbit gamma-globulin. *Proc. Soc. exp. Biol. (N.Y.),* **106**, 822.

HARBOE, M., RAU, B. & AHO, K. (1965) Properties of various anti-γ-globulin factors in human sera. *J. exp. Med.* **121**, 503.

KORMEIER, L.C., ING, J.T. & MANDY, W.J. (1968) Specificity of antiglobulin factors in normal human serum reacting with enzyme digested γ G-globulin. *J. Immunol.* **100**, 612.

NATVIG, J.B. (1966a) Reactions of human anti-antibodies with incomplete anti-D and its sub-units. *Acta path. microbiol. scand.* **66**, 383.

NATVIG, J.B. (1966b) Heterogeneity of anti-γ-globulin factors detected by pepsin digested human γ G-globulin. *Acta path. microbiol. scand.* **66**, 369.

OSTERLAND, C.K., HARBOE, M. & KUNKEL, H.G. (1963) Anti-γ-globulin factors in human sera revealed by enzymatic splitting of anti-Rh antibodies. *Vox Sang.* **8**, 133.

WALLER, M., DECKER, B., TOONE, E.C. & IRBY, R. (1961) Evaluation of rheumatoid factor tests. *Arthritis Rheum.* **4**, 579.

WALLER, M. & BLAYLOCK, K. (1966) Further studies on the antiglobulin factors in human serum to the pepsin digested fragment of the Ri anti-Rh antibody. *J. Immunol.* **97**, 438.

WALLER, M. (1967) Serum agglutinators of erythrocytes sensitized with enzyme digested anti-Rh antibodies. *Vox Sang.* **13**, 233.

WALLER, M., CURRY, N. & RICHARD, A. (1968) Serological specificity of IgG and IgM antiglobulin antibodies in anti-Gm(a) antisera. *Clin. exp. Immunol.* **3**, 631.

WALLER, M., CURRY, N. & MALLORY, J. (1968) Immunochemical and serological studies of enzymatically fractionated human IgG globulins. I. Hydrolysis with pepsin, papain, ficin and bromelin. *Immunochemistry,* **5**, 577.

WALLER, M., RICHARD, A.J. & MALLORY, J. (1969) Immunochemical and serological studies of enzymatically fragmented human IgG globulins. II. Hydrolysis with subtilisin, elastase, trypsin, and chymotrypsin. *Immunochemistry,* **6**, 207.

WALLER, M. (1969) Methods of measurement of rheumatoid factor. *Ann. N.Y. Acad. Sci.* **168**, 5.

WALLER, M. & CURRY, N. (1970) The demonstration of plasmin agglutinators in human sera. *Vox Sang.* (in press).

WILLIAMS, R.C. & KUNKEL, H.G. (1962) Rheumatoid factor, complement and conglutinin aberrations in patients with subacute bacterial endocarditis. *J. clin. Invest.* **41**, 666.

WILLIAMS, R.C. and KUNKEL, H.G. (1963) Antibodies to rabbit γ-globulin after immunizing with various preparations of autologous γ-globulin. *Proc. Soc. exp. Biol. (N.Y.),* **112**, 554.

WILLIAMS, R.C. & LAWRENCE, T.G. (1966) Variations among pepsin digested gamma globulins. *J. Clin. Invest.* **45**, 714.

ABBREVIATION

SHC   sensitized human cell

VASCULITIS IN ASSOCIATION WITH AUSTRALIA ANTIGEN*

By DAVID J. GOCKE, KONRAD HSU, COUNCILMAN MORGAN, STEPHENO BOMBARDIERI, MICHAEL LOCKSHIN, AND CHARLES L. CHRISTIAN

The possible role of infectious agents in the production of various connective tissue disorders in man has long been postulated. In animals there is evidence for the role of viruses in inducing immunologic disease in lymphocytic chorio-meningitis in mice (1), the lupus-like disease of New Zealand black mice (2), the Aleutian disease of mink (3), and the arteritis of horses (4). In man, how-ever, convincing evidence of such a mechanism has been lacking. In the course of studies of the association between hepatitis and Australia antigen (hepatitis-associated antigen) (5, 6) a small number of patients were discovered with typical polyarteritis nodosa who also had Australia antigen in their sera. Further study suggested a special relationship between this human hepatitis antigen and the syndrome of diffuse vasculitis in these patients.

Methods

Australia antigen was detected in serum specimens by the two-dimensional immunodiffusion and counterelectrophoresis techniques previously employed in this laboratory (5, 7). Specificity of positive reactions was confirmed by comparison with reference sera containing Australia antigen or antibody.

Serum complement titers were determined by the method of Kent and Fife (8). The C1q reactions were carried out as described by Agnello et al. (9). Immune complexes were sedimented from serum by centrifugation in a 35–50% sucrose gradient at 157,000 g for 15 hr. Pellet fractions of such gradients were negatively stained with 1% phosphotungstic acid (PTA)[1] pH 7.2 and examined by electron microscopy (RCA 3G, RCA Corp., New York).

Fluorescein-conjugated antisera were prepared as described by Strauss et al. (10). The anti-Australia antigen serum was of human origin and had a gel diffusion titer of 1/1024. Other antisera were of goat origin. Frozen sections were cut at 4 μ, fixed in 95% ethanol for 10 min, washed once for 10 min in phosphate-buffered saline (PBS) pH 7.2, and stained with conju-gated antiserum for 60 min at 37°C. After being washed twice for 10 min in PBS, the specimens were mounted in glycerol and examined with a Reichert fluorescence microscope (American Optical Corp., Buffalo, N. Y.). For control purposes, the specimens were also reacted with fluorescein-conjugated normal human and goat sera to look for nonspecific staining of the patient's tissue. Tissue from patients with other diseases were reacted with the various fluores-cein-labeled antisera to rule out nonspecific staining by the antisera. The specimens were read independently by two experienced observers.

---

* Supported in part by grants AI 01889 and AI 06814 from the U.S.P.H.S.

[1] *Abbreviations used in this paper:* PBS, phosphate-buffered saline; PTA, phosphotungstic acid.

Table I summarizes the clinical characteristics of six patients with biopsy-proven polyarteritis and chronic Australia antigenemia, four of whom have recently been reported (11). All presented with fever accompanied by polyarthralgia, myalgia, rash, urticaria, and hepatic dysfunction. While evidence of hepatic damage was present in all, hepatitis was the primary presenting problem in only one patient. In time, additional features of a diffuse vasculitic syndrome

TABLE I

Clinical Characteristics in Patients with Polyarteritis and Australia Antigen

(*a*) Onset as fever of obscure origin with polyarthralgia, myalgia, rash, urticaria, hepatic dysfunction mild (not the primary problem).

(*b*) Progressed to peripheral neuropatheis, hypertension, eosinophilia, hematuria, azotemia.

(*c*) Tissue diagnosis based on typical fibrinoid necrosis and perivascular infiltration in walls of small arteries.

(*d*) Australia antigen or antibody persistent in all patients.

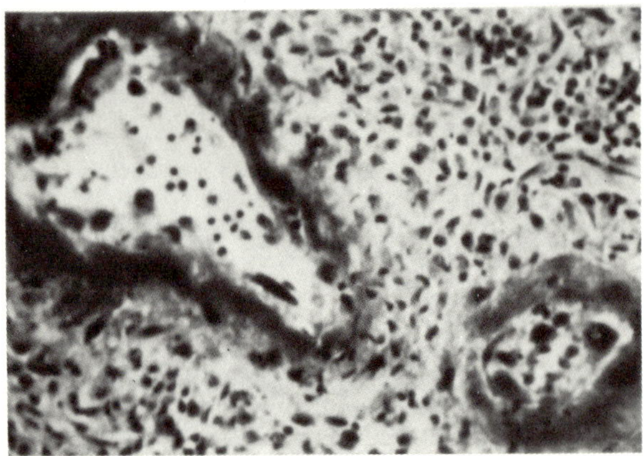

Fig. 1. A liver biopsy specimen illustrating the type of vascular lesions with inflammation and necrosis typical of these patients. (H and E, × 400)

with peripheral neuropathies, hypertension, eosinophilia, hematuria, and azotemia appeared. A tissue diagnosis was eventually made in all cases on the basis of typical fibrinoid lesions and inflammation in the walls of small arteries. Australia antigen or antigen–antibody complexes persisted in the serum throughout the course of their illness. Fig. 1 illustrates the type of vascular lesions seen in these patients. Fibrinoid necrosis and intense inflammatory infiltration of the blood vessel walls was seen in both liver and muscle biopsy specimens.

The possibility that circulating immune complexes were present in these patients was suggested by several bits of evidence (Table II). For example, in patients studied during the early acute phase of their disease, the serum complement level was found to be depressed on a number of occasions. In addition, the C1q reaction (9) in which soluble antigen–antibody complexes are precipitated from serum by interaction with C1q was noted to be positive during the acute stages in three of these patients. In order to pursue the possibility that immune complexes composed of Australia antigen and antibody were present, ultracentrifugal studies were carried out. Serum specimens were centrifuged in

TABLE II

Summary of Six Patients with Polyarteritis Nodosa and Australia Antigen

Patient	Australia antigen		Circulating immune complexes			Immunofluorescence in vessels
	Detected	Duration	$C'H_{50}$	C1q	EM	
A	3 days	18 mon	↓	+	+	+ Au Ag* + IgM* + β_1C*
B	1 mon	30 mon	↓	+	+	Neg. 16 mon after onset
C	23 mon	37 mon	–	–	+	Neg. 2 yr after onset
D	5 yr	5 yr (died)	ND‡	ND	ND	ND
E	4 mon	6 mon (died)	↓	+	+	+Au Ag§ +IgM§
F	5 mon (Ab)	–	–	–	+	Negative

* 3 mon after onset.
‡ ND, not done.
§ 6 mon after onset.

a 30–50% sucrose gradient at 157,000 g for 15 hr. The supernatant fractions were removed from the top and the pellet fraction was negatively stained with 1% PTA (pH 7.2) and examined electron microscopically. Serum pellet preparations from five of the patients contained small clusters of the 40 and 20 mμ particles which are characteristically associated with the Australia antigen by electron microscopy (Fig. 2). The pellet was negative by immunologic techniques for Australia antigen, but the antigen could be recovered from the upper fractions of the gradient.

In patients A and E (Table II) it has also been possible to localize Australia antigen and immunoglobulin within blood vessel walls by immunofluorescent techniques. Fig. 3 illustrates a frozen section of muscle from patient E stained with fluorescein-conjugated human anti-Australia antigen serum. It can be noted that specific fluorescent deposits are seen in a nodular distribution adjacent to the elastic membrane within the blood vessel wall. Fig. 4 is a cross-section from the same patient stained with fluorescein-conjugated goat anti-human IgM antiserum, and again deposits of specific fluorescence within the blood vessel wall are seen. In addition, patient A was found to have deposits of β_1C in blood vessel walls (11). The typical bright-green color of this fluorescence

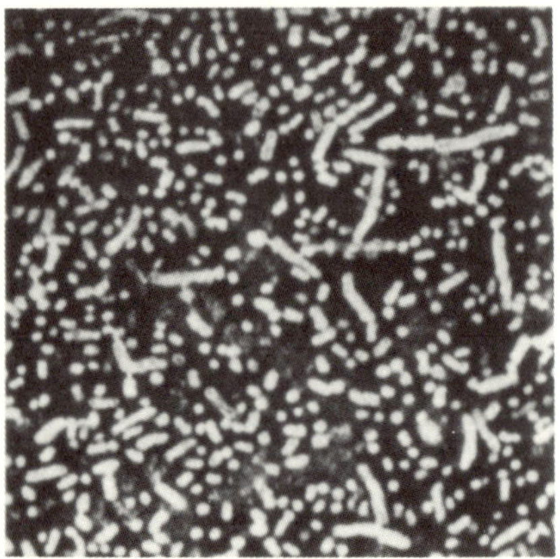

FIG. 2.   Electron micrograph illustrating the 20 and 40 mμ particles found in the pellet fraction after ultracentrifugation of the patient's serum as described in the text. These particles are characteristic of those associated with Australia antigen. ($\times$ 88,000)

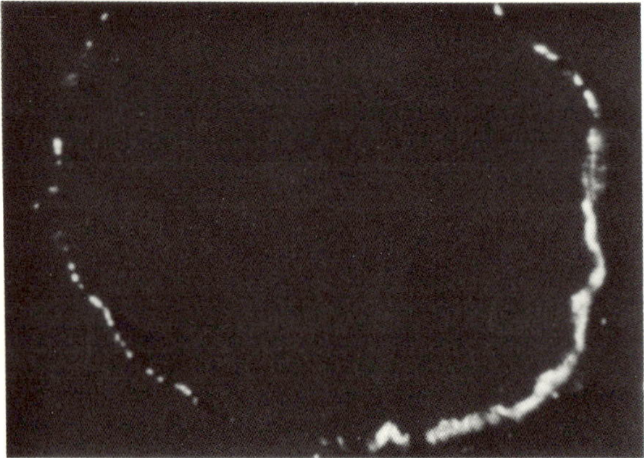

FIG. 3.   A frozen section of liver tissue from patient E stained with fluorescein-conjugated human anti-Australia antigen serum. Specific fluorescent deposits in a nodular distribution can be seen in the blood vessel wall adjacent to the elastic membrane. ($\times$ 400)

was clearly distinguishable from the blue or yellowish autofluorescence of the elastic membrane of the normal blood vessels. Furthermore, not all blood vessels observed in various sections from these patients exhibited specific fluorescent deposits, suggesting that the localization was of a segmental nature. Control slides of the same patient tissues stained with other fluorescein-conjugated antisera failed to show the pattern of fluorescent deposits described. Conversely, the fluorescein-conjugated antisera employed here were applied to specimens from other patients with vascular diseases and to normal tissue without observation of specific fluorescence.

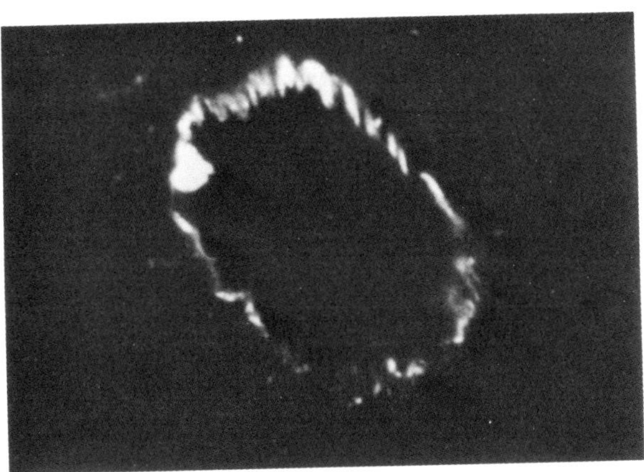

FIG. 4. A frozen section of tissue from patient E stained with fluorescein-conjugated goat anti-human IgM serum showing fluorescent deposits in the blood vessel wall. (× 400)

DISCUSSION

In total, 16 patients with a diagnosis of polyarteritis have now been tested for Australia antigenemia, but an association could be found only in the 6 described here. Thus, not all cases of polyarteritis nodosa can be related to this particular antigen. However, an incidence of 6 in 16 cases is much higher than would be expected by chance alone. The experience of several laboratories has been that Australia antigen is very closely correlated with acute hepatitis and with some forms of chronic hepatitis (5, 12, 13). While unusual associations between Australia antigen and other conditions such as Down's syndrome, leprosy, and hepatoma have been reported (14), these findings occur in certain situations or areas of the world where exposure to the virus of Australia antigen is known to be high. We have not found Australia antigen in 49 patients with lupus erythematosis and other connective tissue disorders, nor has it been encountered as an incidental finding in 153 in-patients tested at random. Finally, while blood transfusion may be the source of infection in some patients with polyarteritis,

147

prospective studies of post-transfusion hepatitis indicate that the expected frequency of Australia antigenemia after transfusion in a group of unselected recipients would be only about 1% (6, 15).

Other reports confirming an association between Australia antigen and polyarteritis have recently appeared (16, 17). In addition, an immune complex mechanism has been suggested as responsible for the polyarteritis and arthralgia syndrome sometimes seen as a prodrome or early feature in patients with acute viral hepatitis (18, 19). Thus, it appears reasonable to suggest in the six patients described here that immune complexes composed of Australia antigen and immunoglobulin were responsible for their syndrome of diffuse vasculitis. Since current evidence indicates that Australia antigen is a product of a viral agent, this may represent the first recognition in man of a systemic vasculitis due to an immunologic reaction to a virus.

BIBLIOGRAPHY

1. Oldstone, M. B., and F. J. Dixon. 1969. Pathogenesis of chronic disease associated with persistent lympocytic choriomeningitis viral infection. *J. Exp. Med.* **129:** 483.
2. Dixon, F. J., T. S. Edgington, and T. Lambert. 1967. Non-glomerular antigen-antibody complex nephritis. Fifth International Pathology Symposium. P. Grabar and P. Miescher, editors. Schwabe and Co., Basel. 17.
3. Henson, J. B., J. R. Gorham, and R. W. Leader. 1963. Hypergammaglobulinemia in mink initiated by a cell-free filtrate. *Nature (London).* **197:**206.
4. Doll, E. R., J. T. Bryans, W. H. McCollum, and M. E. W. Crowe. 1957. Isolation of a filterable agent causing arteritis in horses and abortion in mares. *Cornell Vet.* **47:**3.
5. Gocke, D. J., and N. B. Kavey. 1969. Hepatitis antigen—correlation with disease and infectivity of blood-donors. *Lancet* **2:**1055.
6. Gocke, D. J. 1970. The Australia antigen and blood transfusion. *Vox. Sang.* **19:**327.
7. Gocke, D. J., and C. Howe. 1970. Rapid detection of Australia antigen by counter immunoelectrophoresis. *J. Immunol.* **104:**1031.
8. Kent, J. F., and E. H. Fife. 1963. Precise standardization of reagents for complement fixation. *Amer. J. Trop. Med. Hyg.* **12:**103.
9. Agnello, V., R. J. Winchester, and H. G. Kunkel. 1970. Precipitin reactions of the C1q component of complement with aggregated γ-globulin and immune complexes in gel diffusion. *Immunology.* **19:**909.
10. Strauss, A. J., B. C. Seegal, K. C. Hsu, P. M. Burkholder, W. L. Nastuk, and

K. E. Osserman. 1960. Immunofluorescent demonstration of a muscle-binding, complement fixing serum globulin fraction in myasthenia gravis. *Proc. Soc. Exp. Biol. Med.* **105**:184.

11. Gocke, D. J., K. Hsu, C. Morgan, S. Bombardieri, M. Lockshin, and C. L. Christian. 1970. Association between polyarteritis and Australia antigen. *Lancet* **2**:1149.

12. Blumberg, B. S., A. I. Sutnick, and W. T. London. 1970. Current concepts: Australia antigen and hepatitis. *N. Engl. J. Med.* **283**:349.

13. Shulman, N. R. 1970. Hepatitis-associated antigen. *Amer. J. Med.* **49**:669.

14. Sutnick, A. I., W. T. London, and B. S. Blumberg. 1971. Australia antigen: a genetic basis for chronic liver disease and hepatoma? *Ann. Intern. Med.* **74**:442.

15. Gocke, D. J., H. B. Greenberg, and N. B. Kavey. 1970. Correlation of Australia antigen with posttransfusion hepatitis. *J. Amer. Med. Ass.* **212**:877.

16. Trepo, C., and J. Thivolet. 1970. Antigène Australie, hépatite à virus et périartérite noueuse. *Presse Med.* **78**:1575.

17. Baker, A., J. Cidel, and M. Kaplan. 1971. Australia antigen positive hepatitis complicated by acute polyarteritis. *Gastroenterology.* **60**:183.

18. Alpert, E., R. L. Coston, and P. H. Schur. 1970. Arthritis associated with hepatitis: complement component studies. *Arthritis Rheum.* **13**:303.

19. Fernandez, R., and D. J. McCarty. 1971. The arthritis of viral hepatitis. *Ann. Intern. Med.* **74**:207.

HUMAN ANTIBODIES TO VASCULAR ENDOTHELIUM

K. J. LINDQVIST and C. K. OSTERLAND

INTRODUCTION

In the course of antinuclear factor testing by immunofluorescence using mouse kidney sections as tissue substrate, a linear type of staining pattern was noted, in which specific fluorescence was seen outlining the peripheral border of the renal tubules and the glomerular tufts. Since most of the serum samples being studied came from patients suspected of having some sort of connective tissue disease, early indications were that this pattern frequently occurred with sera from patients with polymyositis or dermatomyositis. In subsequent studies this activity was found in a variety of disease states and some normal sera as well.

In this presentation we describe the antibody nature and tissue specificity of this fluorescent staining pattern. It is clear that the sera under study have antibodies directed against endothelial cell cytoplasm. The antigen appears to be an interspecies antigen, similar to but not identical with a typical Forssman antigen. Whatever the chemical nature of the antigen involved, the antibody specificity directed against endothelium has some added interest in view of the fact that endothelial changes seem to be an important component of a number of vasculitic disorders as well as possibly organ transplant rejection.

MATERIALS AND METHODS

The initial serum samples examined in this series were among those submitted to this laboratory for tests for antinuclear factor (ANF), smooth muscle or striated muscle antibody activities. Consequently, this material came from a population with a high incidence of connective tissue disease. The finding of a peritubular staining pattern (PTS) in some of these sera prompted the further investigation of sera from patients with other diseases and from normal individuals. These latter samples were provided at random by the Barnes Hospital blood bank.

Fluorescent antibody technique

The indirect immunofluorescent technique was used (Coons & Kaplan, 1950). Mouse kidney (or, on occasion mouse, rat or even human liver or kidney) was used as a tissue substrate. Sections 4 μ thick were cut from frozen tissue blocks and were fixed for 10 min in acetone. Endocardial scrapings were treated in a similar fashion. Test sera were screened initially at a 1:5 dilution. The conjugated anti-human-immunoglobulin sera were prepared by the method described by Nairn (1962) and in some cases commercially prepared (Hyland Laboratories, Los Angeles, California) antiserum conjugates were used. The specificity of the reagents used was confirmed by gel diffusion and by specific absorption or blocking procedures. Slides were examined with a Leitz Ortholux microscope equipped with an Osram HBO-200 W light source, UG1 or BG12 exciting and K430 barrier filters.

Isolation of serum components

The proteins producing the endothelial staining pattern were partially purified using ammonium sulphate fractionation, followed by DEAE chromatography or by preparative zone electrophoresis. Fractions were analysed by cellulose acetate electrophoresis and by immunoelectrophoresis.

Demonstration of C'3 fixation

Fresh human serum known to be negative for peritubular staining was mixed with a positive serum that had been heat-inactivated at 56°C for 30 min. The mixture was then used for the immunofluorescent staining procedure with the exception that the fluorescein conjugate used was anti-human C'3.

RESULTS

Fig. 1 illustrates the typical endothelial staining pattern using a mouse kidney substrate. Specific fluorescence is seen around the outer border of renal tubules. This pattern was

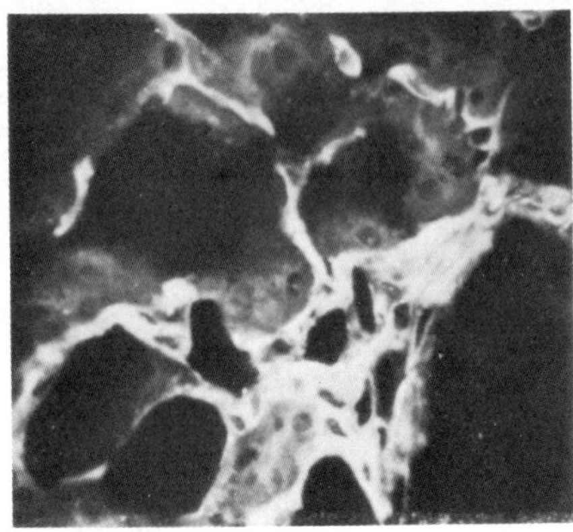

Fig. 1. The peritubular staining pattern. Mouse kidney sections treated first with human serum followed by fluorescein-tagged anti-human γ-globulin.

initially regarded as peritubular basement membrane staining. Since many of the sera examined came from patients with connective tissue diseases, several instances of sera showing both nuclear and endothelial staining were noted. However, no correlation was found between positive ANF tests and endothelial staining.

The frequency of endothelial staining in patients without evidence of connective tissue disease, was determined in 129 sera from hospitalized patients. An incidence of 17·8% was found. In a group of sixty patients with chronic pulmonary tuberculosis the incidence was 26·6% (Lindqvist, Coleman & Osterland, 1970). There was no predeliction for a particular

TABLE 1. Serum from a group O individual absorbed with erythrocytes from various species, and with blood group substances A and B

	Serum after absorption				
	Agglutination tests with				
Serum absorbed with	Human A	Human B	Sheep RBC	Rabbit RBC	Endothelial Staining
No absorption	+	+	+	+	+
Human O, Rh+	+	+	+	+	+
Human A, Rh+	−	+	+	+	+
Human B, Rh+	+	−	+	+	+
Sheep RBC	+	+	−	+	−
Rabbit RBC	+	+	+	−	−
Group A substance*	−	+	+	+	+
Group B substance*	+	−	+	+	−

* Chas. Pfizer & Co., Inc.

sex or age group. An incidence of endothelial staining was found in fourteen of one hundred normal blood-donors.

Relationship to blood groups and heterophile antigens

All human ABO blood group types were represented in the material and there was no relationship between isoagglutinin titres and the presence of endothelial staining. For example of fifty-nine patients with positive reactions who were typed, thirty-four were blood group O, nineteen group A, four group B, and two group AB. Absorption studies using human red cells confirmed the lack of correlation between endothelial antibody and ABO blood group isoagglutinins. Washed human A, B and O, Rh positive and negative erythrocytes were mixed with the serum which had been inactivated for 30 min at 56°C (0·5 ml packed erythrocytes per 0·5 ml serum) and incubated for 30 min at 37°C and overnight at 4°C. This absorption procedure was repeated once, and the serum examined for completeness of absorption by the agglutination test. These experiments did not result in any reduction in the intensity of the peritubular staining pattern (Table 1). Furthermore, no inhibition of staining was observed when N-acetyl-glucosamine, N-acetyl-galactosamine, d-galactose, fucose or mannose was added to serum in amounts up to 100 mg per ml. A mixture of these sugars at a concentration 20 mg of each per ml serum also failed to inhibit the reaction.

The staining activity would be absorbed by red cells and tissue extracts of some heterologous species. The staining was completely abolished after absorption with sheep or rabbit erythrocytes and with blood group B substance derived from gastric mucosa of the horse. Blood group A substance (Chas. Pfizer & Co., Inc.) from hog gastric mucosa had no effect (Table 1). Since the human B cells did not absorb the activity while the equine-derived B substance did, it seems apparent that the absorbing material of the latter is some component of the tissue extract other than B antigen.

Substrate specificity

The particular staining property described here was seen initially using mouse kidney sections as substrate. A lack of organ specificity was obvious since several other mouse tissues could be used as tissue substrate and yield a similar linear type staining pattern. Though the specific fluorescence was observed largely to coincide with vascular structure of the kidney, the appearance in some areas suggested that the basement membrane might be involved. However, when endothelial cells from guinea-pigs were obtained by scraping the endocardium and great vessels and subsequently stained, the cytoplasm of these cells showed bright immunofluorescent staining (Fig. 2). Close observation of staining on other tissues also suggests that the fluorescence was localized to capillary walls and vascular endothelium (Fig. 3).

Mouse, rat, human, guinea-pig and rabbit kidney sections could be stained in a similar fashion but in general, human kidney gave less conspicuous staining and so was not used for routine screening tests. Fixation for 15 min in 95% methanol prevented the staining while 95% ethanol fixation had little or no effect. In contradistinction, human blood group antigens in tissues are said to be sensitive to fixation in 95% ethanol (Szulman, 1960).

Antibody nature of the reaction

The use of fluorescent antisera specific for the major immunoglobulin classes established

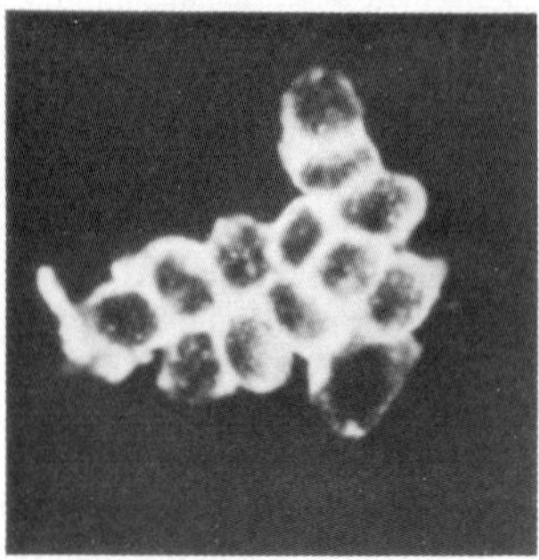

that both γG and γA at least were involved in the reaction. Controls using conjugated antibodies to albumin and fibrinogen gave negative results. A strongly positive serum was fractionated by DEAE-cellulose column chromatography, Sephadex G-200 gel filtration and agarose electrophoresis. Most of the activity was found in the γG globulin fraction. In some cases it appeared that the electrophoretically fast γG had greater activity than the slow.

Fixation of $C'3$

To further ensure the antigen–antibody nature of the reaction, evidence of complement fixation was sought. Since the fixation of $C'3$ is one of the constant secondary phenomena of antigen–antibody interaction, its participation in the process would be a strong indication

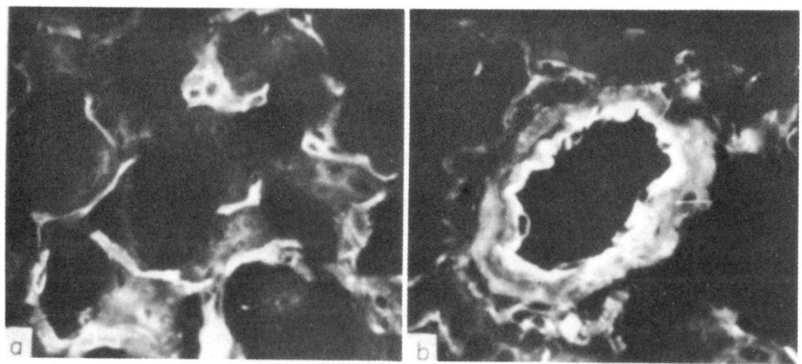

FIG. 3. Specific fluorescence localized to capillaries (a) and vascular endothelium (b). The mouse kidney sections were treated with human serum and fluorescein-tagged antihuman γ-globulin.

that the immunoglobulins responsible for the staining patterns were functioning as antibodies. Evidence of fixation of C'3 was obtained by immunofluorescence (Fig. 4). The controls, normal serum and inactivated anti-endothelial human serum, did not show any staining.

DISCUSSION

Antibody activity, revealed by the fluorescent antibody technique has been detected against vascular endothelium. Since no serum and tissue from the same patient were obtained it is not certain whether this represents auto- or iso-antibody activity. Neither the precise stimulus for production of the antibody, nor its pathogenetic significance is clear. The results show that the antibody activity is present in human serum in a variety of disease states and also in some normal individuals. No evidence was obtained to indicate that basement membrane antigens were involved in the reaction, but with this microscopical technique basement membrane and endothelial staining can look very similar.

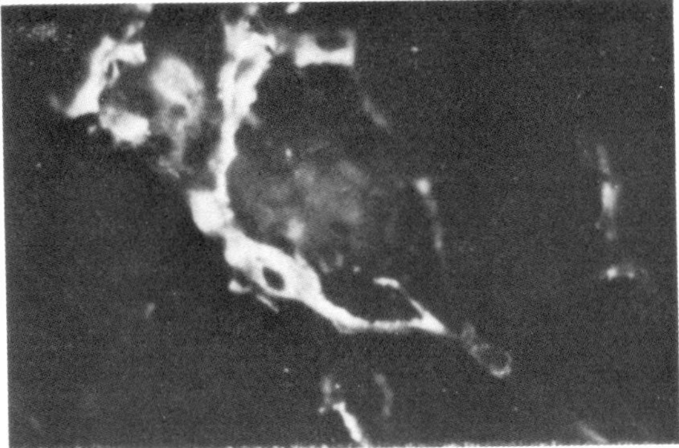

FIG. 4. Mouse kidney sections showing staining of capillary cells using fluorescein-tagged anti-human C'3 serum. Inactivated positive human serum was mixed with fresh human serum and applied to the kidney section, followed by anti C'3 conjugate.

A spontaneously occurring antibody reacting with the cytoplasm of glomerular cells has recently been described (Whittingham, Mackay & Irwin, 1966). The antibody was present in a large proprotion of sera from cases of chronic active hepatitis, and was concomitant with antibodies to smooth muscle. Apparently glomerular cells were the only cells reactive in the immunofluorescence test. The authors suggest that the antiglomerular antibody may account for the mild membranous glomerular lesions occasionally demonstrated in chronic heptatitis. Our experience with smooth muscle staining in chronic active hepatitis is at variance with the observations cited above. Of a large number of serum samples from patients with lupoid hepatitis and smooth muscle antibodies, few showed staining of glomeruli or peritubular endothelial cells.

Immunofluorescent staining of vascular endothelium and erythrocytes has been described using calf thyroid as substrate with sera from patients with infectious mononucleosis and a positive Paul-Bunnell test (Johnson & Holborow, 1963). Wide species reactivity was not found with these sera unlike the reaction described in the present communication. The development in mononucleosis of antibodies against a herpes-like virus has been demonstrated by immunofluorescence tests using cultured Burkitt lymphoma cells (Henle, Henle & Diehl, 1968; Niederman *et al.*, 1968). These antibodies were shown to be distinctive from heterophile antibodies. It might be of interest to examine Burkitt lymphoma cells by immunofluorescence using sera giving the endothelial staining pattern.

The relationship between the antibody giving endothelial staining and isoagglutinins, Forssman antibodies and other heterophile antibodies has not been defined. While the activity seems to be a type of heterospecific antibody, its specificity is atypical and also unlike that of human blood group antibodies. Blood group antigens A and B are widely distributed in nature and in various human tissues including the intimal lining of the capillary bed (Szulman, 1960). In embryological development, vascular intimal cells take origin from the same precursors that give rise to the haematopoietic series and so a rather similar immunochemical makeup might be expected among these cell types. It is notable that high-titred anti-A and anti-B sera did not react with mouse kidney sections. Apparently, such tissues lack the human A and B antigens. Fixation of tissue sections in 95% ethanol, which has been shown to abolish staining of the vascular intima of man by potent anti-A and anti-B sera (Szulman, 1960), had only a small effect on the endothelial staining pattern observed in our material. However, fixation in 95% methanol abolished the staining. Sera giving endothelial staining came from individuals of all ABO blood groups, and absorption with A, B and O cells had no effect on the staining property.

It is also apparent that the antibodies are not of the Forssman type, since rat and rabbit kidney lacking the Forssman antigen (Boyd, 1966) can serve as substrates, and some human sera from group A and AB individuals which possess the Forssman antigen contained antibodies to endothelial cells. The antigen is present on sheep and rabbit red cells and in group B substance isolated from horses, since absorption with these completely abolished the endothelial staining.

The antigen responsible for this staining pattern appears to be present in a variety of animal species. Whether it is present in every human individual or absent in individuals whose serum contains the corresponding antibodies is not certain. While human kidney can be used as the tissue for demonstrating this activity the pattern visualized is not as striking as with mouse or rat kidney. It is not known if the production of the antibodies is stimulated by endogenous factors and host antigen thus representing an autoimmune phenomenon, or if their presence is due to antigenic stimulation of foreign origin, for example infectious agents. The cross-reactivity of the antibodies with tissues and red cells of different species seems to justify their designation as heterophile antibodies (Jenkin, 1963).

Several investigators have described the formation of isoantibodies and autoantibodies by patients who had received organ transplants (Wasaki, Talmage & Starzl, 1967; Porter *et al.*, 1964; Klassen & Milgrom, 1969). Immunologic observations on renal homografts have confirmed that both γ-globulin and C'3 are localized to vascular endothelium during graft rejection (Horowitz *et al.*, 1965). The work of Rapaport, Kano & Milgrom (1968) on the formation of heterophile antibody in patients receiving transplants seems especially pertinent to the endothelial antibodies described here.

The presence of these antibodies in normal persons as well as in a variety of disease states suggests that they bear no direct relationship to clinical disease. In the normal, intact endothelial cell, the antigen may not be accessible to the antibodies; additional factors may be required for these antibodies to assume a pathogenetic role. At present it cannot be stated whether surface or only intracellular antigens are involved.

The demonstrations of anti-endothelial activity in sera from two transplant patients may be significant in view of the reports of antibodies and complement on endothelial cells during graft rejection. It seems plausible that antibodies to vascular endothelium constitute an early immunological attack on grafts and they may be concerned in accelerated graft rejection phenomena (Lindqvist, *et al.*, 1970; Szulman, 1960).

ACKNOWLEDGMENTS

The authors wish to thank Mrs Irene Dorner for her continued cooperation. Mrs C. Gibson provided expert assistance. This work was supported in part by the John A. Hartford Foundation, United States Public Health Service grant AM 08490 and the Arthritis Foundation, Eastern Missouri Chapter.

REFERENCES

BOYD, W.C. (1966) *Fundamentals of Immunology*. Interscience Publishers, New York.

COONS, A.H. & KAPLAN, M.H. (1950) Localization of antigen in tissue cells: improvements in a method for the detection of antigen by means of fluorescent antibody. *J. exp. Med.* **91**, 1.

HENLE, G., HENLE, W. & DIEHL, V. (1968) Relation of Burkitt tumor-associated Herpes-type virus to infectious mononucleosis. *Proc. nat. Acad. Sci.* **59**, 94.

HOROWITZ, R.E., BURROWS, L., PARONETTO, F., DREILING, D. & CLARK, A.E. (1965) Immunologic observations on homografts. II. The canine kidney. *Transplantation*, **3**, 318.

JENKIN, C.R. (1963) Heterophile antigens and their significance in the host-parasite relationship. *Adv. Immunol.* **3**, 351.

JOHNSON, G.D., & HOLBOROW, E.J. (1963) Immunofluorescent test for infectious mononucleosis. *Nature (Lond.)*, **198**, 1316.

KLASSEN, J. & MILGROM, F. (1969) Autoimmune concomitants of renal allografts. *Transplantation Proc.* **1**, 605.

LINDQVIST, K., COLEMAN, R.E. & OSTERLAND, C.K. (1970) Autoantibodies in chronic pulmonary tuberculosis. *J. chron. Dis.* **22**, 717.

NAIRN, R.C. (1962) *Fluorescent Protein Tracing*. E. & S. Livingstone Ltd., Edinburgh and London.

NIEDERMAN, J.C., MCCOLLUM, R.W., HENLE, G. & HENLE, W. (1968) Infectious mononucleosis. Clinical manifestations in relation to E B virus antibodies. *J. Amer. med. Assoc.* **203**, 205.

PORTER, K.A., PEART, W.S., KENYON, J.R., JOSEPH, N.H., HOEHN, R.J. & CALNE, R.Y. (1963) Rejection of kidney homotransplants. *Ann. N. Y. Acad. Sci.* **120**, 472.

RAPAPORT, F.T., KANO, K. & MILGROM, F. (1968) Heterophile antibodies in human transplantation. *J. clin. Invest.* **47**, 633.

SZULMAN, A.E. (1960) The histological distribution of blood group substances A and B in man. *J. exp. Med.* **111**, 785.

WASAKI, I., TALMAGE, D. & STARZL, T.E. (1967) Humoral antibodies in patients after renal homotransplantation. *Transplantation*, **6**, 191.

WHITTINGHAM, S., MACKAY, I.R. & IRWIN, J. (1966) Autoimmune hepatitis. Immunofluorescence reactions with cytoplasm of smooth muscle and renal glomerular cells. *Lancet*, **i**, 1333.

THE IMMUNE COMPLEX GLOMERULONEPHRITIS OF BACTERIAL ENDOCARDITIS

ROBERT A. GUTMAN, M.D., GARY E. STRIKER, M.D.,
BRUCE C. GILLILAND, M.D. AND
RALPH E. CUTLER, M.D.

INTRODUCTION

The pathogenesis of the renal lesions associated with bacterial endocarditis has remained obscure. Early descriptions placed great weight on the presence of gross infarcts and it was later suggested that the glomerulonephritis was the result of micro-emboli, hence the term "focal embolic glomerulonephritis" (4, 10). Many recognized that a diffuse glomerulonephritis was present in patients with bacterial endocarditis (10, 74). In fact, it has long been appreciated that the local[1] renal lesion is trivial, in the sense that renal failure is rare in patients who have only this form, whereas renal insufficiency may accompany the diffuse variety (82). One early hypothesis was that local glomerulonephritis resulted from the lodgement of infected emboli in the glomeruli whereas the diffuse glomerulonephritis represented an allergic phenomenon (74). Bacteria were, in fact, seldom found in the local lesions (2, 39) and the etiology remained unclear.

Circulating antigen-antibody complexes are present in patients with endocarditis (85) and may mediate an immunological injury by being deposited on the glomerular basement membrane (GBM), activating complement and stimulating an inflammatory response (27). There is some evidence that this occurs in patients with bacterial endocarditis. Williams noted a clear relation between hypocomplementemia and clinical evidence of nephritis (85). Granular deposits of immunoglobulin have been noted on the GBM of a few patients with subacute bacterial endocarditis (55, 56) and subepithelial deposits were seen in two patients with staphylococcal endocarditis by electron microscopy (77). If the nephritis of endocarditis is an immune-complex injury, it shares this pathogenetic mechanism with the nephritis of several other diseases including post-streptococcal glomerulonephritis (21, 27, 28), quartan malaria (3, 73, 83), infected ventriculo-atrial shunts (12, 49, 63, 74) and (perhaps) secondary syphilis (15, 33).

In order to examine further the relationship between endocarditis and possible immunological injury to the kidney, we have prospectively studied three patients with serologic and morphologic techniques and have reviewed available clinical and biopsy material in an additional six patients with bacterial endocarditis. The observations suggest that the diffuse glomerulonephritis in patients with endocarditis represents an immune-complex nephritis (21, 28).

METHODS

Selection of Patients (Case Reports in Appendix, Table I)

The first three patients listed in Table I were studied prospectively during a search for patients with bacterial endocarditis who also had clinical evidence of glomerulonephritis. Therefore, detailed serological data and the results of immunofluorescence microscopy were available in addition to the light and electron microscopic examination of renal tissue that was performed in all nine patients. Two of the three studied prospectively were parenteral drug abusers (#2, 3) with severe staphylococcal sepsis, pneumonia, fever, anemia, splenomegaly and microscopic hematuria with red cell casts. Clinical presentation, findings and subsequent course strongly suggested the diagnosis of

This investigation was supported by National Institutes of Health Research Fellowship Grant #1 F03 AM25887-01, National Institutes of Health grants #R01 HE03174 and #I-L01-GM13543 and by a grant (RR-133) from the General Clinical Research Centers Programs of the Division of Resources, National Institutes of Health.

[1] In keeping with current usage, "local" refers to changes involving portions of individual glomeruli. In the older literature, "focal" was often used in the same sense as well as to indicate involvement of some glomeruli.

159

TABLE I

Clinical Characteristics of Nine Patients with Endocarditis with Glomerulonephritis[1]

Patient	Age	Sex	Blood culture	RHD[2]	Drug abuse	Previous antibiotics	Fever	Splenomegaly	Murmur	Destructive endocarditis	Special features	Hematocrit	ESR[3]	Outcome
						Prospectively Studied Patients								
1.	40	M	Negative	No	No	No	Yes	Yes	Aortic regurgitation	Aortic cusp perforation	Pleuritic chest pain	24	132	Died of CHF[4] one year later
2.	34	M	Staphylococcus coagulase positive	No	Yes	No	Yes	Yes	Tricuspid regurgitation	No	Roth spots	24	142	Alive
3.	33	M	Staphylococcus coagulase positive	No	Yes	No	Yes	Yes	Aortic systolic	No	Renal failure	27	145	Required dialysis. Alive
						Retrospectively Studied Patients								
4.	39	M	Negative	No	No	Yes	Yes	Yes	Aortic regurgitation	Aortic cusp perforation	Ill for 6 months before	30	80	Died of CHF while being treated with steroids
5.	53	M	Negative	Yes	No	No	No	Yes	Aortic regurgitation	Aortic cusp perforation	Remained afebrile	35	48	Died in 2 months with CHF before being treated
6.	36	M	Negative	Yes	No	No	Yes	Yes	Mitral regurgitation	Probable ruptured chordae tendinae	Positive ANF. Clubbing. Hemolytic anemia	25	62	Alive
7.	58	M	Negative	No	No	Yes	Yes	Yes	Mitral and aortic regurgitation	Aortic cusp perforation	Purpura. Pancytopenia. Clubbing	32	58	Died of CHF after 22 months
8.	71	M	Group G beta hemolytic streptococcus	Calcific aortic stenosis	No	No	Yes	No	Aortic regurgitation and stenosis	Aortic cusp perforation		40	45	Died of CHF after 25 months
9.	46	M	Negative	Yes	No	Yes	Yes	No	Aortic and mitral regurgitation	Ruptured chordae tendinae	Gross hematuria	46	67	Alive after repair of mitral valve

[1] All patients had hematuria, proteinuria and red cell casts.
[2] Rheumatic Heart Disease.
[3] Erythrocyte Sedimentation Rate (Westegren method).
[4] CHF—Congestive Heart Failure.

endocarditis. Patient #1, whose blood cultures were negative and who had a more indolent course than the other two, developed acute aortic regurgitation after a four-week course of antimicrobial therapy and died one year later of congestive heart failure. At autopsy, bacterial endocarditis with perforation of the aortic valve was found.

The remaining six patients (Table I) were chosen from a review of the renal biopsy files at the University of Washington rather than from autopsy records. This selection process was followed because renal tissue was available for electron microscopic examination. Tissue for immunofluorescence microscopy was also available in one patient. Only patients whose clinical course or necropsy findings provided firm evidence of endocarditis during or shortly before the renal biopsy were selected. Only one of these six patients (#5) had positive blood cultures. He and four others developed valve damage demonstrable at surgery or autopsy. The remaining patient (#8) responded dramatically to antimicrobial therapy and is, therefore, also included in this series. In many cases, renal biopsy had been done because of the confusion regarding diagnosis in a culture-negative individual. The decision to include patients was made without regard to the electron microscopic data which became available later.

Serological Data

Rheumatoid factor (anti IgG) was determined by latex flocculation (72). Serum hemolytic complement was performed on specimens frozen within two hours of sampling at $-70°$ C and stored no longer than two weeks. The end point was 50% lysis of sensitized sheep cells and was expressed as 'H$_{50}$ units (42). Normal range in our laboratory was 80–160 units. Serum immunoglobulins (IgG, IgA, IgM) and C3 component of complement levels were measured by radial diffusion.[2] Antinuclear antibodies were tested by immunofluorescence using rat liver as substrate (89).

Processing of Renal Biopsy Material

All biopsies were taken percutaneously with either a Franklin or disposable Travenol® needle. Tissue from four patients (#1, 2, 3 and 8) was available for fixing in two ways: frozen for immunofluorescence staining, and fixed in glutaraldehyde for routine and electron microscopy. Tissue from the other five patients was not available for immunofluorescence staining.

Anti-gamma globulin and anti-beta 1-c complement sera, conjugated with fluorescein, were purchased.[3] The renal biopsy tissue was quick

[2] Hyland Immunoplates®.
[3] ibid.

frozen, cut at 3 microns and exposed to the conjugated antisera with the appropriate controls (37). All biopsies were processed for light and electron microscopy after fixation in glutaraldehyde.

RESULTS

Clinical Response

Four of the nine patients have survived. One (#3) required dialysis for transient severe renal insufficiency. Patient #8, who responded to antimicrobial therapy with marked improvement in renal function, weight gain and loss of anemia, splenomegaly and clubbing, is currently well. Another patient (#9) required surgical repair of a ruptured chordae tendinae but is now well. The two drug abusers (#2 and 3) are known to have resumed their habit but have thus far remained free of systemic infection and renal disease.

Five of the patients have died of their heart disease. Two (#1 and 4) received appropriate antimicrobial therapy within two weeks of the onset of fever. However, both developed aortic regurgitation and died about a year later. At autopsy, aortic valve perforations were found but there was no evidence of active inflammation or bacterial forms. The renal lesions were healed at the time of autopsy. Patient #5, on the other hand, experienced weight loss, fever, edema, purpura for nine months and later developed an "active" urine sediment before antimicrobial therapy was instituted. The fever and other inflammatory manifestations did not respond until adrenal corticosteroids were added to the drug regimen. He eventually died of congestive heart failure more than two years afer the onset of symptoms. Patient #7, whose illness was diagnosed as a "collagen vascular disease", was treated with steroids for three months during which time he had increasing breathlessness, proteinuria and azotemia before he died of heart failure. The other patient who was not treated with antibiotics (#6) remained afebrile with a rising blood urea nitrogen (BUN), proteinuria, anemia and died after developing aortic regurgitation.

All nine patients were found to have at least one organic heart murmur at some time in their course. Five of the seven with culture-negative endocarditis and one (#4), whose blood contained Group G beta-hemolytic streptococci, had aortic regurgitation. Three patients with nega-

161

TABLE II

Laboratory Findings during the Course of Nine Patients with Bacterial Endocarditis with Glomerulonephritis

Patient	Organism	Treatment	Date	BUN mg/100 ml	Creatinine mg/100 ml	$c_{H_{50}}$	C-3	IgG mg/100 ml	IgA mg/100 ml	IgM mg/100 ml	R.F.	ANF
			Prospectively Studied Patients									
1.	Negative	PCN and Strep	10/28/68	22	1.8							
			10/30	27	2.2						Pos.	
			11/4	44	2.7	0	<60	1400	390	200	1 → 2560	Neg.
			11/8	35	2.2	13						Neg.
			11/18	47	2.8	31	<60	1950	460	255	1 → 1280	Neg.
			11/25	53	2.3	58						
			12/2	37	1.9	60	71	2080	515	160	1 → 1280	Neg.
			3/5/69	14								
			5/6	23		98	94	1400	710	104	1 → 40	
			6/3	12	0.8	123	105	1420	760	66		
			6/20			147	132	1400	800	180	1 → 20	
			†-CHF									
2.	Staphylococcus	Cephalothin Methicillin	3/14/69	77								
			3/16	59	1.6	57	<60	2080	227	360	1 → 160	Neg.
			3/18	27	1.2	101						
			3/20		1.1	106	147	2080	192	84		Neg.
			3/26			104	215	2450	214	230	1 → 160	
			3/28	11	1.0	107						
			4/4			121	265				1 → 1280	Neg.
			9/24			104	170	2200	295	380	1 → 160	

3.	Staphylococcus	Cephalothin	1/22/70	141	11.7								
			1/28	77	11.2 (after dialysis)								
			2,6	29	7.6 (after dialysis)	69	<60	2100	225	100		Neg.	
			2/11	35	10.4 (after dialysis)	50	<60	2200	160	88			
			2/16	45	12.2 (after dialysis)								
			2/18	52	11.5			2500	112	76		Neg.	
			2/25	91	8.5	116	110	2500	128	172			
			3/6			125	125	1720	92	182		Neg.	
			3/13	24	3.1								
			5/10	16		128	118	1600	82	128		Neg.	
			5/19	14	0.8	100							
4.	Group G beta hemolytic streptococcus	PCN and Strep	2/13/63	22									
			3/6	11									
			12/5										
			†-CHF										
5.	Culture negative		5/9/63	17				Diffuse increase in globulins				Pos.	L.E. preparation: tart cells.
		PCN and Strep	6/5		1.3								
			7/19		1.4								
			7/29	45									
			9/4	35	1.4								
			7/4/64	15									
			1/20/65	16	1.2								
			†-CHF										
6.	Culture negative		3/1/65	39									
			3/10	57									
			3/16	49	2.5								
			3/22	68	2.4								
			4/5	84									

†-Advancing uremia and CHF

TABLE II—*Continued*

Patient	Organism	Treatment	Date	BUN mg/100 ml	Creatinine mg/100 ml	$c_{H_{50}}$	C-3	IgG mg/100 ml	IgA mg/100 ml	IgM mg/100 ml	R.F.	ANF
							Prospectively Studied Patients					
7.	Culture negative	Steroids	3/29/66	37	2.1							Neg.
			4/5	49	1.7						Pos.	
			5/3	56	1.6							
			5/23	31	2.5							
			6/7	53	1.8							
			7/17	60	3.0							
			†-CHF									
8.	Culture negative	PCN and Strep	6/3/68	42	3.9							
			6/10	53		91		Diffuse increase in gamma globulin			Pos.	4+
			6/17	57								
			6/24	45	1.9							
			7/17	21	1.4							
			8/6	13							Neg.	Neg.
9.	Culture negative	PCN and Strep	3/3/69	20							Neg.	Neg.
			3/12	21	1.3							
			3/16		1.1						Neg.	
			3/21			125		700	160	100		Neg.
			4/9	26	1.3							
			12/4			119	350	2100	280	149		Neg.

PCN—penicillin; Strep—streptomycin; BUN—blood urea nitrogen; $c_{H_{50}}$—hemolytic activity of complement; C-3—third component of complement; R.F.—rheumatoid factor; ANF—antinuclear factor: CHF—congestive heart failure.

†—patient died.

tive cultures developed mitral regurgitation which had to be repaired in one case. The two drug abusers had hemodynamically insignificant murmurs.

Splenomegaly, which was noted in seven patients, abated with therapy in the five who received antimicrobials. The Roth spots present in one with staphylococcal sepsis and the purpura in one with negative cultures improved with antimicrobial therapy. Clubbing was seen in one patient and also improved following treatment with penicillin and streptomycin.

Seven of the nine patients were anemic when first seen. All five of the anemic treated patients had a significant rise in hematocrit, whereas the two who were untreated did not. An elevated erythrocyte sedimentation rate, noted in all patients, fell appreciably in the seven who were treated with antimicrobial agents, but rose during the three month course of steroid therapy in one case (#7).

Urinary Sediment and Renal Function (Table III)

All nine patients had protein, red cells and red cell casts in the urine early in their illness. These abnormalities persisted from two weeks to seven months in the treated patients. The urine of most patients cleared. Patient #3, who required dialysis, has continued to have significant proteinuria and hematuria with a large number of red cell casts. Patient #1 had microscopic hematuria without proteinuria until his death from congestive heart failure. The two untreated patients (#6 and 7) had persistent hematuria, proteinuria (reaching 500 mg/100 ml in the case of #7) and advancing renal failure.

Six of the nine patients had a BUN greater than 35 mg/100 ml or creatinine above 2.0 mg/ 100 ml when first hospitalized but only one (#3) actually required dialysis. In other cases, treatment was associated with a prompt fall in BUN or creatinine.

Immunological Data (Table II)

All three patients who were studied prospectively had reduced serum complement levels at the time of admission. In each case, the level rose to normal during antibiotic therapy. Rheumatoid factor was present in the sera of five patients. The titer rose during and then fell after antibiotic therapy of two (#1 and 2) on

whom serial observations were made. One of the five patients (#8) tested for antinuclear antibody had a 4+ positive reaction which became negative after antimicrobial therapy. Serum immunoglobulins (IgG, IgA and IgM) measured sequentially in four patients rose at the time complement and rheumatoid factor levels were rising and returned to pre-treatment levels late in the patients' course. Two additional patients (#5 and 8) had diffuse elevations in gamma globulin.

Renal Microscopy (Table III. Fig. 1–11)

Light microscopy revealed a proliferative glomerular lesion in the biopsies of all patients except patient #4 who had no demonstrable glomerular lesion. The extent, distribution and cell type involved in the proliferative process was variable. For example, in one patient, the proliferation, while involving all glomeruli, was not equally severe among glomeruli or individual lobules of a single glomerulus and might, therefore, have been called local or focal glomerulonephritis (Fig. 1). However, careful glomerular cell counting and the use of thin sections led us to decide that all patients except one had diffuse glomerular hypercellularity (Fig. 2). Local necrotic (or embolic) lesions, so called because they consist of discrete local glomerular fibrin deposits (Fig. 3), were seen in addition to the diffuse proliferation in two patients. This lesion, which may represent microscopic fibrin emboli, should be distinguished from other changes which were also "local." For example, four patients had loci of epithelial proliferation (Fig. 4) and three patients had a striking disparity in the distribution of neutrophils among glomeruli.

Fluorescence microscopy was performed in four patients (two with staphylococcal endocarditis and two with culture-negative endocarditis). Granular deposits of IgG and complement were noted in all on the glomerular basement membrane and/or in the mesangial regions (Fig. 5–8).

Electron microscopic examination was carried out on all patients. Three patients, two of whom had staphylococcal endocarditis, had both subepithelial (Fig. 9) and intramembranous deposits (Fig. 10). One of these had small deposits in all areas. The other five patients with electron microscopic abnormalities, four of whom were

TABLE III

Results of Renal Biopsy Examination in Nine Patients with Bacterial Endocarditis

Pt.	Blood Culture	Number of glomeruli	Glomerular changes (number affected)						Distribution of granular deposits of γG & β-1-C globulins		Distribution of electron dense deposits			
			Proliferation			Other features								
			Undetermined	Mesangial	Epithelial	Fibrin	Neurophils	Obsolescent	Peripheral	Mesangial	Subepithelial	Intramembranous	Subendothelial	Mesangial
1.	Negative	11	11	0	5	2	5	0	3+	2+	1+	1+	1+	1+
2.	Staphylococcus coagulase positive	40	0	40	1	0	40	0	4+	3+	3+	3+	0	0
3a.	Staphylococcus coagulase positive	4	4	0	0	0	4	0	—	—	4+	4+	0	1+
b.	Follow-up 6 months later	18	0	13	0	0	0	5	1+	3+	0	1+	0	2+
4.	Group G beta hemolytic strep.	19	0	0	0	0	0	0	—	—	0	0	1+	1+
5.	Negative	12	0	12	0	0	0	0	—	—	0	0	3+	4+
6.	Negative	11	0	11	0	1	3	0	—	—	0	0	3+	2+
7.	Negative	6	6	0	4	0	0	0	—	—	0	0	4+	3+
8.	Negative	17	17	0	4	0	5	0	3+	3+	0	0	2+	3+
9.	Negative	27	0	3	0	0	0	0	—	—	0	0	0	0.

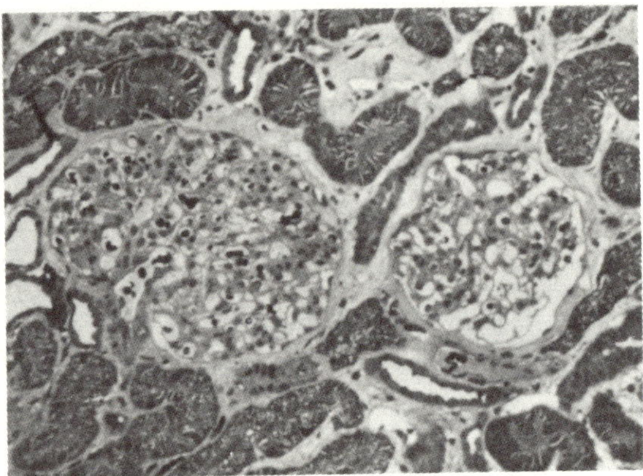

Fig. 1. Light microscopy of renal tissue from patient #9 with culture-negative endocarditis showing mild local proliferative glomerulonephritis. Masson's trichrome stain × 64.

culture-negative, had primarily subendothelial and mesangial deposits (Fig. 11). Several glomeruli were examined in patient #9, whose blood cultures were also negative, but no abnormalities were seen. A follow-up biopsy on one patient (#3) with staphylococcal endocarditis obtained six months after the acute illness revealed deposits primarily in the mesangial re-

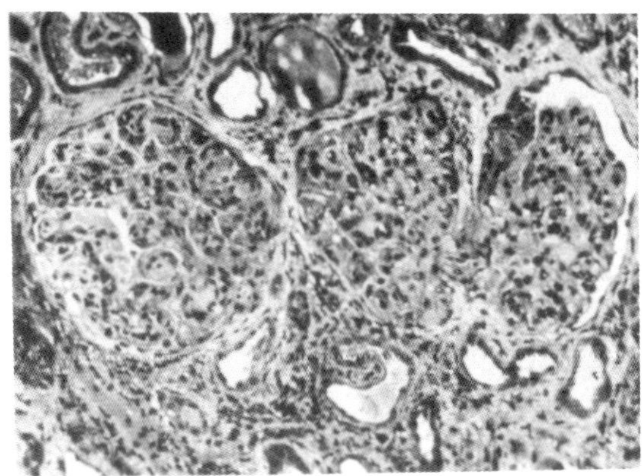

Fig. 2. Light microscopy of renal tissue from patient #2 with staphylococcal endocarditis showing diffuse cellular proliferation in the glomerulus and marked leukocytic infiltration. Masson's trichrome stain × 64.

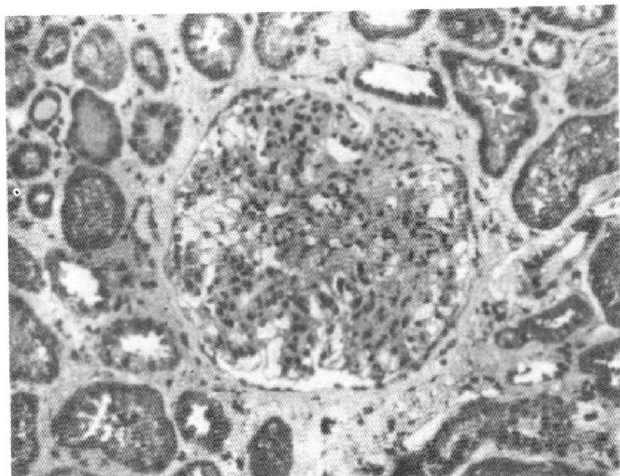

Fig. 3. Light microscopy of renal tissue from patient #6 with culture-negative endocarditis showing diffuse proliferative glomerulonephritis with focal areas of fibrin deposition and necrosis. Masson's trichrome stain × 64.

gions and a few in an intra-membranous location by both light and electron microscopy (Fig. 10).

DISCUSSION

Evidence for Immune Complexes

The diffuse glomerulonephritis associated with endocarditis in our nine patients can be considered to be an antigen-antibody complex disease by most available morphological and immunological criteria (21, 27, 28). There was serologic evidence of active complement consumption which abated once antimicrobial therapy was started. This can be taken as indirect evidence for the presence of antigen-antibody complexes. The histologic study of the renal tissue shows these complexes were present and causing an inflammatory response. The glomerular basement membranes (GBM) of nine of ten patients contained electron dense deposits. Further,

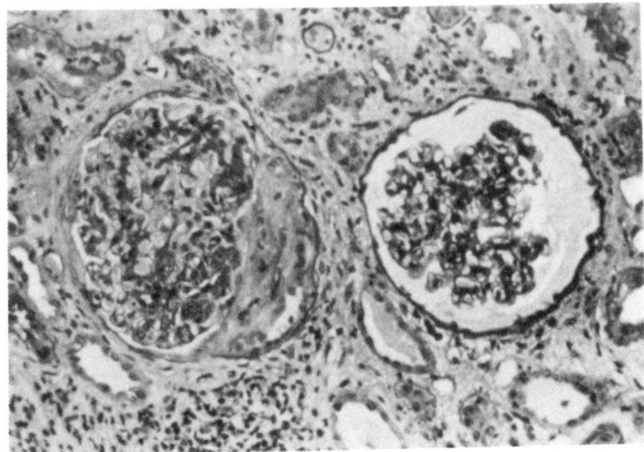

FIG. 4. Light microscopy of renal tissue from patient #8 with culture-negative endocarditis showing diffuse glomerulonephritis with focal epithelial proliferation and crescent formation. Without the use of thin sectioning, the diffuse proliferation is not easily appreciated. Masson's trichrome stain × 64.

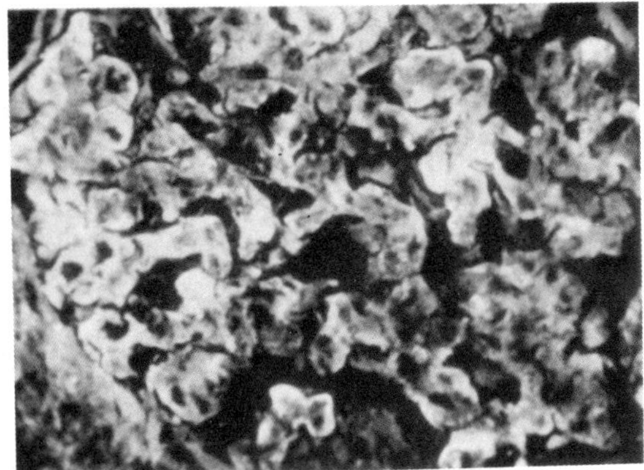

FIG. 5. Fluorescence micrograph of renal tissue from patient #2 showing diffuse, granular deposits of γ-G globulin in mesangial areas and on the peripheral GBM. × 128.

the renal tissue of the four patients examined by immunofluorescence had irregular deposits of IgG and B_{1C}-B_{1A} in the glomerular basement membrane and in the mesangium.

While this observation is not entirely new, it has not been systematically studied. Messner mentions the presence of immune deposits on the GBM in "several" renal biopsies of patients with endocarditis (55). Michael et al presented a single picture of a glomerulus of a patient with endocarditis which was positive for IgG (56), and Tu et al demonstrated large subepithelial deposits on the GBM of two patients with staphylococcal endocarditis by electron microscopy (77). Our three patients with staphylococcal endocarditis also had deposits predominantly on the epithelial side of the GBM and in this regard, are different from the patients who had

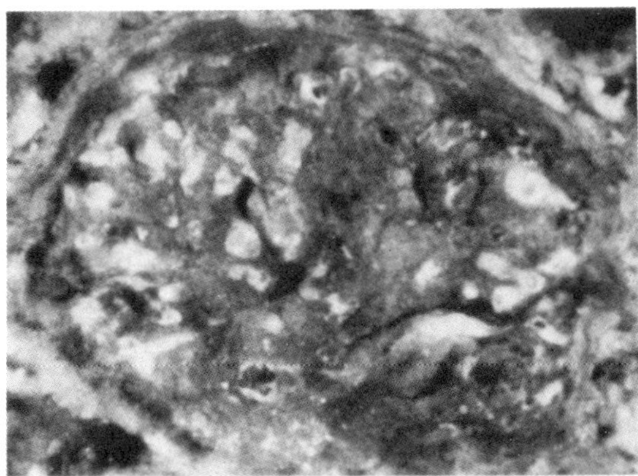

Fig. 6. Fluorescence micrograph of renal tissue from patient #3. The renal biopsy was taken six months after the acute episode. Irregular deposits of IgG are present in several mesangial areas and irregularly on the peripheral GBM. × 128.

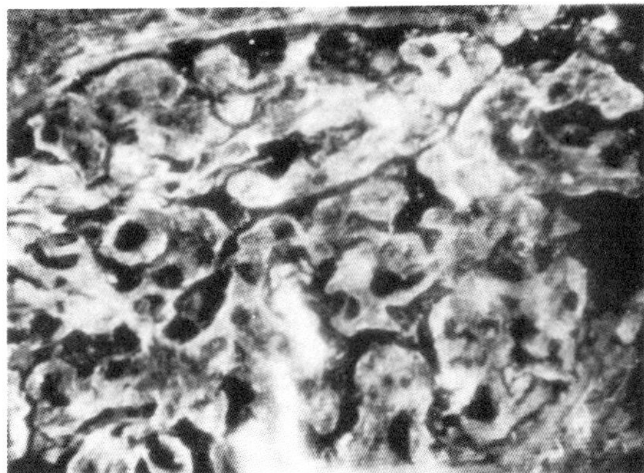

Fig. 7. Fluorescence micrograph of renal tissue from patient #1. Granular deposits of IgG are present on peripheral glomerular capillary basement membranes. × 128.

the more chronic infections. The latter group who, for the most part, had negative blood cultures, more often had deposits within and on the endothelial surface of the GBM, a location similar to that seen in lupus erythematosus (24, 62).

The question of whether the antigen is derived from the foreign organism or from host tissue is an important one. While IgG and complement are identified in many of these GBM deposits, the nature of the antigen is not known. However, the observations that glomerulonephritis may be associated with endocarditis caused by fungal, bacterial or viral infection (16, 57, 66, 80, 90) attests to the non-specificity of the infecting organism in causing this renal response and makes it unlikely that the renal response is due to an antibody which cross-reacts with the GBM and the infectious agent.

Role of Endocarditis

With a few exceptions, endocarditis is unique among bacterial infections because of persistent

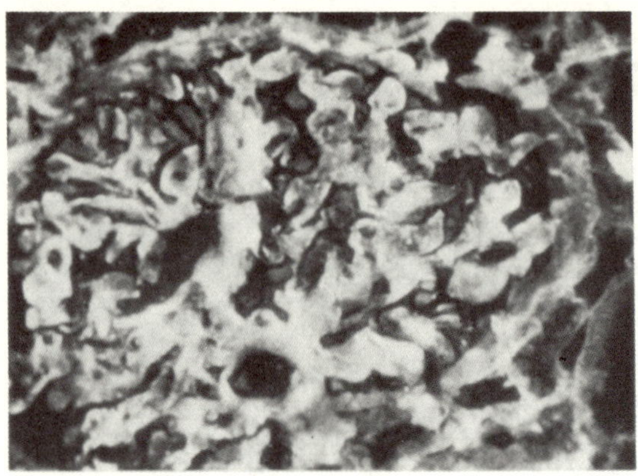

Fig. 8. Fluorescence micrograph of renal tissue from patient #8. IgG is present on the GBM as in patient #1 but in lesser amounts. × 128.

bacteremia (9, 84). Chronicity may be especially important in light of current concepts of immune complex disease. Prolonged or repeated contact of the host with a foreign protein serves both to stimulate antibody production and to provide a supply of antigen for formation of antigen-antibody complexes (27, 28, 29, 36). The production of lesions in all experimental models (29, 26, 79) depends on the formation of soluble circulating complexes under conditions of antigen excess, a condition likely to exist intermittently in bacterial endocarditis. Other human diseases in which immune complexes have been implicated in the associated nephropathy are also of a chronic or relapsing nature. These include infected ventriculo-atrial shunts (12, 49, 63, 75), quartan malaria (3, 73, 83), syphilis (15, 33), osteomyelitis (13) and infectious mononucleosis (64).

Further evidence for a state of chronic immunization in bacterial endocarditis is the appearance of rheumatoid factor and its subsequent disappearance following eradication of bacteria (87). In animal experiments, the repeated injection of various antigens results in a rising titer of rheumatoid factor which disappears on cessation of antigenic stimulation (1, 86, 88). Rheumatoid factor appears in several other chronic human diseases (8) such as tuberculosis (71), syphilis (60), trichinosis (32) and kala azar (48). Patients with lepromatous leprosy, another chronic infection with persistent bacteremia

(31) have as high as a 44% incidence of rheumatoid factor (18) and have also been found to have hematuria, red cell casts and occasionally proliferative glomerulonephritis (Gutman, R. A., Lu, W.-H., Drutz, D. J., unpublished observations).

The other role which endocarditis probably plays is that the vegetations serve as the focus from which embolization, macroscopic and possibly microscopic, occurs.

Staphylococcal Endocarditis

It is now clear that staphylococcal infections, including endocarditis can also lead to glomerulonephritis. We report two additional drug-addicted patients with staphylococcal sepsis, probable endocarditis and immune-complex nephritis who are very similar to the two reported by Tu, Shearn and Lee (77). Heptinstall (39) mentions two patients with staphylococcal disease who had a glomerulonephritis and there are several reports of staphylococcus albus infection of ventriculo-atrial shunts leading to nephritis and the nephrotic syndrome (12, 49, 63, 75). Although most authors have not emphasized the relationship of staphylococcal sepsis, endocarditis (35, 52, 65, 70) and drug addiction (19, 23, 53, 68), a nephritis in drug users has been noted previously (20). The observation that drug addicts have high titer of opsonizing antibodies to several groups of gram-negative bacteria and perhaps to at least one strain of staphylococcus led

Nickerson (59) to emphasize the need for a further search for immune-complex nephritis in such patients. The report of a proliferative glomerulonephritis in dogs with induced staphylococcal endocarditis (40) is experimental confirmation of the relationship between staphylococcal infection and nephritis. It should also be emphasized that the electron microscopic appearance of the GBM of the patients with staphylococcal endocarditis, consisting of large subepithelial deposits, is indistinguishable from that associated with post-streptococcal glomerulonephritis.

Culture-Negative Endocarditis

Negative blood cultures were obtained repeatedly from six of the nine patients in this series. This unusually high incidence of culture-negative endocarditis is certainly not representative of the general experience with endocarditis. Other authors (5, 48, 50, 51, 82) have stressed the relationship between the glomerulonephritis and negative blood cultures in patients with endocarditis. However, our experience was influenced by the fact that renal biopsies in the six patients in whom the diagnosis of BE was made retrospectively were obtained because the diag-

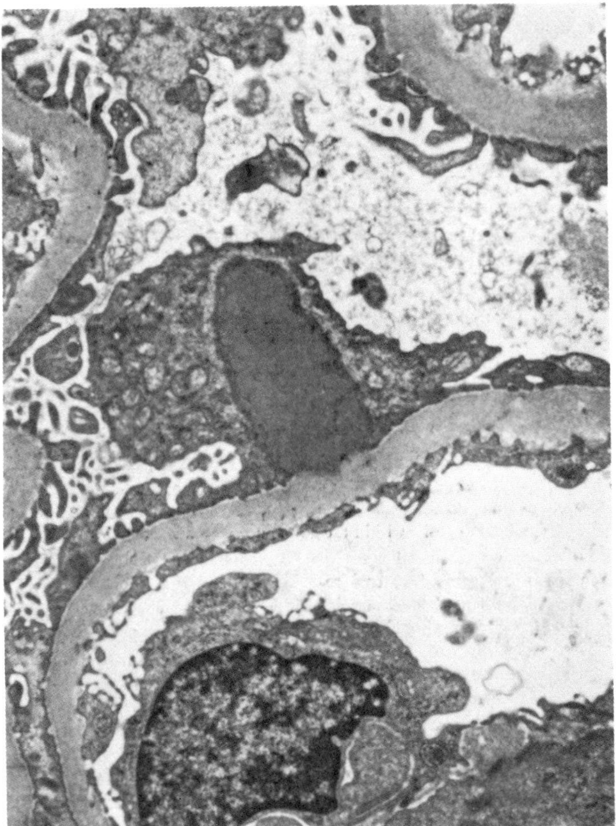

Fig. 9. Electron microscopy of renal tissue from patient #2 with staphylococcal endocarditis showing large subepithelial deposits. × 10,000.

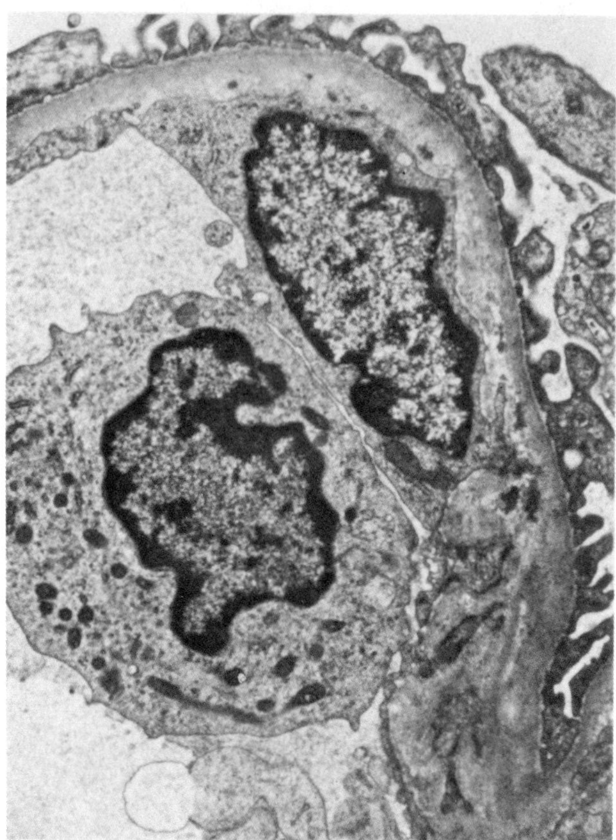

Fig. 10. Electron microscopy of renal tissue from patient #6 with culture-negative endocarditis showing minimal deposits within the glomerular basement membrane. × 15,000.

nosis was unclear. The finding that several responded to antimicrobials suggests that the infecting organism was not a virus, though such a possibility should be considered (16, 57, 80, 90, 91). Recent reports of L-form endocarditis (54, 58) in which routine cultures were negative have led Carpenter to speculate that this phenomenon may be the principal cause for culture-negative endocarditis (17). If this hypothesis is accepted, organisms presumably persist in the circulation or tissue resulting in chronic immunization of the host and, perhaps, providing the necessary antigen moiety of the immune complexes.

Characteristics of the Glomerulonephritis

Most recent reports on the nephritis of bacterial endocarditis have emphasized the coexistence of "focal" and diffuse lesions (2, 39) and felt they had a different etiology. For example, Villarreal and Sokoloff (82) emphasized the "co-existence" of these two lesions in patients with endocarditis but comment that "aside from infarction, embolic glomerulonephritis is the characteristic lesion found in the majority of cases and the occurrence of banal types of glomerulonephritis has also been reported to be of high incidence". Earlier, Bell (10) found the le-

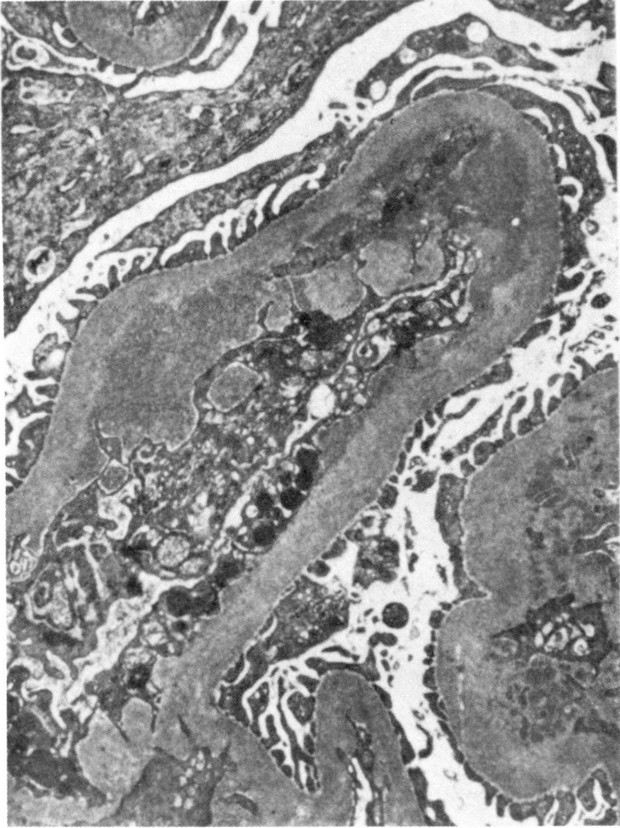

FIG. 11. Electron microscopy of renal tissue from patient #7 with culture-negative endocarditis showing extensive subendothelial and intramembranous deposits. × 10,000.

sions to coexist in 35% of cases but obviously felt they had a different etiology. Baehr spoke of "typical glomerulonephritis" over-shadowing the "focal" lesion (4). Even Heptinstall, in a lucid discussion (39) of the probable role of "allergy" in the glomerulonephritis, fails to clarify the relationship of the two types of glomerulonephritis to one another even though he mentions the occurrence of diffuse and "focal" proliferative glomerulonephritis in the same patients. We also find that the two lesions may be present in the same individual.

The diffuse lesion seems to be best explained on the basis that it is a reaction to circulating antigen-antibody complexes. The light, electron and fluorescence microscopic data and the serologic findings support this view. Although, one of our patients received methicillin, he had clinical evidence of glomerulonephritis before being treated and his biopsy findings did not show the eosinophilic infiltrate characteristic of methicillin nephritis (7, 14).

The nature of the "focal embolic" lesion is less clear. The fact that macroscopic infarcts are known to occur in all organs including the kidneys (78) and that very similar focal or local

173

embolic lesions can be produced experimentally with microspheres and thrombi (46, 87) lends credence to the popular notion that these are truly microembolic lesions. In addition, fibrin can be demonstrated histochemically in most foci. The lack of bacteria in the lesion does not detract significantly from this postulate. The source of fibrin deposits may, of course, be the friable vegetations on the heart valve. It is also conceivable that the so-called "focal embolic" glomerular lesion is but another tissue response to large aggregates of antigen-antibody complexes and fibrin.

The functional sequelae of these two lesions is of considerable importance. The histologic pattern has been shown accurately to reflect the severity and chronicity of the injury in a variety of diseases (69, 76). In this study, diffuse glomerulonephritis was seen in those with the most severe renal dysfunction. In every case in which the creatinine or BUN was elevated, significant interstitial edema was present. Mesangial proliferation was characteristic of those whose biopsies were taken late. It is of interest that the second biopsy in one patient taken six months after successful therapy showed that the electron dense deposits had become localized to the mesangial region. It has been previously noted that the "focal embolic" lesion is infrequently associated with renal dysfunction in the absence of obvious diffuse proliferation (6, 44, 82). In this sense, it appears to be a relatively trivial lesion.

As noted, glomerular basement membrane deposits which consisted of IgG and complement by fluorescence microscopy were seen in the biopsy material from all patients except the one whose lesion was limited to local proliferation. The location of these deposits was of interest because, in general, those with staphylococcal endocarditis had large subepithelial deposits whereas the others tended to have the deposits localized to the endothelial surface. We do not find this of diagnostic importance however, because there was overlap. The difference may simply represent slight variations in size and solubility of the complexes.

Prognosis of the Glomerulonephritis

The renal injury appears to be at least partially reversible if appropriate antimicrobial therapy is instituted (74, 82). Only the two patients in our series who were not so treated died with decreasing renal function and persistent proteinuria and hematuria. The patient with most severe renal dysfunction was treated with steroids at a time when his serum creatinine had stopped rising. While prednisolone may have been important in his recovery, there is reason to believe he was beginning to improve spontaneously. The three patients who died in spite of apparently successful therapy had no renal dysfunction and minimal urinary sediment abnormalities. This experience, then, is quite consistent with that of larger series (10, 22, 61, 74). Bell reported that 15 of 108 patients with bacterial endocarditis developed severe renal insufficiency in the pre-antibiotic era (10). The majority of these had alpha hemolytic streptococcal infection. Although Tumulty and Harvey (78) observed significant renal impairment in seven of 355 patients treated with penicillin after it became generally available, Christie, at about the same time, observed only eight uremic deaths among 269 treated patients (22). Pillsbury (61), in 1950, reported no significant renal insufficiency among his 33 treated cases. In one of the few reports dealing specifically with the prognosis of the renal lesion in treated versus untreated groups, Spain and King reported a 17% incidence of diffuse glomerulonephritis among the 52 untreated patients with bacterial endocarditis in contrast with the complete absence of this complication among 25 treated patients (74). Similarly, the focal lesion was noted in 48% of the untreated compared to 24% of the treated group.

Similarities of Bacterial Endocarditis to Systemic Lupus Erythematosus

Because the glomerulonephritis of endocarditis in culture-negative (as well as positive) patients appears to result from the renal inflammatory response to the deposition of the circulating antigen-antibody complexes, some of the other manifestations of endocarditis may also represent injury to tissue mediated by this same process. It is conceivable that Osler nodes, Roth spots, clubbing, purpura, arthralgias, arthritis and sternal tenderness are the result of an inflammatory response to immune complexes which were deposited in the walls of small peripheral blood vessels. As Kerr (44) discussed in detail, many earlier reports demonstrate the keen awareness of clinicians such as Libman, 1912 (50), Baehr, 1931 (5), Cornil, 1936 (26), Keefer, 1938 (43) and Donzelot, 1949 (30) of a chronic indolent form of endocarditis in which the features of weight loss, clubbing, hematuria and uremia were prominent. Cordeiro applied the term "immunological phase of endocarditis" to similar patients (25). The clinical similarity between the manifestations of some cases of bacterial endocarditis, especially in the absence of positive blood cultures, and systemic lupus erythematosus (SLE) is remarkable. Both can be associated with nephritis, with hypocomplementemia, similar-appearing skin lesions (67), elevated titers of anti-gamma-globulin (RF) and immunoglobulins. The sudden onset of aortic valvular insufficiency in patients with SLE has also been reported (11). The decision to use steroids rather than antimicrobials in one of our patients was clearly caused by the difficulty of separating these two clinical entities. Although antinuclear antibodies occur far more frequently in SLE and are likely to show specificity to DNA (34, 47), exceptions certainly occur in individual patients. In fact, one of our patients had a high antinuclear antibody titer which became negative with antimicrobial therapy. The evidence for a pathogenetic role of immune complexes is rapidly accumulating in a variety of infectious diseases and supports the concept that SLE may simply be a host response to one or several as yet poorly defined infections. In this context, the recent finding of a viral structure on electron microscopy in the renal tissue of patients with SLE (38, 41) is intriguing.

SUMMARY

The clinical course and renal biopsy findings of nine patients who had bacterial endocarditis with glomerulonephritis were studied in order to gain further insight into the nature, morphology and spectrum of the lesion. Two of the patients had staphylococcal endocarditis and six had culture-negative endocarditis. The principal histological reaction is diffuse proliferative glomerulonephritis, probably caused by circulating antigen-antibody complexes. Two patients had, in addition, local deposits of fibrin which may represent emboli. In general, the intensity of the proliferation reflected the severity of the clinical disease. Electron-dense deposits on the glomerular basement membranes (GBM) were seen in eight of the nine. Those patients with staphylococcal endocarditis had predominantly subepithelial deposits whereas subendothelial and intramembranous deposits were most common in those with negative blood cultures. Immunofluorescence microscopy demonstrated the presence of gamma globulin and complement on the GBM in all four patients tested (two with staphylococcal and two with culture-negative endocarditis). Serial serological data available in three patients revealed a fairly uniform pattern: serum complement, reduced initially in four, rose to normal levels during successful therapy. At the same time, rheumatoid factor (R.F.) titer (positive in two) and IgG levels rose and later fell. Three other patients had R.F. in their sera by qualitative testing. These data provide the most comprehensive evidence thus far accumulated that endocarditis like other infectious diseases is capable of causing immune-complex nephritis. Although earlier reports emphasize the tendency for glomerulonephritis to occur in those patients with endocarditis whose blood cultures are negative, the predominance of such paients in this series may simply reflect the tendency to obtain biopsy material in confusing cases. Indeed, two of our patients were presumed to have lupus erythematosus rather than endocarditis. The clinical and pathogenetic similarity of these two diseases was emphasized.

ACKNOWLEDGMENTS

We acknowledge with appreciation the critical review by Dr. Robert G. Petersdorf.

APPENDIX

Case Reports and Biopsy Descriptions

1. (A.H.)

This 40 year old Eskimo man, without previous heart disease, was hospitalized October 28, 1968 because of fever (104.6° F), pleuritic chest pain, heart failure and hematuria of two weeks duration. His heart was enlarged and the precordium was hyperdynamic. Apical systolic and parasternal decrescendo diastolic murmurs were heard. The liver was enlarged and tender. The spleen was palpable 5 cm below the left costal margin. The initial electrocardiogram was normal, but a significant increase in voltage appeared four weeks later. The chest radiograph revealed cardiomegaly and pulmonary venous congestion but no pleural effusion. His initial hematocrit (HCT) was **24%**, white blood cell count (WBC) 8,700/mm³ with 80% polymorphonuclear forms and the erythrocyte sedimentation rate (ESR) was 132 mm/hr. His urine contained 100 mg/100 ml protein, a large number of red cells and red cell casts, and a moderate number of white cells and granular casts. His blood urea nitrogen (BUN) was 22 mg/100 ml, creatinine 1.9 mg/100 ml and serum albumin was 1.9 g/100 ml. Six days after admission, before antibiotic therapy was initiated, his complement level ($^CH_{50}$) was 0 and rheumatoid factor was $1 \rightarrow 2560$. The antistreptolysin O (ASLO) titer remained less than 100. Quantitative determination of immunoglobulins was normal (Table II).

Nine blood cultures were negative. Nevertheless, he was treated with 20 million units of intravenous penicillin G and 2 g of streptomycin per day from 10-31-68 to 11-20-68.

The renal biopsy taken 11-1-68, one day after beginning therapy, revealed 11 diffusely hypercellular glomeruli by light microscopy. Neutrophilic infiltration was prominent. Five of the glomeruli had epithelial proliferation (synechiae) and two had foci of necrosis. Tubular epithelial changes consisted of mitotic figures, thinning and lipid and hyaline droplets. Casts containing red cells and white cells were noted within tubular lumina. The interstitium was moderately edematous and contained many foci of lymphocytes and neutrophils. No vascular changes were noted. Immunofluorescence microscopy (Fig. 8) revealed the presence of gamma globulin and B_{1C}-B_{1A} distributed in a nodular pattern on the peripheral glomerular basement membrane and the mesangium. Electron microscopic examination revealed marked swelling of endothelial cells in the glomeruli as well as numerous neutrophils in glomerular capillary lumina. Small electron dense deposits were noted on the epithelial and endothelial sides of the glomerular basement membrane as well as within its substance and in mesangial regions.

He initially improved but gradually developed heart failure and died August 21, 1969 of severe aortic insufficiency.

Post-mortem examination of the heart revealed dilatation of the heart, particularly the left ventricle. The aortic valve was incompetent, perforated in one leaflet and generally thickened. Microscopically, the valves were fibrotic but contained no inflammatory tissue or bacterial colonies. Electron microscopy of frozen heart and kidney tissue by Dr. George Burch failed to reveal virus particles.⁴ No renal lesions were seen at this time.

⁴ Our appreciation to Dr. Burch for his kind assistance.

2. (D.C.)

This 34 year old black man with a long history of parenteral drug abuse, was hospitalized March 14, 1969 because of progressive weakness, cough and weight loss for two weeks, and chills and fever for three days. He was extremely cachectic, lethargic and acutely ill with a temperature of 102° F. Multiple typical Roth spots were seen in both fundi. His heart was not enlarged but a high-pitched short systolic murmur was heard along the lower portion of the left sternal border. His liver was enlarged and the spleen was palpable 3 cm below the left costal margin. Chest radiograph showed extensive bilateral patchy pneumonitis containing a large number of cavitating nodules. The electrocardiogram was normal. HCT was 24% and WBC was 19,600/mm³ with 30% polymorphonuclear forms. The BUN was 77 mg/100 ml and the creatinine was 1.6 mg/100 ml. Rheumatoid factor titer was $1 \rightarrow 160$. The antinuclear factor was negative. Quantitative immune globulin determination revealed a slightly elevated IgG level and the initial complement level was reduced (Table II). The bilirubin was elevated to 4.4 mg/100 ml and later reached a peak of 7.4 mg/100 ml. His urine contained 300 mg/100 ml protein, innumerable red cells and an occasional red cell cast. Six blood cultures were positive for coagulase positive staphylococci. He was started on intravenous cephalothin and two days later, methicillin was substituted.

Light microscopy (Fig. 2) of the renal biopsy performed two weeks after therapy was started revealed 40 glomeruli, all of which were diffusely hypercellular and contained increased number of neutrophils. In most glomeruli, the intraglomerular cells appeared to be primarily mesangial resulting in accentuation of the lobular pattern. Irregular deposits were seen on the epithelial aspect of the glomerular basement membranes (GBM). The tubules showed many hyaline droplets, areas of degeneration and contained many casts. The interstitium was moderately edematous and contained many plasma cells, lymphocytes and a few neutrophils. Arterioles contained hyaline deposits. Immunofluorescence staining revealed irregular granular deposits of gamma G and B_{1C}-B_{1A} globulins along the GBM. By electron microscopy large subepithelial "humps" were noted as well as numerous osmiophilic densities within the substance of a GBM (Fig. 9).

After three weeks, he began to defervesce, gain weight and his murmur became less intense. During therapy, the complement titer rose to normal levels, the rheumatoid factor titer rose and then fell, and the IgG levels remained elevated (Table

II). Microscopic hematuria persisted throughout hospitalization. He was discharged and lost to follow-up.

3. (M.O.)

This 33 year old white man, a parenteral drug abuser, was transferred from another hospital because of six days of oliguric renal failure and high fever. His blood cultures had been positive for coagulase positive staphylococci and his BUN was over 100 mg/100 ml. During this period of six days of hospitalization, his daily urine output was less than 500 ml and contained 4+ protein and many red cells.

At the time of transfer, he was febrile (102° F) and lethargic. A systolic murmur at the base was heard. The liver was enlarged to the iliac crest and was tender. The spleen was not palpable. There were no petechiae, splinter hemorrhages or Roth spots. The HCT was 27%, WBC 13 300/mm³, ESR 103 mm/hr. His urine contained 100 mg/100 ml protein and 30–40 red blood cells per high power field and several red cell casts. The BUN was 41 and his creatinine was 11.7 mg/100 ml. His serum complement was reduced, the rheumatoid factor was negative and the IgG level slightly elevated (Table II). His ASLO titer was 12.

Shortly after admission, intensive hemodialysis was begun improving the electrolytes and reducing the BUN and creatinine. Intravenous cephalothin was continued. Proteinuria and hematuria persisted and he remained oliguric for a total of four weeks.

A renal biopsy taken February 14, 1970 contained four glomeruli and consisted of cortex and medulla. One glomerulus was obsolescent and the remaining three were enlarged with mesangial cell hyperplasia and marked neutrophilic infiltrate. Subepithelial deposits were seen. The interstitium was very edematous and contained large numbers of neutrophils, plasma cells and lymphocytes. There were foci of tubular necrosis with regeneration. Red blood cells, white blood cells and hyaline casts were present in many tubules. The vessels were normal. Tissue for immunofluorescence staining contained no glomeruli. Electron microscopic examination confirmed the presence of numerous large subepithelial deposits on the GBM.

Following the last hemodialysis on February 16, 1970, his creatinine was 12.2 mg/100 ml and remained at that level for ten days. Prednisolone, 80 mg per day, was started and his oliguria, which had apparently begun to improve, cleared rapidly and within ten days of starting steroid therapy, his serum creatinine had fallen to 6.6 mg/100 ml and reached a level of 4.4 mg/100 ml when he was discharged on March 13, 1970. His serum complement had returned to normal and steroids were therefore discontinued. His renal function continued to improve but proteinuria and red cell casts have persisted.

A second renal biopsy taken six months later contained 18 glomeruli, five of which were obsolescent. Mesangial cell hyperplasia was recognizable in the remainder. Organized synechiae were present in five of these. About one third of the interstitium was fibrotic and contained only a small number of chronic inflammatory cells. The tubules and vessels were not remarkable. By immunofluorescence staining the presence of gamma globulin and B_{1C}-B_{1A} complement was noted primarily in the mesangial regions and some was distributed in a granular pattern on the peripheral GBM (Fig. 6). Electron microscopy revealed electron dense deposits similar to those seen on the first biopsy but the predominant location was in the mesangial region.

4. (E.H.)

This 71 year old white man, with known aortic stenosis and a history of syncope, was admitted February 13, 1962 because of three days of fever and myalgia. He was lethargic and febrile to 104° F. The blood pressure was 100/80 mm Hg and pulse 96/min. Two of four blood cultures were positive for group B beta-hemolytic streptococcus. Five days after admission, the urinalysis revealed minimal proteinuria and many red cells with a few red cell casts.

He was treated with high-dose penicillin and streptomycin and gradually improved. Red cells and casts disappeared from his urine.

Renal biopsy taken one month after therapy was started revealed 19 glomeruli, three of which were obsolescent. The remainder were unremarkable. The interstitium, tubules and vessels were normal for a man of this age. Electron microscopy revealed occasional electron dense deposits in the mesangial region and the subendothelial space near the mesangium.

He was discharged March 29, 1962, two weeks after cessation of antibiotic therapy. Two months after discharge, a new soft aortic diastolic murmur was heard. This murmur grew progressively louder and he developed increasing congestive heart failure requiring rehospitalization. He died one year later. Urinalysis remained normal except for trace protein.

Autopsy revealed a dilated hypertrophied heart. The aortic valve was calcified and very irregular and stenotic, measuring 3 mm in greatest diameter. There was a perforation of the right coronary cusp measuring 5 mm in diameter. The remaining valves were normal.

5. (E.B.)

This 58 year old white man was admitted to the hospital on May 9, 1963 because of a seven-month chronic illness which had begun with pneumonia the previous October. Although penicillin therapy was apparently successful, he became progressively weaker, lost 40 pounds, had recurrent fevers and developed marked purpura. There was no prior history of rheumatic fever or heart murmur.

On physical examination, he was a chronically ill man in no distress. His blood pressure was 117/78 mm Hg, pulse 86/min and temperature 99.8° F. Clubbing was noted. His legs and abdomen were covered with purpuric and non-blanching petechial lesions. No Roth spots or emoblic phenomena were noted. The heart was not enlarged. Murmurs of mitral and aortic regurgitation were heard. The liver was enlarged and tender. The spleen was palpable 6 cm below the left costal margin.

His hematocrit was 32%, ESR 58, reticulocyte count 3.7% corrected to 2.8%, WBC 2,300/mm³ with 60% polymorphonuclear forms. Platelet count was 40.000 'mm³. The urine contained a trace of protein, red cells and red cell casts. BUN was 17 and creatinine 1.3 mg/100 ml. During the patient's long hospitalization, 18 blood cultures were negative. Several sputa were negative for mycobacteria. Cultures of spinal fluid for bacteria and fungi were negative. Cultures of purpuric lesions were negative. The HCT gradually fell to 26%. The Sia water test was negative. Lupus erythematosus preparations contained many "tart cells" but no lupus cells. Rheumatoid factor was positive. Serum electrophoresis revealed a moderate diffuse elevation of gamma globulin. Immunoelectrophoresis revealed an increased gamma and alpha globulin (beta 2A); macroglobulins were only slightly elevated. Chest radiograph showed a normal heart size and old healed hilar granulomatous disease. PPD was positive. Because of the suspicion of bacterial endocarditis, he was treated with large doses of penicillin and streptomycin.

The renal biopsy done August 2, 1963 following ten days of penicillin therapy contained 12 glomeruli all of which showed slight mesangial hypercellularity. The tubular epithelium contained many hyaline droplets. The interstitium contained many foci of lymphocytic and plasma cell infiltrate and some fibrosis. There was slight intimal hyperplasia of the arterioles with splitting and duplication of their internal elastic lamellae. Electron microscopy revealed multifocal mesangial and subendothelial electron dense deposits.

His fever returned and he then developed a seizure disorder. His cerebrospinal fluid contained 89 white cells/mm³, protein 144 mg/100 ml and sugar 54 mg/100 ml. All cultures were negative. Steroids and isoniazid therapy appeared to reduce the fever after cessation of penicillin. The steroids were then tapered.

Between July, 1964 and January, 1965, he was readmitted seven times for advancing congestive heart failure. Each time, he was afebrile and not anemic. He died in February, 1965 during the last admission for congestive heart failure. Post-mortem examination revealed a markedly dilated and hypertrophied left ventricle. The aortic valve had marked calcification of the valve leaflets and old calcified vegetations with a large fenestration of the valve leaflet measuring 0.3 cm in diameter. "Typical endocardial valve pockets 1.5 cm below the aortic valve about the septal wall of the left ventricle" were seen. The remaining valves were normal. No distinctive abnormalities of the kidneys were found at this time.

6. (R.A.)

This 53 year old white man entered the hospital March 1, 1965 because of three weeks of progressive orthopnea. Three years previously, an apical systolic murmur had been heard. Blood pressure was 180/90 mm Hg, pulse 130/min and regular. The neck veins were distended and there were signs of a right-sided pleural effusion with basilar rales. Physical examination during the first two days in the hospital revealed tachycardia, cardiac enlargement to the sixth intercostal space, a systolic heart murmur, splenomegaly and marked peripheral edema.

Hematocrit was 35%, WBC 8,000/mm³ with 70% polymorphonuclear forms. The sedimentation rate was 48 mm/hr. The urine had a specific gravity of 1.010, pH 6, and 15–20 RBC/high power field. There was no proteinuria or casts. BUN was 39 mg/100 ml and the electrolytes were normal. ASLO titer was 100.

Throughout hospitalization, he remained completely afebrile and never developed leukocytosis. However, his general condition deteriorated after the congestive heart failure was brought under control with digitalis and diuretics. On the second hospital day, he became mildly paretic on the left. On the tenth hospital day, his hematocrit was noted to be 38% with an elevated reticulocyte count (4.1%). The Coombs test was negative. The urinalysis at this time revealed a large number of red cells and red cell casts. Proteinuria developed and the blood urea nitrogen rose to 51 mg/100 ml.

A renal biopsy (Fig. 3) taken at this time (11th hospital day) showed 11 glomeruli all of which

178

showed some mesangial hypercellularity. In addition, three glomeruli contained glomerular tuft
proliferation, one with a synechia and another
with focal necrosis. Many hyaline droplets and a
few vacuoles were seen in tubular epithelial cells.
Tubular lumina contained white cells, red cell
casts and white cell casts. There was moderate
interstitial edema and a diffuse inflammatory infiltrate consisting primarily of plasma cells and lymphocytes and a few neutrophils. The arteries show
mild duplication of the internal elastic lamellae.
Electron microscopy (Fig. 10) revealed multiple
small subepithelial and mesangial deposits and increase in mesangial matrix.

From then until the 20th hospital day, eleven
blood cultures were obtained and all were negative. On the 11th hospital day, a murmur of aortic
regurgitation was heard for the first time. His
blood urea nitrogen continued to rise and he died
suddenly on April 19, 1969 with his BUN in the
range of 85 mg/100 ml.

Examination of the heart at autopsy revealed
an enlarged left ventricle and concomitant enlargement of the left atrium and right ventricle. There
was evidence of generalized coronary atherosclero-
sis. Gross and microscopic evidence of a massive
acute anterior wall myocardial infarction was seen.
Both the aortic and mitral valves showed evidence
of old rheumatic heart disease with thickening of
the free margin of the mitral valve and shortening
of the chordae. The aortic valve was calcified
with rigid fusion between the right and left coronary cusps. In addition, the mitral valve contained
a 1 × 5 cm excrescence and on the front surface of
each of the aortic valve leaflets were friable raised
areas up to 1.5 cm in size which were similar in
appearance. Additionally, there was a 0.7 × 0.3 cm
fenestration in the area of the fusion of the aortic
valve. At the base of the non-coronary cusp of the
aortic valve was a 0.5 × 0.3 cm ulceration having
a depressed center containing blood clot. Microscopic examination of the granulation on the aortic valve revealed the presence of gram-positive
cocci.

7. (R.W.)

This 39 year old white man developed painless
hematuria with albuminuria in September, 1965.
Two months later, he was noted to be febrile and
murmurs of aortic stenosis and regurgitation were
heard for the first time. Four blood cultures were
negative. He was treated with a short course of
penicillin but the fever persisted.

In March, 1966, he was readmitted because of
severe dyspnea. He was a pale, chronically ill man
in obvious respiratory distress. The blood pressure
was 130/60 mm Hg, pulse 120/min and he was
afebrile. No petechiae or Roth spots were noted.
Pulmonary rales were heard. The heart was enlarged. A gallop was heard along with a harsh
aortic systolic and blowing diastolic murmurs.
Quincke's sign was present. His liver and spleen
were enlarged and 2+ edema of the lower extremi-
ties was noted.

Hematocrit was 30%, WBC 7,900/mm³, ESR 80
mm/hr. The urine contained 100 mg/100 ml protein, a large number of red cells and several red
cell casts. The BUN was 37 mg/100 ml and the
creatinine 2.1 mg/100 ml. One urine culture and
nine blood cultures were negative. ASLO titer was
50 and rheumatoid factor (latex fixation) was
weakly positive. Lupus erythematosus preparations were negative.

A renal biopsy contained six glomeruli which by
light microscopy revealed diffuse intraglomerular
hypercellularity and increased numbers of neutrophils. Epithelial proliferation (crescents) were also
seen in four glomeruli. The tubular epithelium
contained hyaline droplets and lipid. A few hyaline casts were seen. There was moderate interstitial edema and multifocal areas of infiltration by
lumphocytes, neutrophils and plasma cells. There
were no vascular changes. Electron microscopy
(Fig. 11) revealed many large subendothelial and
mesangial deposits, swelling and hyperplasia of endothelial cells and the presence of neutrophils with
capillary lumina.

He was treated with diuretics and later prednisolone, 60 mg/day, for one month but the clinical
abnormalities persisted. His hematocrit was 27%,
sedimentation rate 102 mm/hr and white cell
count 15,800/mm³. His urine contained 300 mg/100
ml protein, red cells and red cell casts. His BUN
was 31 and creatinine 2.5 mg/100 ml respectively.
Bedrest, diuretics and salt restriction improved his
symptoms.

In July 1966, he was admitted for the last time
because of shortness of breath. He was in severe
congestive heart failure. His hematocrit was 31%,
WBC 21,000/mm³, BUN 60 mg/100 ml and potas-
sium was 6.2 mEq/liter. The urine contained over
500 mg/100 ml protein. In spite of therapy for
pulmonary edema and hyperkalemia, he died.

Autopsy revealed extensive destruction of the
aortic valve which contained numerous bacterial
colonies within the substance of the valve. Culture
of the valve was positive for streptococcus viri-
dans and a nonhemolytic streptococcus. There was
diffuse glomerulonephritis and an old splenic infarction.

8. (D.M.)

This 36 year old white male was admitted June
2, 1968 because of fever and weakness. He had

179

known rheumatic heart disease and had had a closed mitral commissurotomy in December, 1965. For one year, he had noticed increasing fatigability and for two months, dark urine. His blood pressure was 120/70 mm Hg, pulse 110/min and respiratory rate 36/min. There were no petechiae or Roth spots at first but two conjunctival petechiae appeared later in his course. There was definite clubbing. His heart was enlarged and in normal sinus rhythm. There was a right ventricular heave and murmurs of mitral stenosis and mitral regurgitation were noted. The liver and spleen were enlarged. His hematocrit was 25%, reticulocyte count 6.1 corrected to 3.6%, white count of 6,800/mm³ and ESR 62 mm/hr. The urine contained 100 mg/100 ml protein, many red cells, few white cells and several red cell casts. The BUN was 42 and creatinine 3.9 mg/100 ml respectively and gradually fell over the course of three weeks while on antimicrobial therapy (Table II). The complement level was 91 $^CH_{50}$ units (normal 100–130). Serum electrophoresis revealed a diffuse gamma globulin elevation. Antinuclear factor was 4+ but no LE cells were seen. ASLO titer was 100 units. Latex fixation was weakly reactive. The Coombs test, direct and indirect, was negative. Urine culture grew an insignificant number of organisms. Six blood cultures and two bone marrow cultures were negative.

The renal biopsy taken June 8, 1968 contained 17 glomeruli (Fig. 4). Two were obsolescent, 11 were diffusely hypercellular and four showed focal areas of hypercellularity. Two glomeruli contained crescents and no glomerular basement membrane deposits were demonstrable by light microscopy. The tubular epithelium contained mitotic figures, was focally necrotic and contained lipid, hyaline and vacuolar inclusions. Their lumina contained red cells, hyaline and granular casts. There was minimal edema of the interstitium but there were several foci of neutrophilic and plasma cell infiltrate. No vascular changes were noted. Fluorescence microscopy revealed granular deposits of IgG and B_{1C}-B_{1A} localized largely to mesangial portions of the glomeruli. Electron microscopy showed electron dense deposits localized primarily to the mesangial region of the glomerulus but also seen in subendothelial portions of the peripheral glomerular basement membrane.

He was treated with penicillin and streptomycin for 15 days and then discharged on oral penicillin for two weeks. By September, 1968, he was feeling quite well and had resumed full activity. The clubbing had abated. The spleen was no longer palpable but the heart murmurs persisted. He was able to enter stage III of the multistage exercise test which is equivalent to functional class I or II. His hematocrit was 42% and ESR 4 mm/hr. His creatinine clearance had risen from 52 ml/min to 112 ml/min. Serum creatinine was 1.0 mg/100 ml. The urinalysis was normal in that no protein was present and there were only 1–2 RBC/high power field. When next seen in June, 1969, he remained perfectly well while being maintained on digoxin, diuretics and salt restriction. The ANF titer and rheumatoid factor had become negative. By March 1971, he required open heart repair because of re-stenosis of the mitral valve.

9. (W.W.)

This 46 year old white man was admitted to the hospital on March 3, 1969 because of gross hematuria. He had rheumatic heart disease with aortic stenosis and regurgitation and for five years, had had progressive dyspnea on exertion with angina. He had been taking prophylactic penicillin for several years. His blood pressure was 120/84 mm Hg, pulse 84/min and temperature 99.6° F. There were no petechiae or funduscopic abnormalities. His heart was enlarged and hyperdynamic with the point of maximal impulse at the sixth intercostal space of the mid-clavicular line. Murmurs of aortic stenosis and insufficiency were heard. The liver was slightly enlarged and the spleen was not palpable. There was no edema.

The initial HCT was 46%, WBC 14,400/mm³ and ESR 67 mm/hr. His urine contained 25 mg/100 ml protein and the sediment had 10–15 red cells per high power field, "many" white cells and a few red cell casts.

The renal biopsy (Fig. 1) taken March 20, 1969 revealed 27 glomeruli, two of which were obsolescent. Only three showed some hypercellularity which was localized primarily to the mesangial region. Several red cell casts were present in the tubules. The interstitium contained an occasional small focus of lymphocytes. Multiple small hyaline deposits were seen in arterioles. The major changes by electron microscopy were hyaline deposits in the mesangial region and ischemic glomerular basement membrane changes. No osmiophilic deposits were seen in the tissue examined by electron microscopy.

In spite of 11 negative blood cultures, therapy for bacterial endocarditis with penicillin and streptomycin was given for two weeks. His temperature fell from 100.4° F to levels below 99° F, the ESR rate fell and the complement level was measured at 125 $^CH_{50}$ units (Table II). His clinical condition improved and he returned to work after discharge on March 31, 1969.

One week later, he became suddenly and severely short of breath, with chest pain and congestive heart failure. A loud murmur of mitral regurgitation was heard for the first time. Cardiac cath-

180

eterization revealed mitral regurgitation. Following open heart surgery for repair of ruptured chordae tendinae of the otherwise completely normal mitral valve and replacement of the aortic valve with a Starr-Edwards prothesis, he has done well and returned to work.

REFERENCES

1. Abruzzo, J. L. and Christian, C. L.: The induction of a rheumatoid factor-like substance in rabbits. J. Exp. Med., *114:* 791, 1961.
2. Allen, A. C.: The Kidney. 2nd Ed., Grune and Stratton, New York, 1962, p. 195.
3. Allison, A. C., Hendrickse, R. G., Edington, G. M., Houba, V., De Petris, S. and Adeniyi, A.: Immune complexes in the nephrotic syndrome of African children. Lancet, *1:* 1232, 1969.
4. Baehr, G.: Glomerular lesions of subacute bacterial endocarditis. J. Exp. Med., *15:* 330, 1912.
5. Baehr, G.: Renal complications of endocarditis. Trans. Assoc. Amer. Phys., *46:* 87, 1931.
6. Baehr, G. and Lande, H.: Glomerulonephritis as a complication of subacute streptococcus endocarditis. J. A. M. A., *75:* 789, 1920.
7. Baldwin, D. S., Levine, B. B., McCluskey, R. T. and Gallo, G. R.: Renal failure and interstitial nephritis due to penicillin and methicillin. New Eng. J. Med., *279:* 1245, 1968.
8. Bartfield, H.: Incidence and significance of seropositive tests for rheumatoid in non-rheumatoid disease. Ann. Intern. Med., *52:* 1059, 1960.
9. Beeson, P. B., Brannon, E. S. and Warren, J. V.: Observations on the sites of removal of bacteria from blood in patients with bacterial endocarditis. J. Exp. Med., *81:* 9, 1945.
10. Bell, E. T.: Glomerular lesions associated with endocarditis. Amer. J. Path., *8:* 639, 1932.
11. Bernhard, G. C., Lange, R. L. and Hensley, G. T.: Aortic disease with valvular insufficiency as a principal manifestation of systemic lupus erythematosus. Ann. Intern. Med., *71:* 81, 1969.
12. Black, J. A., Challacombe, D. N. and Ockenden, B. G.: Nephrotic syndrome associated with bacteremia after shunt operations for hydrocephalus. Lancet, *2:* 921, 1965.
13. Boonshaft, B., Maher, J. F. and Schreiner, G. E.: Nephrotic syndrome associated with osteomyelitis without secondary amyloidosis. Arch. Intern. Med., *125:* 320, 1970.
14. Brauninger, G. E. and Remington, J. S.: Nephropathy associated with methicillin therapy. J. A. M. A., *203:* 103, 1968.
15. Braunstein, G. D., Lewis, E. J., Galvanek, E. G., Hamilton, A. and Bell, W. R.: The nephrotic syndrome associated with secondary syphilis. An immune deposit disease. Amer. J. Med., *48:* 643, 1970.
16. Burch, G. E. and Colcolough, H. L.: Progressive coxsackie viral pancarditis and nephritis. Ann. Intern. Med., *71:* 963, 1969.
17. Carpenter, C. C. J. and Wallace, C. K.: Bacterial endocarditis: current concepts. Johns Hopkins Med. J., *124:* 339, 1969.
18. Cathcart, E. S., Williams, R. C., Ross, H. and Calkins, E.: The relationship of the la-
tex fixation test to the clinical and serologic manifestations of leprosy. Amer. J. Med., *31:* 758, 1961.
19. Cherubin, C. E.: The medical sequelae of narcotic addiction. Ann. Intern. Med., *67:* 23, 1967.
20. Cherubin, C. E., Baden, M., Kavaler, F., Lerner, S. and Cline, W.: Infective endocarditis in narcotic addicts. Ann. Intern. Med., *69:* 1091, 1968.
21. Christian, C. L.: Immune complex disease. New Engl. J. Med., *280:* 878, 1969.
22. Christie, R. V.: Penicillin in subacute bacterial endocarditis. Brit. Med. J., *1:* 1, 1948.
23. Cluff, L. E., Reynolds, R. C., Page, D. L. and Breckenridge, J. L.: Staphylococcal bacteremia and altered host resistance. Ann. Intern. Med., *69:* 859, 1968.
24. Comerford, F. R. and Cohen, A. S.: The nephropathy of systemic lupus erythematosus. Medicine, *46:* 425, 1967.
25. Cordeiro, A., Costa, H. and Laginha, F.: Editorial: immunologic phase of subacute bacterial endocarditis. A new concept and general considerations. Amer. J. Cardiol., *16:* 477, 1965.
26. Cornil, L., Mosinger, M. and Joure, A-X: Les lésions rénales dans les endocardites malignes. Arch. Méd. gén. colon., *5:* 33, 1936.
27. Dixon, F. J.: The role of antigen-antibody complexes in disease. Harvey Lectures, *58:* 21, 1963.
28. Dixon, F. J.: Editorial. The pathogenesis of glomerulonephritis. Amer. J. Med., *44:* 493, 1968.
29. Dixon, F. J., Feldman, J. D. and Vazquez, J.: pathogenesis of a laboratory model resembling the spectrum of human glomerulonephritis. J. Exp. Med., *113:* 899, 1961.
30. Donzelot, E., Kaufmann, H. and Escalle, Y.: Etude des portides du sérum sanquin dans les endocardites infectieuses subaiqües. Arch. Mal. Coeur, *42:* 405, 1949.
31. Drutz, D. J., Lu, W-H. and Chen, T. S.: The continuous bacteremia of lepromatous leprosy. Abstract. Clin. Res., *17:* 120, 1969.
32. Epstein, W. V., Engleman, E. P. and Ross, M.: Evaluation of a qualitative precipitation reaction for the detection of the rheumatoid factor. Ann. Rheumat. Dis., *16:* 448, 1957.
33. Falls, W. F., Ford, K. L., Ashworth, C. T. and Carter, N. W.: The nephrotic syndrome in secondary syphilis. Report of a case with renal biopsy findings. Ann. Intern. Med., *63:* 1047, 1965.
34. Friou, G. J.: Antinuclear antibodies: diagnostic significance and methods. Arth. and Rheum., *10:* 151, 1967.
35. Geraci, J. E., Hanson, K. C., Giuliani, E. R.: Endocarditis caused by coagulase negative staphylococci. Mayo Clin. Proc., *43:* 420, 1968.
36. Germuth, F. G., Senterfit, L. B. and Pollack, A. D.: Immune complex disease. I. Experimental acute and chronic glomerulonephritis. Johns Hopkins Med. J., *120:* 225, 1967.
37. Goldman, M.: Fluorescent antibody methods. Academic Press, New York, 1968, p. 173–183.
38. Györkey, F., Min, K-W., Sincovics, I. G. and Györkey, P.: Systemic lupus erythematosus and myxovirus. New Engl. J. Med., *280:* 333, 1969.

39. Heptinstall, R. H.: Pathology of the Kidney. 1st Ed., Little, Brown and Co., Boston, 1966, p. 325–331.

40. Highman, B., Altland, P. D. and Roshe, J.: Staphylococcal endocarditis and glomerulonephritis in dogs. Circ. Res., *7:* 982, 1959.

41. Hurd, E. R., Eigenbrodt, E., Ziff, M. and Strunk, S. W.: Cytoplasmic tubular structures in kidney biopsies in systemic lupus erythematosus. Arth. and Rheum., *12:* 541, 1969.

42. Kabat, E. A. and Mayer, M. M.: Experimental Immunochemistry. 2nd Ed., Charles C Thomas, Springfield, 1961, p. 149–153.

43. Keefer, C. S.: Subacute bacterial endocarditis: active cases without bacteremia. Ann. Intern. Med., *11:* 714, 1937–1938.

44. Kerr, A. Jr.: Subacute Bacterial Endocarditis. Charles C Thomas, Springfield, 1955, p. 66, 67, 89, 162.

45. Koffler, D., Schur, P. H. and Kunkel, H. G.: Immunological studies concerning the nephritis of systemic lupus erythematosus. J. Exp. Med., *126:* 607, 1967.

46. Koletsky, S. and Rivera-Velez, J. M.: Renin-angiotensin system in microembolic renal hypertension. Arch. Path., *85:* 1, 1968.

47. Krishnan, C. and Kaplan, M. H.: Immunopathologic studies of systemic lupus erythematosus. II. Antinuclear reaction of γ-globulin eluted from homogenates and isolated glomeruli of kidneys from patients with lupus nephritis. J. Clin. Invest., *46:* 569, 1967.

48. Kunkel, H. G., Simon, H. J. and Fudenberg, H.: Observations concerning positive serological reactions for rheumatoid factor in certain patients with sarcoidosis and other hyperglobulinemic states. Arth. and Rheum., *1:* 289, 1958.

49. Lam, C. N., McNeish, A. S. and Gibson, A. A. M.: Nephrotic syndrome associated with complement deficiency and staphylococcus albus bacteremia. Scot. Med. J., *14:* 86, 1969.

50. Libman, E.: Characterization of various forms of endocarditis. J. A. M. A., *80:* 813, 1923.

51. Libman, E. and Friedberg, C. K.: Subacute Bacterial Endocarditis. 2nd Ed., Oxford, New York, 1948, p. 68–76.

52. Lisan, P., Uricchio, J. F., Marino, D. J., Deshmukh, M. and Likoff, W.: Staphylococcal endocarditis. Amer. Heart. J., *59:* 184, 1960.

53. Louria, D. B., Hensle, T. and Rose, J.: The major medical complications of heroin addiction. Ann. Intern. Med., *67:* 1, 1967.

54. Louria, D. B., Kaminski, T., Grieco, M. and Singer, J.: Aberrant forms of bacteria and fungi found in blood or cerebrospinal fluid. Arch. Intern. Med., *124:* 39, 1969.

55. Messner, R. P., Laxdal, T., Quie, P. G. and Williams, R. C. Jr.: Rheumatoid factors in subacute bacterial endocarditis—bacterium, duration of disease or genetic predisposition. Ann. Intern. Med., *68:* 746, 1968.

56. Michael, A. F., Herdman, R. C., Fish, A. J., Pickering, R. J. and Vernier, R. L.: Chronic membranoproliferative glomerulonephritis with hypocomplementemia. Transplantation Proc., *1:* 925, 1969.

57. Monteiro, G. E. and Lillicrap, C. A.: Case of mumps nephritis. Brit. Med. J., *4:* 721, 1967.

58. Neu, H. C. and Goldreyer, B.: Isolation of protoplasts in a case of enterococcal endocarditis. Amer. J. Med., *45:* 784, 1968.

59. Nickerson, D. S., Williams, R. C. Jr., Boxmeyer, M. and Quie, P. G.: Increased opsonic capacity of serum in chronic heroin addiction. Ann. Intern. Med., *72:* 671, 1970.

60. Peltier, A. and Christian, C. L.: The presence of the "rheumatoid factor" in sera from patients with syphilis. Arth. and Rheum., *2:* 1, 1959.

61. Pillsbury, P. L. and Fiese, M. J.: Subacute bacterial endocarditis. Follow-up study of thirty patients treated with penicillin. Arch. Intern. Med., *85:* 675, 1950.

62. Pollack, V. E. and Pirani, C. L.: Renal histological findings of systemic lupus erythematosus. Mayo Clin. Proc., *44:* 630, 1968.

63. Rames, L., Wise, B., Goodman, J. R. and Piel, C. F.: Renal disease with staphylococcal albus bacteremia. A complication in ventriculoatrial shunts. J. A. M. A., *212:* 1671, 1970.

64. Randall, R. E. Jr., Bridi, G. S. and Still, W. J. S.: Glomerulonephritis following infectious mononucleosis. Abstract. 3rd Meeting, American Society of Nephrology, 1969, p. 56.

65. Resenekov, L.: Staphylococcal endocarditis following mitral valvotomy with special reference to coagulase-negative staphylococcal albus. Lancet, *2:* 597, 1959.

66. Roberts, W. C. and Rabson, A. S.: Focal glomerular lesions in fungal endocarditis. Ann. Intern. Med., *56:* 610, 1962.

67. RuDusky, B. M.: Recurrent Osler's nodes in systemic lupus erythematosus. Angiology, *29:* 33, 1964.

68. Sapira, J. D.: The narcotic addict as a medical patient. Amer. J. Med., *45:* 555, 1968.

69. Schainuck, L. I., Striker, G. E., Cutler, R. E. and Benditt, E. P.: Structural-functional correlations in renal disease. II. The correlations. Human Path., *1:* 631, 1970.

70. Shinefield, H. R. and Ribble, J. C.: Current aspects infections and diseases related to staphylococcal aureus. Ann. Rev. Med., *16:* 263, 1965.

71. Singer, J. M., Plotz, C. M., Peralto, F. M. and Lyons, H. C.: Presence of anti-gamma globulin factors in sera of patients with active pulmonary tuberculosis. Ann. Intern. Med., *56:* 545, 1962.

72. Singer, J. M. and Plotz, C. M.: The latex-fixation test. I. Application to the serologic diagnosis of rheumatoid arthritis. Amer. J. Med., *21:* 888, 1966.

73. Soothill, J. F. and Hendrickse, R. G.: Some immunologic studies of the nephrotic syndrome of Nigerian children. Lancet, *2:* 269, 1967.

74. Spain, D. M. and King, D. W.: The effect of penicillin on the renal lesions of subacute bacterial endocarditis. Ann. Intern. Med., *36:* 1086, 1952.

75. Stickler, G. B., Shin, M. H., Burke, E. C., Holley, K. E., Miller, R. H., and Segar, W. E.: Diffuse glomerulonephritis associated with infected ventriculoatrial shunt. New Eng. J. Med., *279:* 1077, 1968.

76. Striker, G. E., Schainuck, L. I., Cutler, R. E. and Benditt, E. P.: Structural-functional correlations in renal disease. I. A method for assaying and classifying histopatholic changes in renal disease. Human Path., *1:* 615, 1970.

77. Tu. W. H., Shearn, M. A. and Lee, J. C.: Acute diffuse glomerulonephritis in acute staphylococcal endocarditis. Ann. Intern. Med., *71:* 335. 1969.
78. Tumulty, P. A. and Harvey, A. M.: Experience in the management of subacute bacterial endocarditis treated with penicillin. Amer. J. Med., *4:* 37, 1948.
79. Unanue, E. R. and Dixon, F. J.: Experimental glomerulonephritis:immunological events and pathogenetic mechanisms. Adv. Immunological events and pathogenetic mechanisms. Adv. Immunol., *6:* 1, 1967.
80. Utz. J. P., Houk, V. N. and Alling, D. W.: Clinical and laboratory studies of mumps. IV viruria and abnormal renal functions. New Eng. J. Med., *270:* 1283, 1964.
81. Vassalli, P., Simon, G. and Rouiller, C.: Electron microscopic study of glomerular lesions resulting from intravascular fibrin formation. Amer. J. Path., *43:* 578, 1963.
82. Villarreal. H. and Sokoloff, L.: The occurrence of renal insufficiency in subacute bacterial endocarditis. Amer. J. Med. Sci., *220:* 655, 1950.
83. Ward. P. A. and Kibukamusoke. J. W.: Evidence for soluble immune complexes in the pathogenesis of the glomerulonephritis of quartan malaria. Lancet, *1:* 283. 1969.
84. Werner, A. S., Cobbs. C. G., Kaye, D. and Hook. E. W.: Studies on the bacteremia of bacterial endocarditis. J. A. M. A., *202:* 199. 1967.

85. Williams. R. C. Jr. and Kunkel. H. G.: Rheumatoid factor, complement, and conglutinin aberrations in patients with subacute bacterial endocarditis. J. Clin. Invest., *41:* 666. 1962.
86. Williams, R. C. Jr. and Kunkel. H. G.: Antibodies to rabbit γ-globulin after immunizing with various preparations of autologous γ-globulin. Proc. Soc. Exp. Biol. Med., *112:* 554. 1963.
87. Williams. R. C. Jr. and Kunkel. H. G.: Rheumatoid factors and their disappearance following therapy in patients with subacute bacterial endocarditis. Abstract. Arth. and Rheum.. *5:* 126. 1962.
88. Willkens. R. F., Anderson. R. V. and Gilliland, B. C.: Response of sensitized rabbits to intra-articular gamma globulin. Arth. and Rheum.. *11:* 418. 1968.
89. Willkens, R. F. and Decker. J. L.: Rheumatoid arthritis with serological evidence suggesting systemic lupus erythematosus:clinical. serological and chromatographic studies. Arth. and Rheum.. *6:* 720. 1963.
90. Yuceoglu. A. M., Berkovich, S. and Minkowitz. S.: Acute glomerulonephritis associated with ECHO virus type 9 infection. J. Ped.. *69:* 603. 1966.
91. Yuceoglu. A. M., Berkovich, S. and Minkowitz. S.: Acute' glomerulonephritis as a complication of varicella. J. A. M. A.. *202:* 879. 1967.

MECHANISMS INVOLVED IN THE DEPOSITION OF IMMUNE COMPLEXES IN TISSUES*

By CHARLES G. COCHRANE

The observations that immune complexes circulate in the bloodstream in experimental and human diseases stimulated considerable research into their role in immunologic injury. Studies of experimental models in the late 1950s demonstrated that the presence of complexes in the circulation coincides temporally with the development of lesions in glomeruli, arteries, endocardium, spleen, and elsewhere. As complexes were demonstrable in the lesions using fluorescent antibody techniques, it was reasonable to assume that they reached their target sites after passage through the bloodstream. The immune complex in the circulation, in fact, provided the most plausible explanation of the question of how antibody molecules could be transported from the lymphoid organs, where they were fabricated, to the target tissue.

One of the major areas to be investigated at that point was the mechanism whereby the circulating complexes left the bloodstream to be deposited in tissues. Were the complexes phagocytized by endothelial cells or did they have a particular affinity for cells or structures in the vessel walls? Did the complexes possess an electrostatic charge that allowed binding to occur in vessels? Was there an active mechanism that induced changes in the blood vessels leading to deposition of the complexes?

Work being conducted in several laboratories was directed at these questions. Immune complexes infused intravenously in animals could be shown to induce injury histologically, but interestingly, the results were variable and the lesions were not always the same as those seen in the primary model, immune complex disease (serum sickness) in rabbits. Also, in our hands and others, fluorescent antibodies, when employed, often revealed a pattern of immune complexes in glomeruli different from that seen in experimental serum sickness. Germuth and Pollack (1) infused antibody into rabbits having antigen already present in the circulation. The antigen was eliminated at much the same rate as in serum sickness and the rabbits developed mild swelling of glomerular endothelial cells and occasional foci of arterial inflammation in vessels of the stomach,

* Publication No. 481 from the Scripps Clinic and Research Foundation. The work was supported by the United States Public Health Service Grant AI-07007, National Multiple Sclerosis Society Grant 459, and a Grant-in-Aid from the American Heart Association and the Council for Tobacco Research.

duodenum, or peripancreatic tissues. Functional evidence of glomerular injury, i.e. proteinuria, was not tested. The coronary arteries, most frequent targets in serum sickness, were not involved. About half the rabbits showed one or a combination of these lesions. McCluskey and coworkers (2–4) injected immune complexes into mice and rats which developed glomerular, endocardial, and, to a lesser extent, arterial lesions within 36 hr of the first injection. The glomerular lesions contained large numbers of neutrophils and thus differed from the acute lesions in serum sickness of rabbits. In our laboratory, the results obtained from injecting preformed immune complexes in over 80 rabbits and 200 mice were inconsistent and variable. In mice, lesions were found in the glomeruli on occasions, but these appeared to be caused by immune precipitates in glomerular capillary lumina and mesangial cells as seen by immune fluorescence. A granular pattern of fluorescence distributed along the glomerular basement membrane, the hallmark of serum sickness, was not seen. In rabbits, mild swelling of glomerular endothelial cells was not accompanied by deposited immune complexes along the basement membrane and thus the mild lesions could not be attributed positively to immune complexes. In addition, Michael et al (5) infused aggregated gamma globulin in mice leading to uptake of aggregates by mesangial cells, i.e., in a location not associated with typical glomerular injury. The difficulty in obtaining histologic changes and significant fluorescent patterns consistently with passively transferred, preformed immune complexes suggested that some essential factor was missing in the experimental protocol. This prompted a series of investigations dealing with the mechanisms responsible for deposition.

Evidence of an active process required for deposition of circulating colloidal particles was obtained by Benacerraf et al. (6). Mice injected intravenously with colloidal carbon were then given histamine, 5-hydroxytryptamine (serotonin), epinephrine, or preformed immune complexes. In each case, carbon deposited in the intimal layer of large arteries, endocardium of the heart, and in the walls of venules in various sites. The immune complexes were thought to liberate vasoactive amines in vivo, leading to deposition of the carbon. In our laboratory, immune complexes themselves (7, 8) could be made to deposit in the walls of venules in guinea pigs by simultaneous infusion of agents that increased vascular permeability or liberated vasoactive amines from the mast cells. The immune complexes could be detected in the vessel walls in a fine granular pattern with the fluorescent antibody technique, almost identical to the pattern seen in vessels in serum sickness (Fig. 1). Anaphylatoxin, passive anaphylaxis, and the known histamine liberator octylamine all produced release of histamine from mast cells in vivo and the deposition of circulating immune complexes. Pretreatment with antihistamines prevented increased vascular permeability and deposition of circulating complexes.

Examination of the affected blood vessels histologically indicated that the immune complexes were trapped along a limiting membrane. Using particles visible with the electron microscope, the membrane was identified as the vascular basement membrane (7). This suggested that a process of filtration existed in which the basement membrane prevented passage of the immune complexes through the vessel wall during a state of increased permeability.

In keeping with the notion that immune complexes deposit by a process of filtration was the finding that only large immune complexes became entrapped

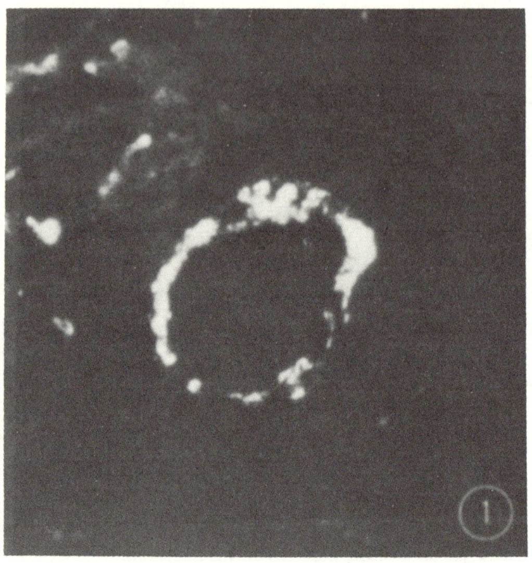

Fig. 1. Fluorescent photomicrograph of a small vessel in the lung of a guinea pig showing the deposition of bovine serum albumin (BSA)–anti-BSA complexes in the vessel wall. This section was treated with fluorescent anti–rabbit gamma globulin. Treatment with fluorescent anti-BSA or anti–guinea pig C'3 gave a similar fluorescent pattern. Electron photomicrographs in previous studies showed the complexes and other markers to lie between and beneath endothelial cells, up against the limiting basement membranes. $\times$ 350.

in vessel walls (9). Complexes of various sizes, i.e. prepared by varying the quantities of antigen, were assayed for their ability to deposit in vessel walls. Only large immune complexes were found in vessel walls. When immune complexes were sedimented in a sucrose gradient and the various fractions assayed, only those complexes greater in size than 19S were deposited in vessel walls. The data are shown in Fig. 2. Individual protein molecules were also able to become lodged in vessel walls provided they were of adequate size. Hemocyanin from the keyhole limpet in its associated form (7×10^6 mol wt) was capable of depositing, while in its dissociated form (0.8×10^6 mol wt) it would not deposit (9). Native IgG would not deposit, while if aggregated by heat it would. The critical size was greater than that of molecules of 19S, as IgM and thyroglobulin would not deposit.

A series of experiments was then performed to find if a release of vasoactive agents increased vascular permeability, and if filtration of large immune complexes occurred in acute immune complex disease (serum sickness) of rabbits. Evidence was obtained indicating immune complexes were depositing from the circulation. Colloidal carbon, injected intravenously, became localized along

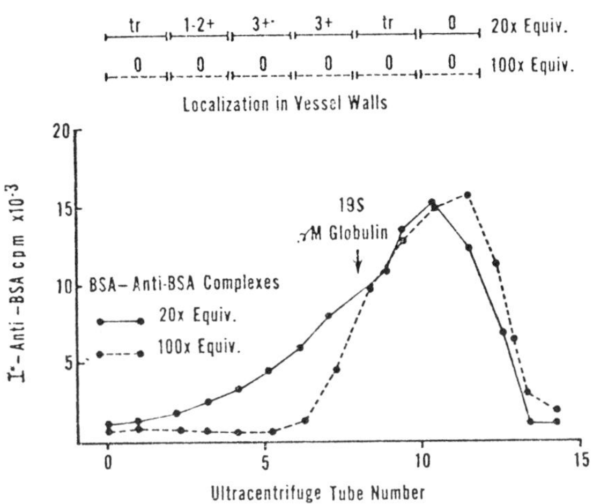

Fig. 2. Patterns of sedimentation of anti-I*BSA complexes with BSA using two quantities of BSA. Sedimentation carried out in a linear sucrose gradient, 10–37%, 4 hr, at 50,000 rpm. Purified human γM served as marker. Those made using a large excess of BSA (100 × equivalence) yielded slowly sedimenting complexes, while those prepared in moderate antigen excess (20 × equivalence) demonstrated both slowly sedimenting and more rapidly sedimenting components. Fractions collected after centrifugation and injected into guinea pigs showed localizing complexes only in tubes taken from complexes prepared at 20 × equivalence and greater than 19S in size (from reference 9).

with the complexes in the developing intimal lesions (10). The carbon filtered between endothelial cells and lined up along the internal elastic lamina of the coronary arteries. This elastic lamina (or a membrane closely associated with it) apparently acted as the filtration barrier, and lost its integrity only when neutrophils entered the reaction (11).

Evidence of an active mechanism of inducing vascular permeability was also observed. Antagonists of vasoactive amines given during the time immune complexes appeared in the circulation prevented in great part the deposition of immune complexes in arteries and glomeruli (Table I). In addition, when the most important reservoirs of vasoactive amines in the circulation of rabbits, i.e. platelets (12, 13), were depleted in rabbits subjected to serum sickness, deposition of immune complexes and the development of arterial and glomerular lesions were markedly suppressed (Table I).

The size of the immune complex is also important in determining whether deposition and development of lesions occur. In a correlative study, the deposition of circulating complexes and the development of glomerular and arterial lesions in acute immune complex disease of rabbits was found almost exclusively in animals forming large complexes, i.e., greater than 19S in size (9) (Table II). The sedimentation patterns of complexes in serum of rabbits that were sufficiently large to deposit in vessels, as opposed to those that were too small, are

TABLE I

*Incidence and Severity of Serum Sickness Lesions in Treated and Control Rabbits**

	Treated rabbits (% positive)		Control rabbits (% positive)
	Antihistamine anti-serotonin 11 rabbits	Platelet depletion 16 rabbits	10 rabbits
Coronary artery			
Endothelial proliferation	9	44	90
Medial necrosis	9	19	80
Glomeruli			
Immunofluorescent deposits‡	0 to + (fine)	0 to + (fine)	+ to ++ (coarse)
Endothelial swelling and proliferation§	1.0+	1.7+	2.2+

Values tabulated are averages for each group.

* Data from Kniker and Cochrane (10).

‡ Grading of immunofluorescent deposits of IgG, antigen (BSA): 0 to +++.

§ Grading of glomerular endothelial swelling and proliferation 0 to 3+.

shown in Fig. 3. In chronic immune complex disease in rabbits, a similar correlation has been observed (14).

The data suggest that a complex series of events takes place leading to deposition of circulating complexes. Increased vascular permeability occurs, brought about most probably by the release of vasoactive agents from their reservoirs in the circulation or the tissues. In the rabbit, the circulating reservoirs. i.e., platelets, are probably most important for disease in glomeruli and arterial intima where mast cells do not exist. Then in the presence of increased permeability, the large macromolecular immune complexes deposit along a filtering membrane. Inflammation ensues.

Hydrodynamic forces also play a role in the deposition of circulating complexes. Arterial lesions in acute immune complex disease of rabbits occur most commonly along heart values, at the entrance of the coronary arteries. and at branches and bifurcations of the aorta. In addition, if a coarctation is induced artificially in the lower aorta, lesions develop around the constricted zone (10). This is of great interest since it has been shown that platelets clump and adhere with leukocytes to endothelium around these areas of turbulence (15).

TABLE II

Relationship of the Sedimentation Characteristics of Circulating Immune Complexes to the Development of Lesions in Serum Sickness *

Rabbits	Avg. amt. BSA–^{131}I bound to globulin at maximum‡	Pattern of BSA–^{131}I sedimentation§	Glomerular lesions	Total amt. proteinuria	Maximal complement depletion
	%			mg	
9	43.3	Heavy	2.3+	567	78
5	41.6	Light	0 to ±	0	67

* Data taken from Cochrane and Hawkins (9).

‡ Per cent (average) of BSA–^{131}I bound to globulins determined by precipitation of the globulins with ammonium sulfate at 50% saturation.

§ Pattern of sedimentation of BSA–^{131}I complexed to globulin as determined in sucrose gradient. Heavy = BSA–^{131}I sedimentation pattern extends below 19S marker. Light = BSA–^{131}I sedimentation pattern does not reach 19S marker (see Fig. 2).

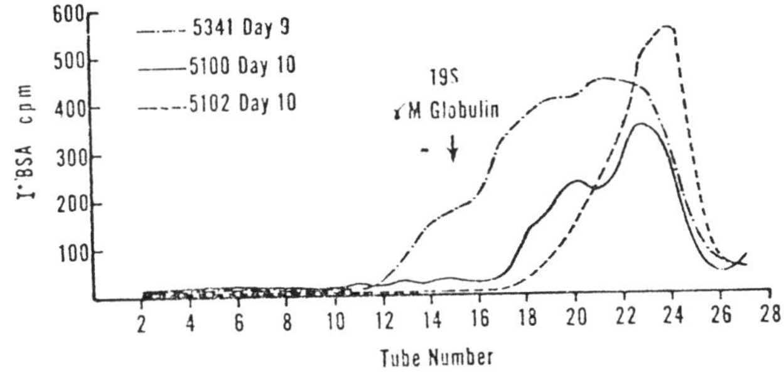

Fig. 3. Sedimentation patterns of I*BSA in sera obtained from three rabbits at the times shown after injection of I*BSA. Centrifugation carried out in linear sucrose density gradient 10–37% at 50,000 rpm for 4 hr. No. 5100 demonstrates a typical "light" pattern and No. 5341 a "heavy" pattern. No. 5102 failed to develop antibodies and showed a sedimentation pattern of free BSA in normal serum (from reference 9).

Release of Vasoactive Amines from Platelets.—Clearly a subject of pressing interest has been the immunologic mechanisms responsible for the release of histamine from platelets. To date, four immunologic reactions have been observed that lead to release of vasoactive amines:

(*a*) Immune complexes have been found by many investigators to bring about the release of amines from rabbit platelets in the presence of plasma (16–23). The reaction is augmented greatly in antibody excess (17–19, 22). The require-

189

ment of fresh plasma has been shown in several laboratories (16, 20, 22). Strong evidence favoring the participation of complement components emerged from the use of plasma from genetically C6-deficient rabbits. Immune complexes failed to induce release of histamine and serotonin from rabbit platelets in the presence of C6-deficient plasma, and the ability was restored by addition of semipurified rabbit C6 (22). The requirement of complement has been questioned (23) in view of an apparent requirement of Mg^{++} but not Ca^{++}. The observation may be explained by the activation of C3 proactivator by the immune complexes (see reference 24) which would allow participation of the terminal components. During the reaction of platelets and immune complexes in plasma, clumping of platelets to the complexes occurred by C3 immune adherence, and, through the action of terminal components, lysis of the platelets followed. The lysis was evident with the electron microscope and by measuring the release of several enzymes from cytoplasmic and granular compartments of the platelets. Acid phosphatase, β-glucuronidase (α-granules), and lactic dehydrogenase (cytoplasmic enzyme) were released. ^{86}Rb, previously incorporated into the cytoplasm of the platelets, was also released. The reaction was one of passive lysis, not requiring active participation of the platelet (22, 25).

(*b*) A second mechanism of histamine release from platelets was observed. When C6-deficient plasma was mixed with immune complexes and platelets, release of histamine and serotonin could be induced by adding a few neutrophils (26). Immune adherence but not lysis of platelets resulted, and the reaction required active participation of the platelet. Inhibition of the glycolytic pathway of the platelet prevented release of vasoactive amines. Release of granular and cytoplasmic enzymes did not occur.

(*c*) If a particulate antigen such as zymosan was used together with antibody to its surface determinants, complement components through C3 were required to induce immune adherence of platelets and the particles, and the release of histamine and serotonin occurred (25, 27, 28). Complement components beyond C3 were not required. The release by this mechanism also required the active participation of the platelet, and lysis was not observed (27, 28). Presumably, the surface of the particle together with antibody and C3 offer an adequate stimulus to initiate release of vasoactive amines from the platelet.

(*d*) A fourth mechanism of immunologic release of constituents from rabbit platelets was described independently by Siraganian et al (29) and Schoenbechler and Sadun (30). This mechanism involves a synergy between sensitized leukocytes and platelets. If leukocytes from recently sensitized rabbits are washed and then mixed with platelets in the presence of antigen, histamine and serotonin are released from the platelets. Plasma is not required. While washed leukocytes and platelets were originally employed from rabbits infected with *Schistosoma mansoni*, protein antigens have also been used to elicit this reaction (20, 21, 25). The leukocyte involved was thought at first to be mononuclear in type although direct evidence of its participation was uncertain (31, 32). More recently, the basophil has been implicated as the leukocyte most likely involved in the synergistic action. This has been demonstrated in several ways. Leukocytes from sensitized rabbits were fractionated on a column of glass beads or on a gradient of Ficoll by sedimentation (33). The fractionated cells were then assayed for total content of histamine, morphologic characteristics, and ability to stimulate release of histamine from platelets on exposure to antigen. The ability to release histamine from platelets corresponded to the leukocytes that contained histamine, i.e., the basophils (34). Further studies have correlated the presence of basophils from sensitized rabbits with the presence of the platelet-activating capacity (35). Basophils in these studies have been visualized directly. In experiments in our laboratory, the serum of rabbits having strong reactivity was transferred to normal recipient rabbits, and the recipients were then endowed with reactivity in a manner similar to that reported by Colwell et al. (36). The serum also was rich in homocytotropic antibody as determined by its capacity to transfer passive cutaneous anaphylaxis to normal recipients. Fractionation of antiserum by anion exchange chromatography and gel filtration indicated that the antibody responsible was a fast gamma and larger in size than IgG (i.e., in the range of 200,000 Daltons). In addition, the leukocyte-sensitizing antibody eluted together with homocytotropic antibody activity from the columns. In other experiments, when leukocytes from a sensitized rabbit were treated with anti-IgE (anti-homocytotropic antibody[1]) and platelets added, histamine was released from the platelets. Prior treatment of the leukocytes with this antibody led to desensitization: when the leukocytes from sensitized rabbits were first exposed to anti-IgE, followed by washing, antigen could no longer stimulate them to induce the release of histamine of platelets.

A soluble factor released from the leukocytes that induces clumping of platelets and release of histamine has been described by Henson (28, 32). The factor was labile and readily inactivated by platelets contaminating the leukocyte suspension. This may explain the difficulty noted by others (37) in its detection. It release from sensitized leukocytes with antigen was inhibited when glucose in the medium was replaced by 2-deoxyglucose or when Mg ethylenediaminetetraacetate (EDTA) or acetyl salicylate were added (32). Pretreatment of the cells with antigen induced a state of desensitization. The release of histamine from the platelets by the soluble factor was also inhibited by replacement of glucose by 2-deoxyglucose (10^{-3} M) diisopropyl fluorophosphate (2×10^{-3} M), Mg ethylene glycol Bis(β-aminoethyl ether) N,N,N',N' tetraacetic acid (EGTA) (5×10^{-3} M), adenosine (10^{-3} M), and acetyl salicylate (10^{-3} M). The soluble factor induced clumping of the platelets and release of histamine and serotonin but not enzymes associated with platelet granules

---

[1] Antibody to homocytotropic antibody was generously given by Dr. Nathan Zvaifler.

(acid phosphatase and β-glucuronidase) or cytoplasm (lactic dehydrogenase). By electron microscopy, the platelets were not lysed in confirmation of the observed specific release. The presence of a soluble intermediate has recently been confirmed (38), although lysis of platelets was reported as evidence by release of ^{86}Rb.

A scheme of this mechanism of release of vasoactive amines from platelets is shown in Fig. 4.

Leukocyte-Dependent Release

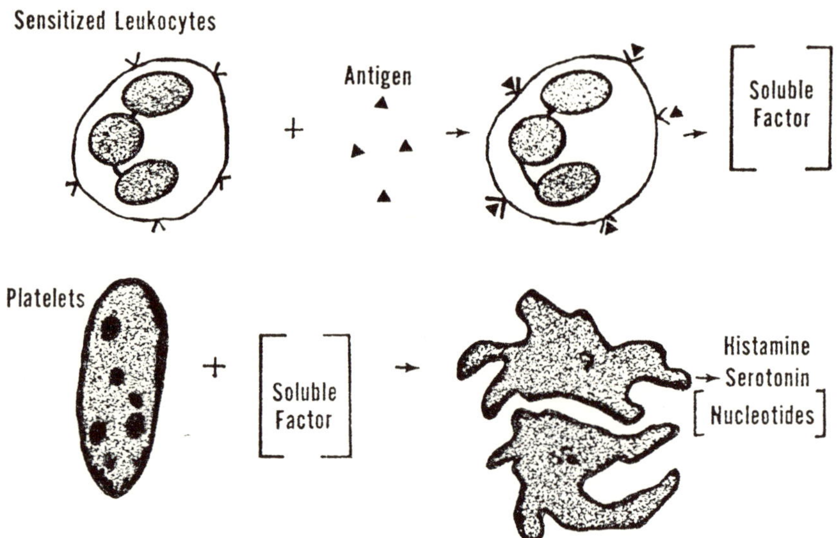

Fig. 4. Schematic presentation of the leukocyte-dependent mechanism of histamine release from platelets in rabbits. The sensitized basophils, having sensitizing antibody on the surface, are reacted with antigen. The basophils then give off a soluble factor that reacts with platelets to cause clumping and release of their vasoactive amines and, to a lesser degree, nucleotides.

Lack of Participation of Complement Components in the Release of Vasoactive Amines from Platelets in Acute Immune Complex Disease (Serum Sickness) in Rabbits.—Experiments have been conducted to determine if the complement-dependent mechanisms of histamine release play a role in the deposition of circulating immune complexes in rabbits. Rabbits were depleted of C3 and terminal components of complement by the injection of cobra venom factor (39). Immune complexes appeared in the circulation and, despite depletion of complement, they deposited in glomeruli to induce injury (Table III) (40). Arteries were also affected, but in the absence of sufficient C3, neutrophils did not accumulate to produce necrotizing arteritis. The fact that the immune complexes are in antigen excess in acute immune complex disease may be important in this observation. The complement-dependent mechanisms of release of vasoactive amines from platelets are significantly augmented in antibody excess and diminished in antigen excess as noted above.

TABLE III

*Effect of C3 Depletion in Acute Immune Complex Disease (Serum Sickness) of Rabbits**

	Glomerulitis (No. positive total)	Avg. amt. proteinuria	Necrotizing arteritis (No. positive total)
		mg/day	
C3 depleted‡	13/13	664	0/6§
Control	43/45	456	20/34

* Data from Henson and Cochrane (40).

‡ C3 depleted by injections of cobra venom factor just before appearance of circulating immune complexes.

§ Arterial intimal proliferation and edema present in all six rabbits, but neutrophil accumulation did not occur in C3-depleted rabbits.

TABLE IV

Correlation of Leukocyte-Dependent Release of Histamine from Platelets and Glomerular Injury in Acute Immune Complex Disease (Serum Sickness) of Rabbits

No. of rabbits*	Glomerulonephritis	Rabbits with leukocyte-dependent release
17	Present	16
8	Absent	1‡

* All rabbits exhibited circulating immune complexes. Amount of complexes was comparable between the two groups.

‡ Complexes of "light" type in sedimentation pattern (see Fig. 2).

Correlation of the Leukocyte-Dependent Mechanism of Histamine Release from Platelets and the Deposition of Immune Complexes and Development of Injury.— A correlative study of the presence of the leukocyte-dependent (LDHR)[2] mechanism of histamine release from platelets and the deposition of immune complexes and injury is shown in Table IV. Only animals with circulating immune complexes are included. As noted, when circulating complexes deposited and injury resulted, the LDHR was detected in all but one instance (18). By contrast, rabbits with immune complexes but without deposition and the development of injury failed in all but one case to demonstrate the LDHR. It is of great interest that the single rabbit with circulating immune complexes and

---

[2] *Abbreviations used in this paper:* BSA, bovine serum albumin; LDHR, leukocyte-dependent mechanism of histamine release from platelets.

the LDHR was found to have complexes of the "light" type (see above, also Table II and Fig. 3) that were too small to be entrapped in vessel walls. This correlation implicated the LDHR as being the important immunologic method of releasing vasoactive amines thereby increasing vascular permeability and bringing about deposition of the circulating complexes. The LDHR may also be detected in rabbits with chronic immune complex disease.

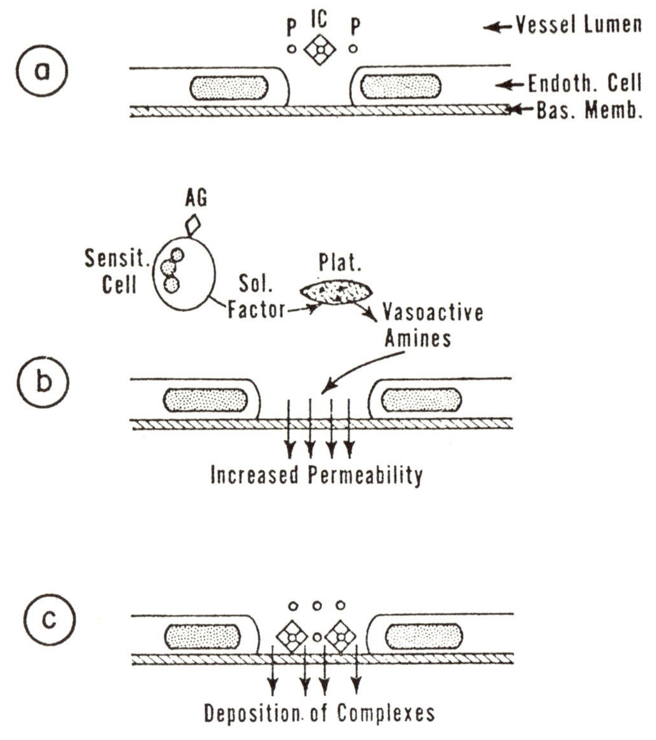

Fig. 5. Theoretical summary of the mechanism responsible for the deposition of immune complexes from the circulation in acute immune complex disease. Explanation given in text.

As discussed previously, Germuth and Pollack (1), by infusing antibody into rabbits with circulating antigen, were able to induce at least mild lesions in glomeruli and certain arteries in about half the recipients, while the injection of preformed complexes made with hyperimmune antibody was ineffectual in this regard.[3] An explanation may lie in the possibility that the infused antibody

[3] Cochrane, C. G., and W. O. Weigle. 1958. W. T. Kniker and C. G. Cochrane. 1964. Unpublished observations.

allowed a sensitization of leukocytes to take place for the LDHR reaction, while combining the hyperimmune antibody with an excess of antigen in vitro did not allow sensitization of leukocytes to take place. Also, since this leukocyte-sensitizing antibody disappears with repeated antigenic exposure, the hyperimmune antibody might not have contained sufficient sensitizing antibody.

Summary.—A summary of the mechanisms by which deposition of immune complexes may occur in acute immune complex disease (serum sickness) of rabbits is shown in Fig. 5. (*a*) Immune complexes and protein molecules circulate in a blood vessel. (*b*) In the presence of basophil leukocytes with adherent IgE antibody, the antigen induces release of the soluble intermediate. This intermediate activates platelets to clump and to release vasoactive amines. These amines then cause an increased permeability of blood vessels, especially in areas where the platelets clump and impinge upon blood vessels. (*c*) With the increased permeability, macromolecular ($>$19S) immune complexes become entrapped along filtering membranes in the vessel wall to induce injury.

SUMMARY

The mechanisms reponsible for the deposition of circulating immune complexes have been analyzed. An active process appears to be responsible in both a laboratory model in guinea pigs and in acute immune complex disease (serum sickness) in rabbits.

In rabbits, after the injection of antigen to induce serum sickness, immune complexes appear in the circulation. In addition, homocytotropic (IgE) antibody is formed which binds to the surface of basophils. Leukocyte suspensions containing these basophils, when combined with specific antigen, release a soluble factor that causes clumping of platelets and release of their vasoactive amines. An excellent correlation was found between the presence of this mechanism of release of vasoactive amine and the deposition of immune complexes in serum sickness of rabbits. Antagonists of vasoactive amines or depletion of platelets, the major circulating reservoir of these amines, suppressed the deposition of circulating immune complexes and inhibited glomerulitis and arteritis. Upon entering the walls of vessels, the complexes became lodged immune complexes, greater than 19S in size, were deposited along the membranes.

The data suggest that at a time when immune complexes appear in the circulation of an immunized rabbit, vasoactive amines are released from platelets in areas where turbulence of blood occurs. Sensitized basophils participate in the release of vasoactive amines from the platelets. The amines induced increased vascular permeability which leads to deposition of large complexes from the circulation in vessel walls by a process of filtration. The deposited complexes then induce inflammatory injury.

REFERENCES

1. Germuth, F. G., Jr., and A. D. Pollack. 1958. The production of lesions of "serum sickness" in normal animals by the passive transfer of antibody in the presence of antigen. *Bull. Johns Hopkins Hosp.* **102**:245.

2. McCluskey, R. T., and B. Benacerraf. 1959. Localization of colloidal substances in vascular endothelium. A mechanism of tissue damage. II. Experimental serum sickness with acute glomerulonephritis induced passively in mice by antigen–antibody complexes in antigen excess. *Amer. J. Pathol.* **35**:275.

3. McCluskey, R. T., B. Benacerraf, J. L. Potter, and F. Miller. 1960. The pathologic effects of intravenously administered soluble antigen–antibody complexes. I. Passive serum sickness in mice. *J. Exp. Med.* **111**:181.

4. McCluskey, R. T., B. Benacerraf, J. L. Potter, and F. Miller. 1960. The pathologic effects of intravenously administered soluble antigen–antibody complexes. II. Acute glomerulonephritis in rats. *J. Exp. Med.* **111**:195.

5. Michael, A. F., A. J. Fish, and R. A. Good. 1967. Glomerular localization and transport of aggregated proteins in mice. *Lab. Invest.* **17**:14.

6. Benacerraf, B., R. T. McCluskey, and D. Patras. 1959. Localization of colloidal substances in vascular endothelium. A mechanism of tissue damage. I. Factors causing the pathologic deposition of colloidal carbon. *Amer. J. Pathol.* **35**:75.

7. Cochrane, C. G. 1963. Studies on the localization of antigen–antibody complexes and other macromolecules in vessels. I. Structural studies. *J. Exp. Med.* **118**:489.

8. Cochrane, C. G. 1963. Studies on the localization of antigen–antibody complexes and other macromolecules in vessels. II. Pathogenetic and pharmacodynamic studies. *J. Exp. Med.* **118**:503.

9. Cochrane, C. G., and D. Hawkins. 1968. Studies on circulating immune complexes. III. Factors governing the ability of circulating complexes to localize in blood vessels. *J. Exp. Med.* **127**:137.

10. Kniker, W. T., and C. G. Cochrane. 1968. The localization of circulating immune complexes in experimental serum sickness. The role of vasoactive amines and hydrodynamic forces. *J. Exp. Med.* **127**:119.

11. Kniker, W. T., and C. G. Cochrane. 1965. Pathogenic factors in vascular lesions of experimental serum sickness. *J. Exp. Med.* **122**:83.

12. Humphrey, J. H., and R. Jaques. 1954. The histamine and serotonin content of the platelets and polymorphonuclear leukocytes of various species. *J. Physiol. (London).* **124**:305.

13. Waalkes, T. P., and H. Coburn. 1959. The role of platelets and the release of serotonin and histamine during anaphylaxis in the rabbit. *J. Allergy.* **30**:394.

14. Wilson, C. B., and F. J. Dixon. 1971. Quantitation of acute and chronic serum sickness in the rabbit. *J. Exp. Med.* **134**(3, Pt. 2):7 s.

15. Mustard, J. F., E. A. Murphy, H. C. Roswell, and H. G. Downie. 1962. Factors influencing thrombus formation *in vivo*. *Amer. J. Med.* **33**:621.

16. Humphrey, J. H., and R. Jaques. 1955. The release of histamine and 5-hydroxytryptamine (serotonin) from platelets by antigen–antibody reactions (*in vitro*). *J. Physiol. (London).* **128**:9.

17. Barbaro, F. J. 1961. The release of histamine from rabbit platelets by means of

antigen–antibody precipitates. I. The participation of the immune complex in histamine release. *J. Immunol.* **86**:369.

18. Barbaro, F. J. 1961. The release of histamine from rabbit platelets by means of antigen–antibody precipitates. II. The role of plasma in the release of histamine. *J. Immunol.* **86**:377

19. Gocke, D. J., and A. G. Osler. 1965. *In vitro* damage of rabbit platelets by an unrelated antigen–antibody reaction. I. General characteristics of the reaction. *J. Immunol.* **94**:236.

20. Gocke, D. J. 1965. *In vitro* damage of rabbit platelets by an unrelated antigen–antibody reaction. II. Studies on the plasma requirement. *J. Immunol* **94**:247.

21. Bryant, R., and R. Des Prez. 1968. Mechanisms of immunologically-reduced rabbit platelet injury. *Clin. Res.* **16**:318.

22. Henson, P. M., and C. G. Cochrane. 1969. Immunological induction of increased vascular permeability. II. The mechanisms of histamine release from rabbit platelets involving complement. *J. Exp. Med.* **129**:167.

23. Siraganian, R. P., A. G. Secchi, and A. G. Osler. 1968. The allergic response of rabbit platelets. II. Dependence on magnesium. *J. Immunol.* **101**:1140.

24. Götze, Otto, and Hans J. Müller-Eberhard. The C3-activator system: an alternate pathway of complement activation. *J. Exp. Med.* **134**(3, Pt. 2):90 s.

25. Henson, P. M., and C. G. Cochrane. 1969. *In* Cellular and Humoral Mechanisms of Anaphylaxis and Allergy. H. Z. Movat, editor. S. Karger AG, Basel. 129.

26. Henson, P. M. 1970. Mechanisms of release of constituents from rabbit platelets by antigen–antibody complexes and complement. II. Interactions with neutrophils. *J. Immunol.* **105**:490.

27. Henson, P. M. 1970. Mechanisms of release of constituents from rabbit platelets by antigen–antibody complexes and complement. I. Lytic and nonlytic reaction. *J. Immunol.* **105**:476.

28. Henson, P. M. 1969. The role of complement and leukocytes in the immunologic release of vasoactive amines from platelets. *Fed. Proc.* **28**:1721.

29. Siraganian, R. P., A. G. Secchi, and A. G. Osler. 1968. *In* Biochemistry of the Acute Allergic Reaction. K. F. Austen and E. L. Becker, editors. Blackwell Scientific Publications Ltd., Oxford. 229.

30. Schoenbechler, M. J., and E. H. Sadun. 1968. *In vitro* histamine release from blood cellular elements of rabbits infected with *Schistosoma mansoni*. *Proc. Soc. Exp. Biol. Med.* **127**:601.

31. Schoenbechler, M. J., and Barbaro, J. F. 1968. The requirement for sensitized lymphocytes in one form of antigen-induced histamine release from rabbit platelets. *Proc. Nat. Acad. Sci. U.S.A.* **4**:1247.

32. Henson, P. M. 1970. Release of vasoactive amines from rabbit platelets induced by sensitized mononuclear leukocytes and antigen. *J. Exp. Med.* **131**:287.

33. Siraganian, R. P., and A. G. Osler. 1971. Destruction of rabbit platelets in the allergic response of sensitized leukocytes. II. Evidence for basophil involvement. *J. Immunol.* In press.

34. Greaves, M. W., and J. Mongar. 1968. The histamine content of rabbit leukocytes and its release during *in vitro* anaphylaxis. *Immunology.* **15**:733.

35. Benveniste, J., and P. M. Henson. 1971. Leukocyte-dependent mechanism of

histamine release from rabbit platelets: transfer of responsible antibody. *Fed. Proc.* **30**:654. (Abstr.)

36. Colwell, E. J., J. R. Ortaldo, M. J. Schoenbechler, and J. F. Barbaro. 1970. *In vivo* passive sensitization of normal rabbit leukocytes with homocytotropic antibody. *Fed. Proc.* **29**:639. (Abstr.)

37. Barbaro, J. F., and M. J. Schoenbechler. 1970. The nature of the reaction of antigen with lymphocytes from rabbits infected with *Schistosoma mansoni* on the release of histamine from rabbit platelets. *J. Immunol.* **104**:1124.

38. Siraganian, R. P., and A. G. Osler. 1971. Destruction of rabbit platelets in the allergic response of sensitized leukocytes. I. Demonstration of a fluid phase intermediate. *J. Immunol.* In press.

39. Cochrane, C. G., H. J. Müller-Eberhard, and B. S. Aikin. 1970. Depletion of plasma complement *in vivo* by a protein of cobra venom: its effect on various immunologic reactions. *J. Immunol.* **105**:55.

40. Henson, P. M., and C. G. Cochrane. 1971. Immune complex disease in rabbits. The role of complement and of a leukocyte-dependent release of vasoactive amines from platelets. *J. Exp. Med.* **133**:554.

INTERACTION OF CELLS WITH IMMUNE COMPLEXES: ADHERENCE, RELEASE OF CONSTITUENTS, AND TISSUE INJURY*

By PETER M. HENSON

The pathogenic effects of immune complexes generally follow their deposition in the walls of blood vessels in different parts of the body. A mechanism for this deposition in experimental immune complex of the rabbit has been described previously.[1] It involves a role for IgE antibody, basophils, and platelets in the induction of increased vascular permeability, which then leads to trapping of large immune complexes along filtering surfaces. This process is independent of the complement system beyond the activation of C2 (1).

The next step to consider in the pathogenesis of immune complex diseases is the mechanism whereby the deposited complexes produce damage to the tissues. The role of neutrophils in the injury will first be discussed. A consideration of two in vitro mechanisms by which neutrophils release injurious constituents to the extracellular medium will follow. Finally, the ability of different immune reactants to stimulate these release processes will be described.

(A) THE ROLE OF NEUTROPHILS IN THE TISSUE INJURY PRODUCED BY IMMUNE COMPLEXES

There are at least two broad categories of immune complex-induced tissue injury, those dependent upon neutrophils and those which do not involve action of this type of cell. These categories can be illustrated by consideration of acute immune complex disease in rabbits.

(1) The Arteritis of Acute Immune Complex Disease.—This arteritis (Fig. 1) is a necrotizing vasculitis and is characterized by massive neutrophil accumulation with consequent damage to the internal elastic lamina, penetration of neutrophils into the media, and adventitia and subsequent necrosis of these

* Publication No. 487 from the Department of Experimental Pathology, Scripps Clinic and Research Foundation. The work was supported by the U. S. Public Health Service Grant AI-07007, a Grant-in-Aid from the American Heart Association and the San Diego County Heart Association.

[1] Cochrane, Charles G. 1971. Mechanisms involved in the deposition of immune complexes in tissues. *J. Exp. Med.* **134**(3, Pt. 2):75 s.

FIG. 1.   Acute immune complex disease in the rabbit. (*a*) Arteritis: the characteristic neutrophil infiltration is apparent. These cells (arrows) have penetrated to all layers of the vessel wall. The lumen is at the top. (*b*) Glomerulonephritis: neutrophils cannot be seen in this esion which is characterized by swelling and proliferation of endothelial cells. × 450.

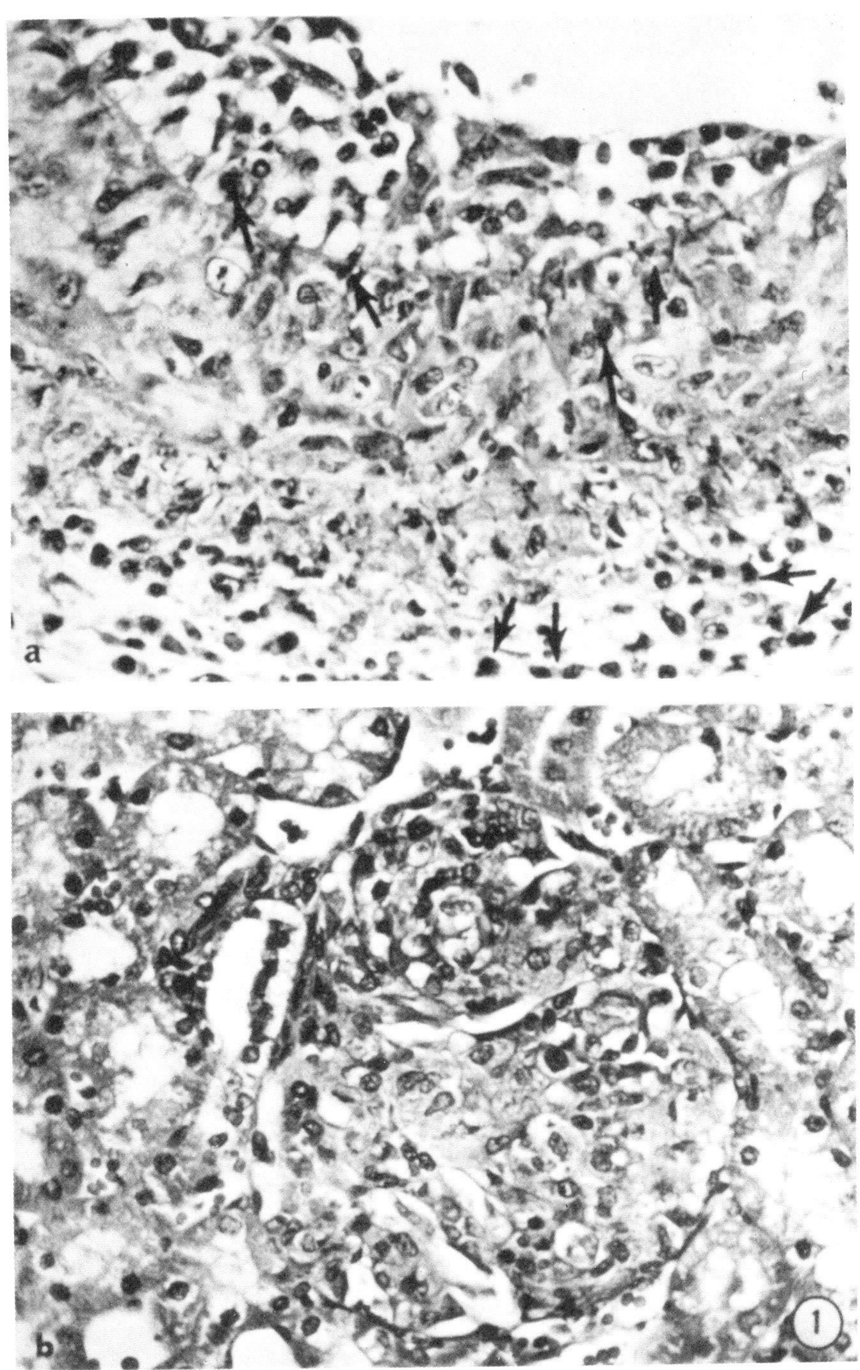

structures. The neutrophil accumulation and tissue damage, but not the deposition of complexes, can be prevented by depletion of circulating complement (C3 and later-acting components) with the anti-complementary factor from cobra venom (1) or by depletion of circulating neutrophils (2). It is presumed that the neutrophils accumulate by complement-mediated processes (chemotaxis and perhaps especially immune adherence), phagocytose the immune complexes, and release injurious constituents capable of digesting structures within the vessel wall.

(*2*) *The Glomerulonephritis of Immune Complex Disease.*—In contrast, the glomerulonephritis of the acute disease model (Fig. 1) is not characterized by neutrophil infiltration and is unaffected by depletion of either complement (1, 3) or neutrophils (2). Neutrophil-independent pathogenic mechanisms, whose nature is at present unknown, are therefore involved in the development of this glomerulonephritis. On the other hand, the glomerular lesions of chronic immune complex disease of the rabbit or the diseases thought to be associated with immune complexes in man frequently contain neutrophils (Fig. 2 *c*). In this situation, therefore, where deposition of large quantities of complexes occurs,[2] neutrophils and their products may contribute to the tissue damage.

(*3*) *Glomerulonephritis Produced by Anti–Glomerular Basement Membrane Antibodies.*– The situation in which complexes of antigen and antibody are dispersed along a surface is even more clearly represented by the glomerulonephritis produced by antibody directed against the glomerular basement membrane. This occurs experimentally in nephrotoxic nephritis in the rabbit or naturally in Goodpasture's disease in man (4). Antibody binds along the membrane and in the experimental system produces injury by both neutrophil-dependent and independent processes (5). When the former predominates, as depicted in Fig. 2 *a*, neutrophils fill the glomerular capillary lumen, having pushed aside the endothelial lining and become closely adherent to the antibody and complement bound to the basement membrane. As in the arteritis of acute immune complex disease, depletion of circulating complement or

---

[2] Wilson, Curtis B., and Frank J. Dixon. 1971. Quantitation of acute and chronic serum sickness in the rabbit. *J. Exp. Med.* **134**(3, Pt. 2):7 s.

Fig. 2.   Neutrophils adherent to immune reactants along glomerular basement membranes. (*a*) Nephrotoxic nephritis in the rabbit. A glomerular capillary loop is depicted, 5 hr after injection of sheep anti–glomerular basement membrane antiserum. Neutrophils (N) have filled the capillary lumen, pushed aside the endothelial cell (*e*), and have become closely adherent to the basement membrane (arrow). × 6300. (*b*) A neutrophil in this glomerular capillary from the same rabbit has lost most of its granules. The foot processes of the epithelial cell have fused, indicating early damage to the vessel wall. × 8300. (*c*) Neutrophils in a human glomerulus from a case of poststreptococcal glomerulonephritis. The neutrophils are again in close contact with the basement membrane which in this case shows evidence of immune complex deposits (*d*). × 12,000. Photograph courtesy of Dr. J. D. Feldman.

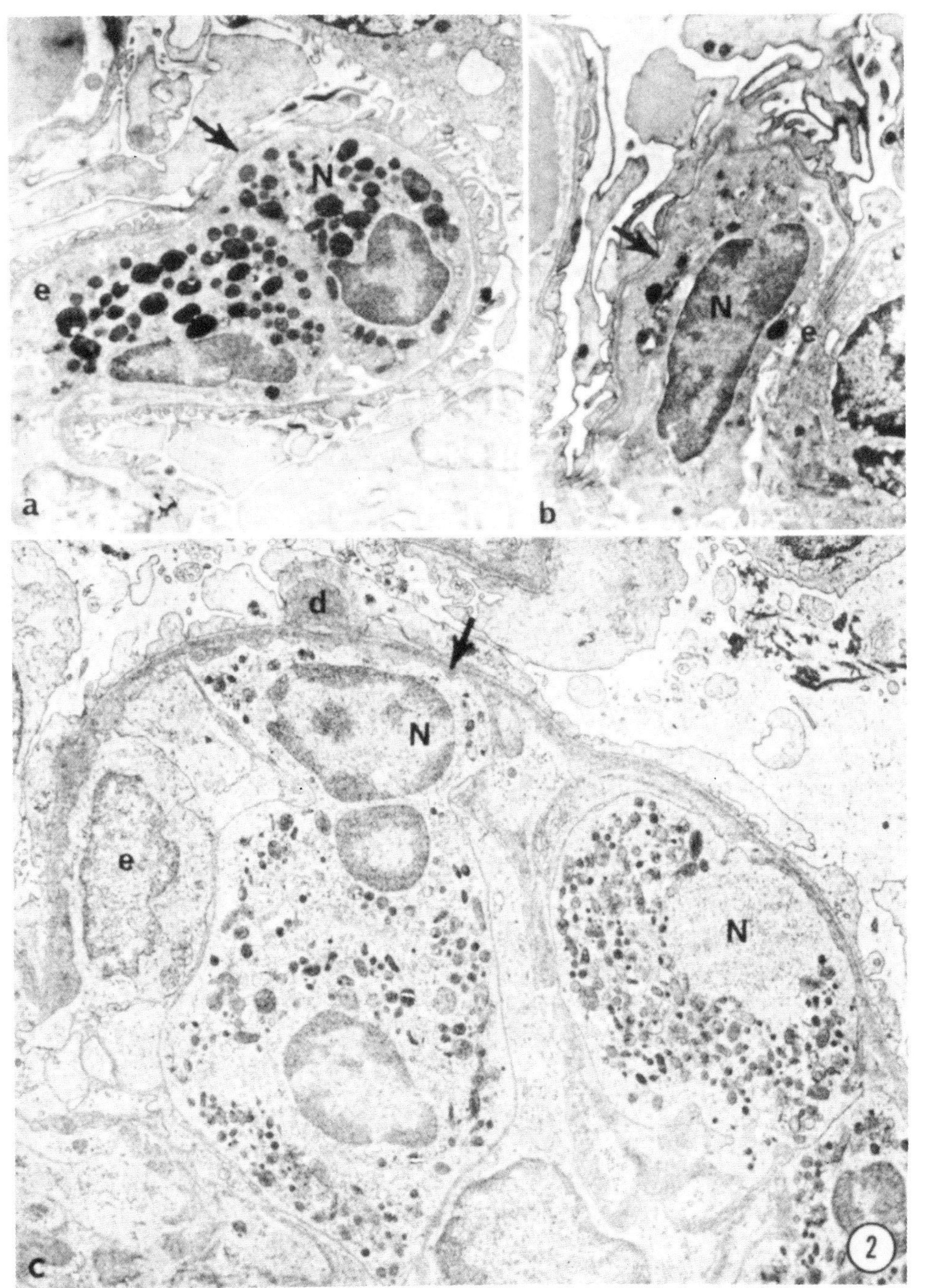

neutrophils prevents the neutrophil accumulation and the subsequent tissue injury (6). However, in this situation, the neutrophils are adherent to immune reactants along a surface which they cannot phagocytose. Nevertheless, release of constituent enzymes is postulated to lead to digestion of basement membrane and, moreover, a neutrophil-derived proteolytic enzyme and fragments of the basement membrane have been detected in the urine (7).

TABLE I

Release of Enzymes from Human Neutrophils after Adherence to Immune Complexes

Stimulus*	Per cent release of enzymes	
	β-glucuronidase	LDH‡
Phagocytosable		
Ag + Ab	10.2	2.6
Ab	2.5	2.4
ZC	11.1	2.2
Z EDTA C	2.8	2.0
—	2.2	2.7
Nonphagocytosable		
Filter + Ag + Ab	13.3	2.7
Filter + Ag	3.1	3.1
Filter + normal human IgG	4.1	2.0

* Ag, tetanus toxoid; Ab, human IgG anti-tetanus. Ag + Ab, 30 μg of precipitates at equivalence. ZC, zymosan incubated with human serum as complement source and then washed (2.0 mg). Z EDTA C, zymosan incubated with serum and 0.01 M EDTA. Filters were incubated with tetanus, washed, incubated with antibody, and again washed, and 5 × 10⁶ neutrophils were drawn gently down onto them. Incubated for 60 min at 37°C.

‡ LDH, lactic dehydrogenase.

(B) RELEASE OF CONSTITUENTS FROM NEUTROPHILS

In the continuing study of the pathogenesis of immune complex–induced tissue injury, it therefore became important to examine the mechanisms of release of constituents from neutrophils. Extracellular release of lysosomal materials from neutrophils after phagocytosis of immune complexes (8–12), bacteria (10, 13, 14), starch (15), or zymosan particles (16) has been described in a number of laboratories. In our experiments, two model systems have been employed, simulating the two in vivo situations described above (Table I). In one, neutrophils were allowed to phagocytose immune complexes or particles with antibody or complement fixed to them, and the release of enzymes to the outside of the cell was examined. In the other, the immune complexes were bound along a nonphagocytosable surface, in this case a micropore filter, and the reaction and release processes of adherent neutrophils were observed.[3]

---

[3] Henson, P. M. Manuscript submitted for publication.

For these studies, pure populations of cells (90–98% neutrophils) were obtained from the peripheral blood of human beings or rabbits and the reactions were carried out in a Tyrode's solution containing added albumin. Control preparations of rabbit neutrophils incubated for 1 hr at 37°C had the

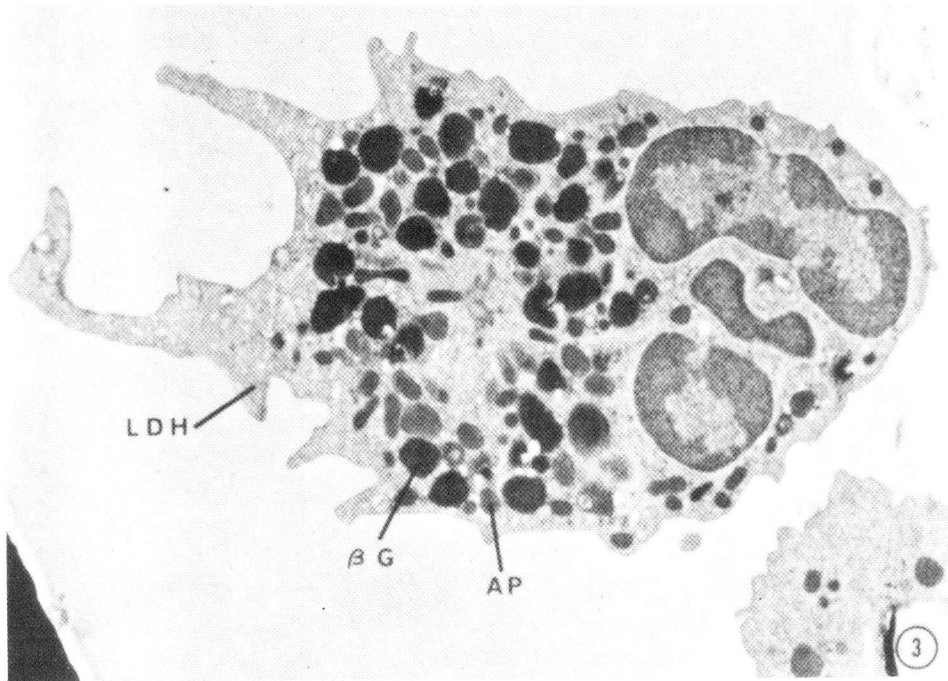

Fig. 3.   Rabbit neutrophil from the blood, washed and incubated for 1 hr at 37°C. This control cell has not lost its complement of granules. The origin of the enzymes which were assayed (see text) are indicated. Lactic dehydrogenase (LDH) from the cytoplasm, β-glucuronidase (βG) from the primary granule, and alkaline phosphatase (AP) from the secondary granule. Fixed with glutaraldehyde and osmic acid, embedded in Vestopal W, and stained with uranyl acetate and lead citrate. × 12,500.

appearance shown in Fig. 3. The two major types of granules are clearly seen in this photograph. Release of enzymes from each type has been examined. β-glucuronidase was chosen as an enzyme which resides in the primary or "azurophil" granule and alkaline phosphatase as an enzyme of the secondary or "specific" granule (17, 18). In addition, to indicate cell death and release of cytoplasmic constituents, liberation of lactic dehydrogenase was also measured and was in most cases low, indicating that little cell lysis was occurring.

(1) Release of Enzymes from Neutrophils on Nonphagocytosable Surfaces.—

Fig. 4 *a* depicts a human neutrophil adherent to the surface of a micropore filter coated with antigen and antibody. The filter had been incubated first in a solution of antigen (tetanus toxoid), washed, and then reacted with human IgG anti-tetanus antibody. After further washing, 5×10^6 neutrophils were gently drawn down onto the surface and the filter with adherent neutrophils was incubated at 37°C. The neutrophil may be seen to be very closely adherent to the surface in a similar manner to the previously described adherence along the basement membrane.

(*a*) *Release of lysosomal constituents*: Neutrophils adherent to antigen and antibody released β-glucuronidase into the external medium (Table I) but not the cytoplasmic enzyme lactic dehydrogenase. In contrast, cells on filters with antigen only did not liberate their lysosomal enzymes. In similar experiments performed with rabbit neutrophils, a wide variety of lysosomal constituents, including cathepsins and permeability factors, were released when neutrophils reacted with immune complexes on these filters. In similar experiments with neutrophils upon a collagen membrane, D. Hawkins (personal communication) has also found that neutrophils release lysosomal enzymes to the external environment. It may be noted that a greater percentage of enzymes was consistently released by all types of stimuli from rabbit neutrophils than from human cells. Nevertheless, the processes of release appeared to be identical in each species.

(*b*) *Release of alkaline phosphatase*: Alkaline phosphatase, an enzyme from the secondary granule, was not detected in the supernatant fluid after the reaction. Nevertheless, release of the enzyme to the exterior of the cells did occur. This enzyme appears to be insoluble or to have the property of binding to membranes (19) and it remains adherent to the outside of the neutrophil cell membrane, where it could be detected histochemically (Fig. 4).

(*c*) *Mechanism of release*: Release of enzymes from neutrophils adherent to antigen and antibody on a nonphagocytosable surface appears to result from a direct degranulation to the outside of the cell. This degranulation has been observed for both human (Fig. 4) and rabbit (Fig. 5) neutrophils. It is postulated that the external cell membrane is stimulated by adherence to the fixed antibody such that granules fuse with it and discharge to the outside as

---

FIG. 4. Human neutrophils adherent to antigen and antibody on a nonphagocytosable surface (micropore filter). (*a*) The close adherence of the neutrophil to the convoluted surface of the filter is apparent. The free surface of the cell is to the top right. $\times$ 15,300. (*b*) A similar neutrophil after 5 min incubation showing the presence of alkaline phosphatase activity (18). The black precipitate of lead phosphate can be seen outside the cell, adherent to the neutrophil membrane where it is in contact with the antigen and antibody on the filter. No activity is present on the free surface of the cell (top right). The arrow indicates discharge of a granule. $\times$ 15,600. (*c*) A control preparation in which the reaction for alkaline phosphatase was performed in the absence of enzyme substrate. No precipitate has occurred. $\times$ 15,600.

206

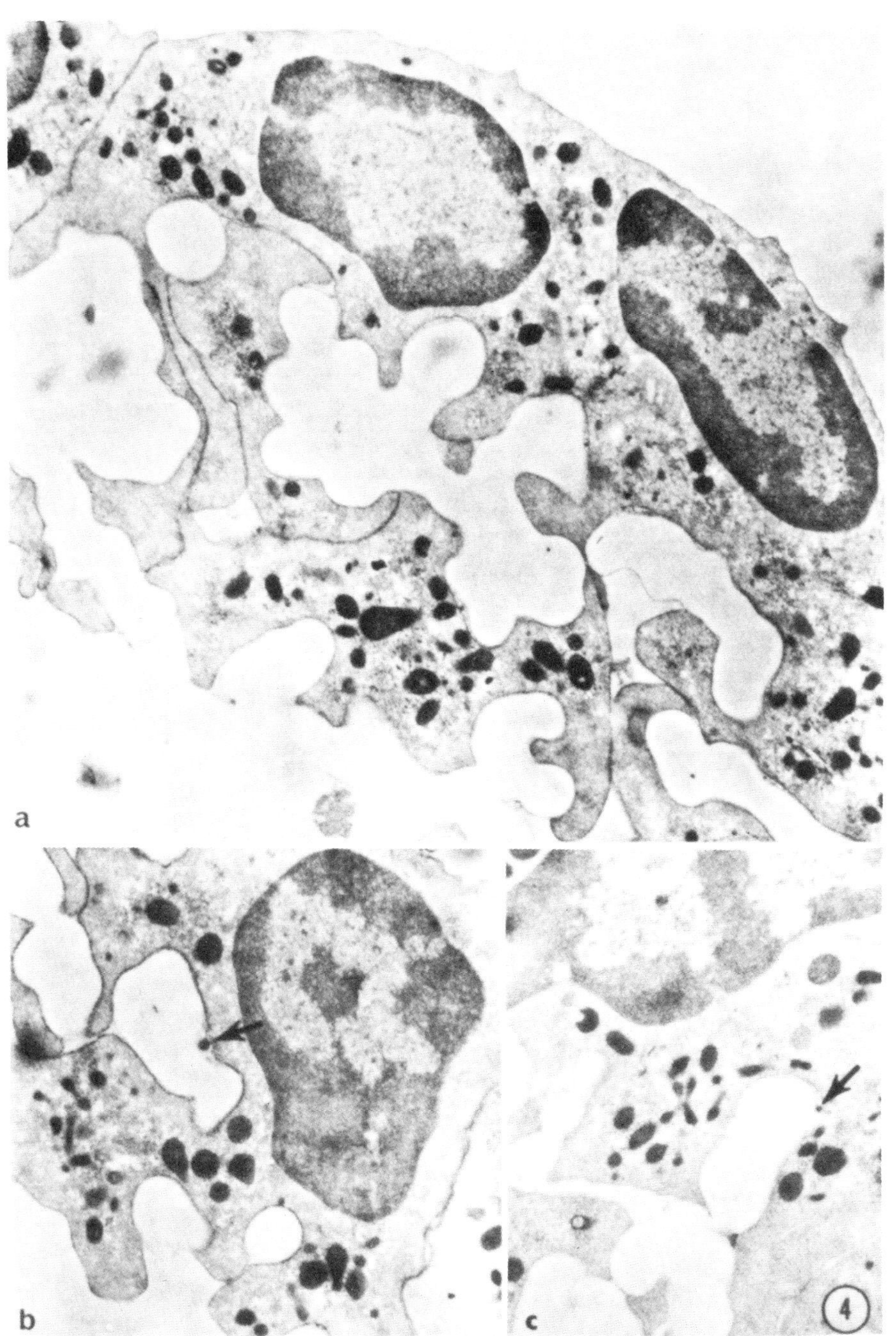

207

if to a phagocytic vacuole. The process may thus be considered one in which the complete phagocytic process is "frustrated" by the large size of the surface.

    (*d*) *Sequential discharge of secondary and primary granules*:   Examination of

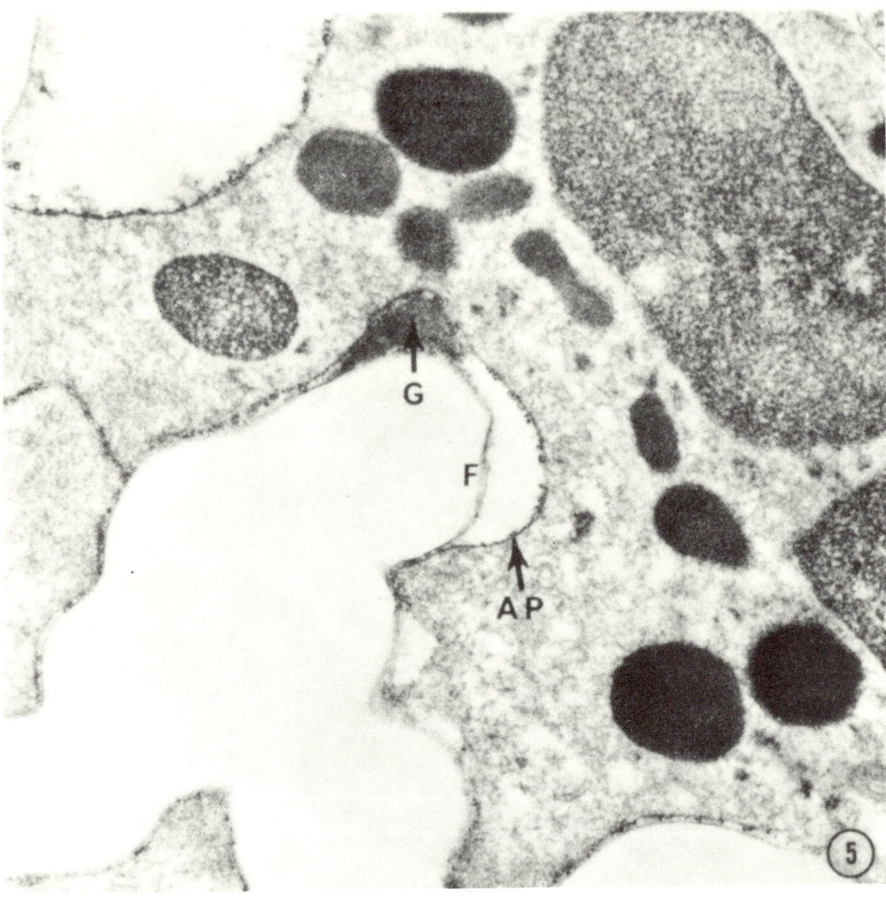

Fig. 5.   Discharge of a secondary granule (G) to the outside of a rabbit neutrophil adherent of antigen and antibody on a micropore filter (F) after 5 min incubation. Alkaline phosphatase reaction product (AP) is visible along the cell membrane. × 39,700.

the time at which the different enzymes were released suggested that secondary granules (alkaline phosphatase) were discharged at an earlier time than the primary granules (β-glucuronidase) (Fig. 6). After 5 min of incubation, secondary granules but not primary granules have been seen degranulating to the outside of the cell (Fig. 5). These experiments confirm the work of Bainton (20) who clearly demonstrated an earlier release of alkaline phosphatase than

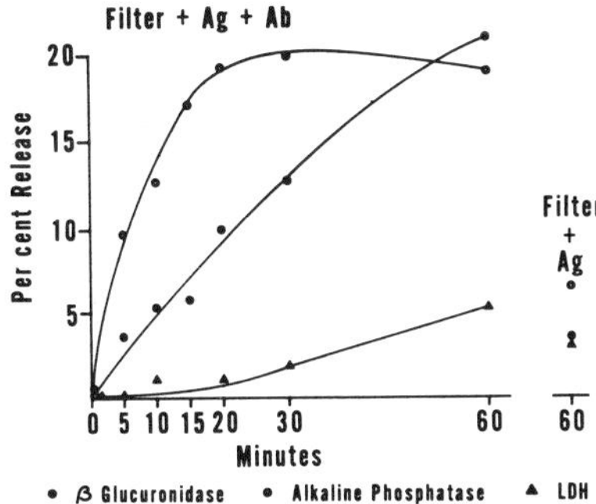

FIG. 6.   Release of enzymes from rabbit neutrophils on nonphagocytosable surfaces with increasing time of incubation. Ag, bovine serum albumin (BSA); Ab, rabbit IgG anti-BSA; LDH, lactic dehydrogenase. The alkaline phosphatase was released more rapidly than the β-glucuronidase.

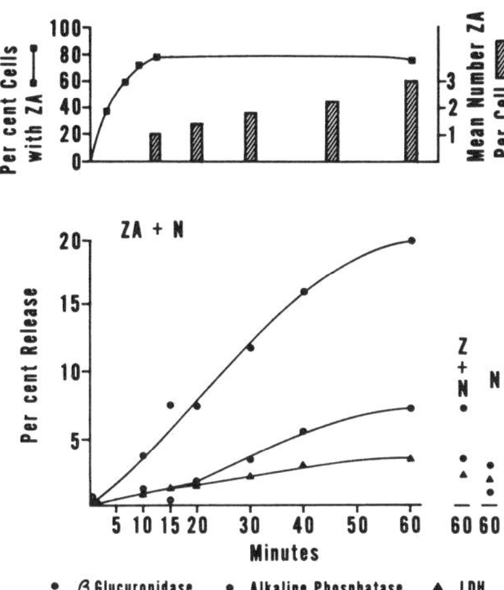

FIG. 7.   Release of enzymes from rabbit neutrophils phagocytosing zymosan particles. ZA, 2 mg zymosan incubated with rabbit IgG anti-zymosan antibody and then washed; N, 10^7 neutrophils; LDH, lactic dehydrogenase. The alkaline phosphatase was only poorly released.

myeloperoxidase (which comes from the primary granule) into phagocytic vacuoles of neutrophils. The mechanisms whereby granules may be discharged at different rates is at present unknown but from a functional standpoint it is of interest that, as suggested by Bainton (20), secondary granules may release enzymes with pH optima near neutrality before the pH within a vacuole (or inflammatory lesion) is reduced.

(e) *Degranulation in vivo*: Neutrophils adherent to antibody and complement along basement membranes in vivo have not yet been observed in the process of discharging granules. Nevertheless, cells may be seen in lesions of nephrotoxic nephritis which have almost completely lost their complement of granules (Fig. 2 b). The process described in vitro may then also contribute in vivo to the release of injurious consitituents from neutrophils.

(2) *Release of Enzymes from Neutrophils during Phagocytosis.*—Phagocytosis of either immune complexes or antibody-coated particles induces release of enzymes from the neutrophil primary granules (Table I) (12).[1] As depicted in Fig. 7, phagocytosis of zymosan–antibody complexes was a very effective stimulus for the release of β-glucuronidase from the primary granule to the exterior of the cells. The minimal release of lactic dehydrogenase and the exclusion of Trypan blue by the cells indicates that this release did not result from lysis of the cells.

(a) *Release of alkaline phosphatase*: When alkaline phosphatase was examined, however, a striking difference was noted between the release stimulated by a nonphagocytosable surface and by a phagocytosed particle. As shown in Fig. 7, phagocytosis of zymosan antibody induced little extracellular release of this enzyme (whether in the medium or bound to the external cell membrane) and, in addition, it was liberated over the same time-course as β-glucuronidase.

(b) *Mechanism of extracellular release*: Morphologic and histochemical studies in the electron microscope helped explain this difference (Fig. 8). In confirmation of Bainton's experiments (20), alkaline phosphatase was liberated into the phagocytic vacuoles after only a short period (2–5 min) of incubation, even though it was not released to the outside. It could be detected there, bound to the surface membrane of the vacuole. It is postulated that the release of enzymes during phagocytosis is a two-stage phenomenon, first a degranulation into the phagocytic vacuole and then an opening of the vacuole, probably transiently, to the outside of the cell. The soluble enzymes, such as β-glucuronidase, escape, but the alkaline phosphatase remains in the vacuole bound to its surface membrane. Direct discharge of granules to the cell surface has not been observed.

One situation in which phagocytic vacuoles may open to the extracellular medium is during the process of phagocytosis of an additional particle, which may be taken into an already existing vacuole before the neutrophil pseudopodia have closed behind it. Evidence for this process has been obtained (Fig. 8). Moreover, the release of enzymes correlates well with the uptake of additional zymosan particles (Fig. 7), not with phagocytosis of the first particle.

A corollary of this hypothesis would suggest that phagocytosis of large particles would induce greater release than that of small particles, since the latter

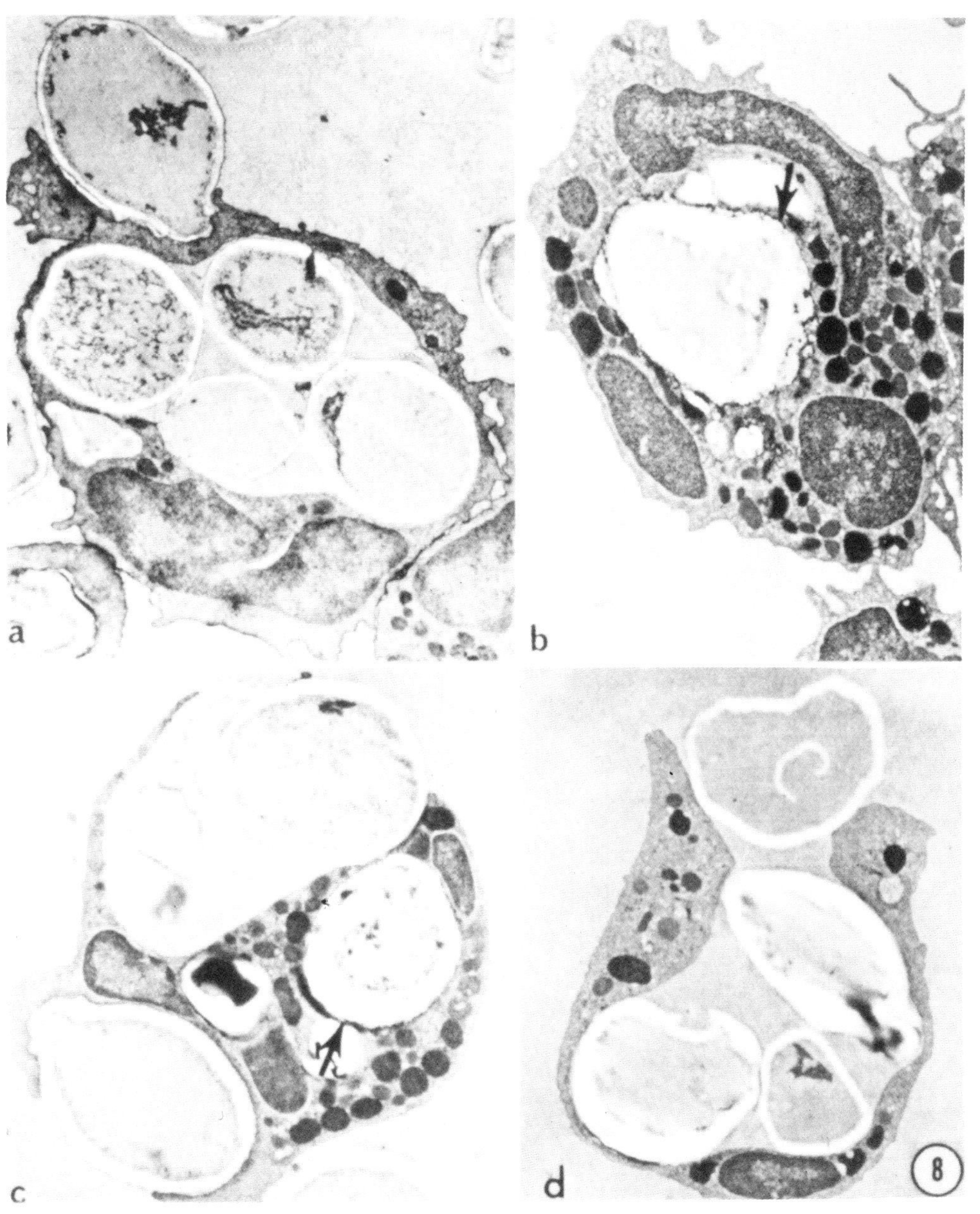

Fig. 8.   Rabbit neutrophils phagocytosing zymosan particles. (*a*) Neutrophil containing six particles of zymosan complement (see text) and adherent to a seventh. × 7300. (*b*) Neutrophil after 10 min incubation with zymosan antibody showing alkaline phosphatase activity. The reaction product (arrow) may be seen along the surface of the phagocytic vacuole which contains one zymosan particle. × 5100. (*c* and *d*) Neutrophils after 30 min incubation with ZA. Stages in the uptake of an additional particle into an already formed phagocytic vacuole are shown. A number of granules remain in *c* but have mostly disappeared in *d*. The latter cell shows an opening of the vacuole, presumably containing lysosomal enzymes, to the outside. Many instances of this phenomenon have been observed. Arrow in *c* same as in *b*. × 8200 and 7600, respectively.

would be more likely to be sequestered in individual vacuoles and the neutrophil would more readily enclose the particle before incorporation into already existing vacuoles. Studies with IgG globulin bound to latex particles of different sizes have revealed that this is indeed the case. Particles of 2, 1, 0.5, and 0.1 μm in diameter induced release of 22, 19, 16, and 9% β-glucuronidase, respectively, where equal surface area (and, therefore, equal amounts of IgG) were presented to the neutrophils. This finding, therefore, confirms the original observations of Cohn and Hirsch (21) who found less than 10% release of lysosomal enzymes to the exterior of neutrophils (heterophils) phagocytosing small particles (bacteria).

Two other related mechanisms of release may also contribute to the reaction and have occasionally been observed. Phagocytosis of one particle by two neutrophils leads to degranulation into a vacuole which is essentially open to the exterior[1] (22). In addition, during phagocytosis, degranulation into a developing vacuole sometimes occurs before the vacuole is completely closed. However, these are likely to be secondary granules (see above), and yet alkaline phosphatase was found in only low levels outside the cell and not generally along the surface of developing vacuoles before they were closed off. Moreover, the release of enzymes correlated with the uptake of not the first, but of additional zymosan particles. These observations do not suggest a major role for these two mechanisms although they probably add to the total release.[1]

(c) *Release in vivo*: Although it has not yet been clearly demonstrated that uptake of particles into preexisting phagocytic vacuoles containing lysosomal enzymes does occur in vivo, Fig. 9 shows that it may be possible. This depicts an Arthus reaction produced with ferritin antigen and shows that precipitates of large size may be formed which may lead to suitably large vacuoles for the postulated release process.

(3) *Comparison of Release of Constituents from Neutrophils Adhering to Phagocytosable Particles or Nonphagocytosable Surfaces.*—Fig. 10 summarizes our concept of the predominant mechanisms of release in these two circumstances. On the surface, there is a degranulation to the external membrane of the cells which is in contact with the immune complexes. After phagocytosis, there is a degranulation into the phagocytic vacuole which later opens to the outside during ingestion of additional particles, a process which is more likely to occur with larger than with smaller particles.

The relative sensitivities of these processes in vitro are shown in Table II To achieve 13% release of β-glucuronidase, 31 μg of antibody in immune complexes in suspension was required. However, on the nonphagocytosable surface, less than 2 μg of antibody was effective. (In fact, more antibody is present on the filter but neutrophils are drawn down onto only a small portion of the total area available.) Immune complexes along surfaces within the body may,

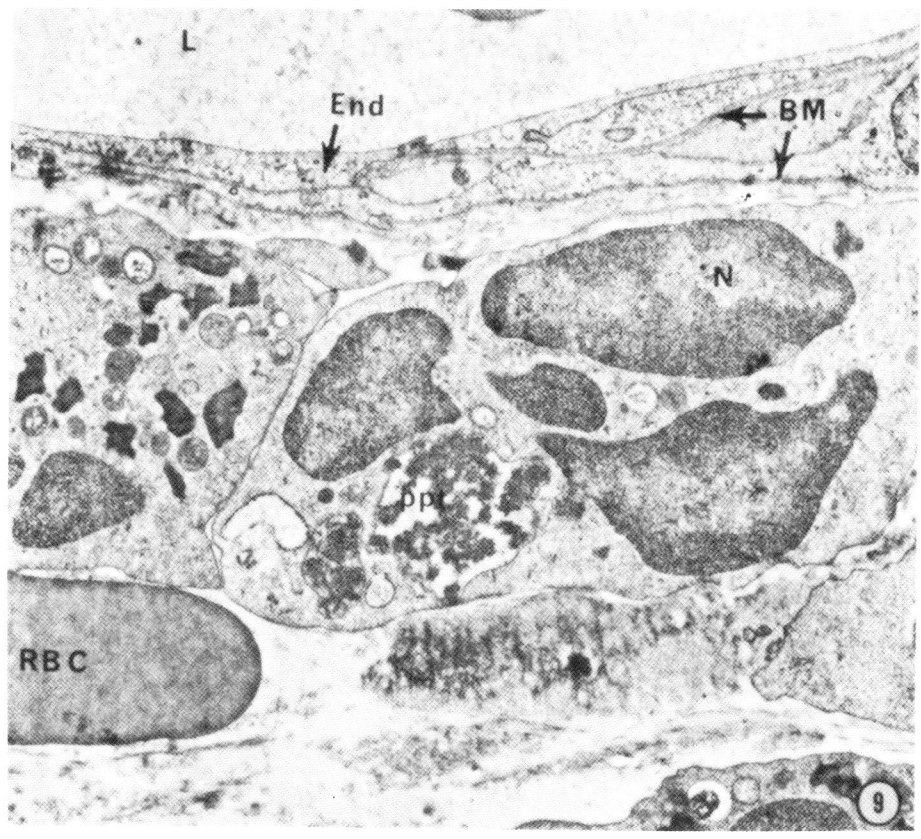

Fig. 9. A reversed passive Arthus reaction in the rabbit bladder wall. Neutrophils (N) are visible in the vessel wall and have phagocytosed immune complexes (ferritin–anti-ferritin). One large vacuole containing such a precipitate (ppt) can be seen and is almost open to the outside of the cell. RBC, red blood cell; *BM*, basement membrane; End, endothelial cell; L, lumen. × 14,500.

therefore, be more effective stimuli to tissue injury than when free in the blood stream.

In inflammatory lesions in vivo, neutrophil degeneration and lysis may play an important role by contributing additional neutrophil enzymes and permeability factors. This cell death could occur for many reasons, but may in part be caused by materials released by active (not degenerative) processes from neutrophils which arrived first at the site of injury and there interacted with the immune complexes by the mechanisms described.

(C) THE STIMULUS TO NEUTROPHILS FOR RELEASE OF
CONSTITUENTS TO THE OUTSIDE

The initial reaction between neutrophils and immune complexes is one of adherence. This adherence is mediated by either antibody or complement

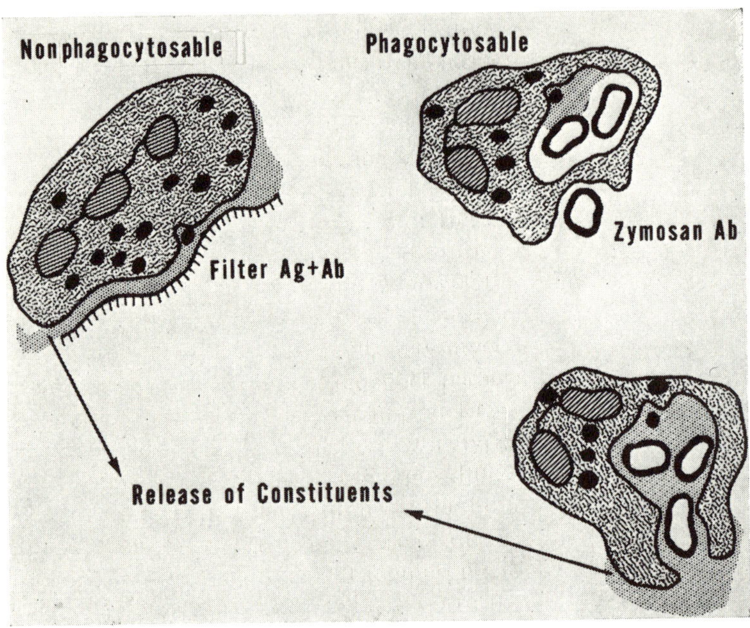

FIG. 10. Two mechanisms of release of granule constituents from neutrophils reacting with immune complexes which may be phagocytosed, or which are bound to nonphagocytosable surfaces.

(23–28) and may be clearly demonstrated by "rosette" formation if the particle is too large for easy phagocytosis or if the neutrophils are metabolically inhibited so that the subsequent phagocytosis is prevented (Fig. 11).

(1) Complement.—The fixation of complement components to erythrocytes or zymosan results in adherence of neutrophils and phagocytosis of the particles. Clear evidence from a number of laboratories (24–26, 28, 29) has implicated C3 as the complement component of major importance in these phenomena of adherence, phagocytosis, and release of constituents.

The ability of complement to induce release of enzymes from neutrophils on nonphagocytosable surfaces has also been examined. Incubation of antigen

214

and antibody bound to micropore filters in normal fresh serum allowed complement fixation. Neutrophils adherent to these complexes exhibited increased release of lysosomal constituents. By use of C6-deficient or C3-depleted sera, it was possible to implicate C3 in this reaction also.[1]

(2) Immunoglobulins.—The receptors on neutrophils (and also those on monocytes and macrophages) which allow adherence to C3 are different from those which permit adherence to IgG antibody (25, 26, 30). The former can be removed by trypsin or, in the case of rabbit neutrophils, prevented from reacting with C3 by the addition of chelating agents. In contrast, adherence of neutrophils to IgG antibody on a particle such as an erythrocyte is inhibited in the presence of excess free, monodisperse IgG, which has no effect on the adherence to complement.

TABLE II

Amounts of Antibody Required to Stimulate Release of Enzymes from Rabbit Neutrophils

	IgG antibody	Per cent release of enzymes	
		β-glucuronidase	LDH
	μg		
Ag Ab precipitates	31	13.2	6.1
Z Ab	5	13.7	5.5
Ag Ab on filter	<2	15.0	6.0

What are the classes of immunoglobulins which induce these reactions? To answer this question, the ability of neutrophils to release β-glucuronidase upon adherence to (or phagocytosis of) aggregated immunoglobulins was examined.[4]

(3) Reaction of Neutrophils with Immunoglobulin Classes and Subclasses.— Purified human myeloma proteins were aggregated with bisdiazo-benzidine (BDB) (31) or by heat. Table III shows the results of incubating aggregated immunoglobulins with human neutrophils. Each myeloma protein was tested in duplicate on a number of occasions with neutrophils from different normal subjects. It may be seen that with these insoluble aggregates (500 μg incubated with 5×10^6 neutrophils for 1 hr at 37°C), IgG$_1$, IgG$_2$, IgG$_3$, and IgG$_4$ all induced release of β-glucuronidase, and adherence of neutrophils to the microscopically visible precipitates was observed. There was also some suggestion that IgG$_4$ was less active but this was in part due to greater variation from myeloma to myeloma of this subclass.

Of great interest was the finding that neutrophils adhered to aggregates of all IgA examined and that these myeloma proteins proved very efficient in

---

[4] Henson, P. M., R. J. Bell, and H. L. Spiegelberg. Manuscript in preparation.

stimulating release of enzymes. IgM macroglobulins were unable to induce either adherence or release of β-glucuronidase and IgD was also inactive.

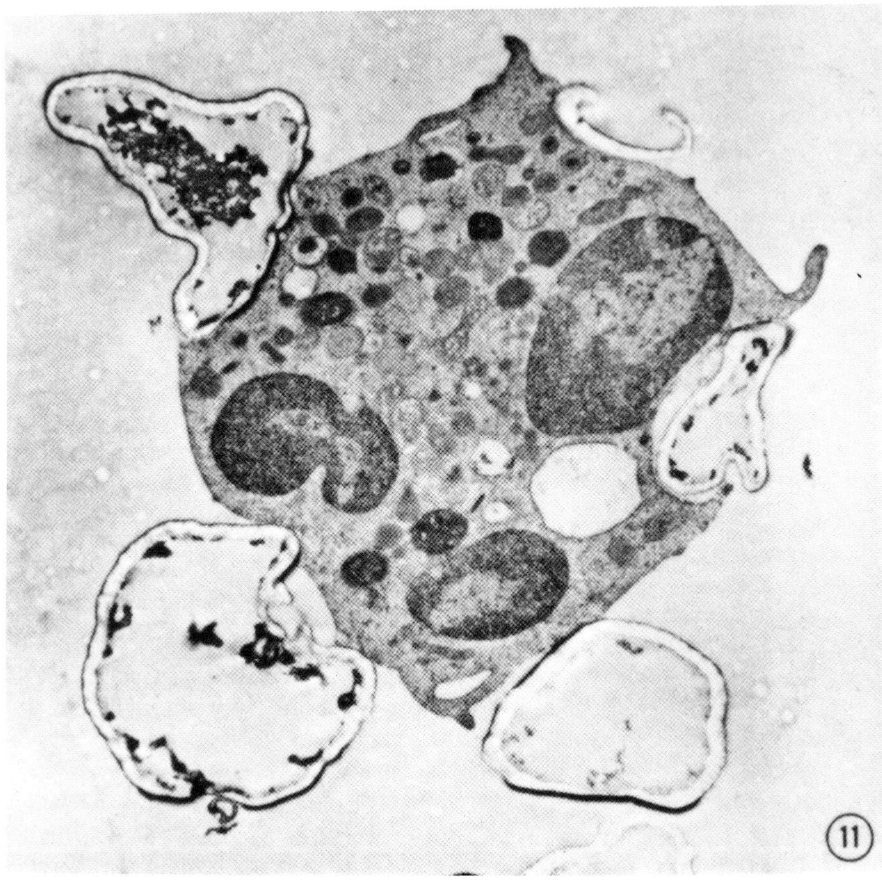

F_{IG}. 11.   Adherence of zymosan–anti-zymosan complexes to the surface of a rabbit neutrophil. The phagocytosis which would normally ensue has been inhibited with 10^{-3} M iodoacetate. $\times$ 13,900.

Table IV shows that for each myeloma, 500 μg was an effective stimulus and 50 μg was not. Since the maximum contamination of any of the myeloma proteins used was 5% and most contained much less, the possibility that the IgA was reacting with neutrophils by virtue of contamination with IgG was excluded. Although the reaction of neutrophil suspensions with insoluble immunoglobulin aggregates resulted in release of enzymes, if soluble aggregates, prepared with less aggregating agent, were employed, no release oc-

TABLE III

Release of Enzymes from Washed Human Neutrophils by Aggregated Immunoglobulins in Suspension

| Myeloma proteins | No. | Per cent release of enzymes* | | | Adherence to precipitates |
| | | β-glucuronidase | | LDH | |
		Mean	Range		
IgG$_1$	(3)	14.6	(6.3–24.7)	2.3	+
IgG$_2$	(4)	9.4	(3.8–14.5)	2.2	+
IgG$_3$	(2)	12.1	(9.0–14.0)	2.5	+
IgG$_4$	(3)	8.3	(3.4–12.4)	2.1	+
IgA$_1$	(4)	10.3	(6.1–18.4)	2.3	+
IgA$_2$	(2)	10.7	(8.7–12.7)	3.0	+
IgD	(2)	1.2	(0.3–2.2)	1.7	
IgM	(4)	1.5	(0.6–2.0)	2.8	0
—		1.1	(0–3.1)	2.1	

* Aggregated immunoglobulins (500 μg aggregated with BDB) were incubated with 5 × 10^6 neutrophils for 60 min at 37°C, and the percentage of enzymes released into the supernatant fluid was measured.

TABLE IV

Percentage of β-Glucuronidase Released from Human Neutrophils by Aggregated Immunoglobulins

| Immunoglobulin | Degree of aggregation | μg aggregated immunoglobulins | | | |
		500	200	100	50
IgG$_1$	Soluble*	3.0	3.0	2.7	2.3
	Insoluble	20.3	9.1	5.2	3.4
IgG$_2$	Insoluble	13.8	8.3	6.1	3.7
IgG$_3$	Insoluble	13.3	10.0	6.6	4.1
IgG$_4$	Insoluble	12.4	7.7	6.3	5.4
IgA$_1$	Insoluble	14.6	10.4	8.0	3.5

* Soluble aggregates of immunoglobulins (2.5 mg/ml) were produced with 12 μg/ml BDB and insoluble aggregates with 50 μg/ml BDB.

curred (Table IV). This again demonstrates the requirement for large particles for this type of release reaction.

In contrast to the lack of release when neutrophils reacted with soluble immunoglobulins in suspension, when such soluble aggregated myeloma proteins were fixed to the surface of micropore filters, adherent neutrophils did release β-glucuronidase (Table V). This occurred if the neutrophils were in contact with only 15 μg (or less) of protein. Once again, all four subclasses of IgG and both IgA₁ and IgA₂ were capable of inducing enzyme release while IgM was ineffective and IgD was only weakly active, if at all.

These results indicated that human neutrophils have receptors on their surface for, and are capable of being directly stimulated by, both IgG and IgA immunoglobulins. IgM does not react in this way and had previously been shown not to induce adherence by itself (26), but due to its complement-fixing activity would cause adherence secondarily by means of the C3 which is fixed. IgG₄ and IgA do not fix complement by the normal process but, nevertheless, as described above, do have the ability to react directly with the neu-

TABLE V

Release of Enzymes from Washed Human Neutrophils by Aggregated Immunoglobulins on Nonphagocytosable Surfaces

Myeloma[a] proteins	No.	Per cent release of enzymes		LDH
		β glucuronidase		
IgG₁	(3)	13.6	(12.1–16.4)	2.1
IgG₂	(2)	11.7	(9.9–13.2)	1.9
IgG₃	(2)	10.5	(8.3–12.7)	1.8
IgG₄	(3)	8.1	(4.5–12.0)	1.9
IgA	(3)	12.3	(7.2–16.4)	2.3
IgA₂	(1)	7.0	(5.3–8.6)	2.5
IgD	(2)	4.0	(0–5.7)	2.7
IgM	(3)	2.7	(0–5.5)	1.9
BSA		2.6	(1.8–3.9)	2.1

trophils. It has been reported (32) that binding of IgG₁ and IgG₃ by neutrophils as measured by inhibition studies was more efficient than that of IgG₂ and IgG₄. The studies described herein provided a semiquantitative assessment of the ability of neutrophils to react directly with the immunoglobulins and showed a reaction with all four subclasses of IgG, although IgG₁ and IgG₃ did appear to be more active.

The adherence of neutrophils to the immune complex (whether induced by complement or by immunoglobulins) is but the first step in the sequence of biochemical events leading to phagocytosis and/or release of enzymes. The release process is an active one and requires neutrophil energy metabolism, the action of serine esterases, and the presence of calcium ions. Moreover, its control may be mediated by cyclic–adenosine monophosphate.[5] However, much has still to be determined before the release process can be selectively

[5] Weissmann, Gerald, Robert B. Zurier, Paul J. Spieler, and Ira M. Goldstein. Mechanisms of lysosomal enzyme release from leukocytes exposed to immune complexes and other particles. *J. Exp. Med.* **134** (3, Pt. 2):149 s.

inhibited in vivo in order to prevent the liberation of injurious materials into inflammatory lesions.

(D) SUMMARY AND CONCLUSIONS

Neutrophils are essential mediators of tissue damage in many forms of immune complex–induced injury. In vitro, they have been shown to release some of their content of injurious constituents upon reaction with immune complexes (Fig. 10). If the complexes are distributed along a nonphagocytosable surface, degranulation to the exterior of the cell is observed. When the complexes were phagocytized, however, degranulation into the phagocytic vacuole, and some loss of enzymes into the surrounding medium, occurred. This may have resulted from a momentary opening of the vacuole to allow ingestion of additional particles, as was demonstrated with the electron microscope. This phenomenon was particularly noticeable when the particles were relatively large. Far more immune complex is required to induce release when in a phagocytosable form than when on a nonphagocytosable membrane.

Neutrophils may be attracted to sites of immune complex deposition in many parts of the body (arteries, heart, skin, brain, kidney, joints) by complement-mediated processes. In some situations, e.g. in the joint fluid, they would encounter free immune complexes, phagocytose them, and release enzymes. In many others, in which immune complexes may be distributed along surfaces, such as in the glomerulus, adherence of neutrophils may also lead to release of injurious constituents (proteases, collagenase, elastase, permeability factors) capable of digesting and injuring the tissues.

The author would like to thank Mrs. D. Durham for preparing the sections for electron microscopy and Mrs. K. Prescott, Mrs. P. Wright, and Miss S. Rader for the illustrations.

REFERENCES

1. Henson, P. M., and C. G. Cochrane. 1971. Immune complex disease in rabbits. The role of complement and of a leukocyte-dependent release of vasoactive amines from platelets. *J. Exp. Med.* **133**:554.

2. Kniker, W. T., and C. G. Cochrane. 1965. Pathogenic factors in vascular lesions of experimental serum sickness. *J. Exp. Med.* **122**:83.

3. Rhyne, M. B., and F. G. Germuth. 1961. The relationship between serum complement activity and the development of allergic lesions in rabbits. *J. Exp. Med.* **114**:633.

4. Lerner, R. A., R. J. Glassock, and F. J. Dixon. 1967. The role of anti–glomerular basement membrane antibody in the pathogenesis of human glomerulonephritis. *J. Exp. Med.* **126**:989.

5 Cochrane, C. G., and P. M. Henson. 1971. Complement and immunologic reactions *in vivo. J. Immunol.* In press.

6. Cochrane, C. G., E. R. Unanue, and F. J. Dixon. 1965. A role of polymorphonu-

clear leukocytes and complement in nephrotoxic nephritis. *J. Exp. Med.* **122:** 99.

7. Hawkins, D., and C. G. Cochrane. 1968. Glomerular basement membrane damage in immunological glomerulonephritis. *Immunology.* **14:**665.

8. Movat, H. Z., T. Uriuhara, and D. R. L. Macmorine. 1964. A permeability factor released from leukocytes after phagocytosis of immune complexes and its possible role in the Arthus reaction. *Life Sci.* **3:**1025.

9. Janoff, A., and J. D. Zeligs. 1968. Vascular injury and lysis of basement membrane *in vitro* by neutral protease of human leukocytes. *Science (Washington).* **161:** 702.

10. Tew, J. G., W. M. Hess, and D. M. Donaldson. 1969. Lysozyme and β-lysin release stimulated by antigen-antibody complexes and bacteria. *J. Immunol.* **102:**743.

11. Parish, W. E. 1969. Effects of neutrophils on tissues. Experiments on the Arthus reaction, the flare phenomenon, and post-phagocytic release of lysosomal enzymes. *Brit. J. Dermatol.* **81:**28.

12. Hawkins, D., and S. Peeters. 1971. The response of polymorphonuclear leukocytes to immune complexes *in vitro. Lab. Invest.* In press.

13. Martin, R. R., J. G. Crowder, and A. White. 1967. Human reactions to staphylococcal antigens. A possible role of leukocyte lysosomal enzymes. *J. Immunol.* **99:**269.

14. Crowder, J. G., R. R. Martin, and A. White. 1969. Release of histamine and lysosomal enzymes by human leukocytes during phagocytosis of staphylococci. *J. Lab. Clin. Med.* **74:**436.

15. Pruzansky, J. J., and R. Patterson. 1967. Subcellular distribution of histamine in leukocytes. *Proc. Soc. Exp. Biol. Med.* **124:**56.

16. May, C. O., B. B. Levine, and G. Weissmann. 1970. Effects of compounds which inhibit antigenic release of histamine and phagocytic release of lysosomal enzymes on glucose utilization by leukocytes in humans. *Proc. Soc. Exp. Biol. Med.* **133:**758.

17. Baggiolini, M., J. G. Hirsch, and C. de Duve. 1969. Resolution of granules from rabbit heterophil leukocytes into distinct populations by zonal sedimentation. *J. Cell Biol.* **40:**529.

18. Bainton, D. F., and M. G. Farquhar. 1968. Differences in enzyme content of azurophil and specific granules of polymorphonuclear leukocytes. II Cytochemistry and electron microscopy of bone marrow cells. *J. Cell Biol.* **39:**299.

19. Henson, P. 1971. Excretion of insoluble alkaline phosphatase by neutrophils stimulated by antigen and antibody on a nonphagocytosable surface. *Fed. Proc.* **30:**511. (Abstr.)

20. Bainton, D. F. 1970. Sequential discharge of polymorphonuclear leukocyte granules during phagocytosis of microorganisms. *J. Cell Biol.* **47** (2, Pt. 2): 11a. (Abstr.).

21. Cohn, Z. A., and J. G. Hirsch. 1960. The influence of phagocytosis on the intracellular distribution of granule-associated components of polymorphonuclear leukocytes. *J. Exp. Med.* **112:**1015.

22. Zucker-Franklin, D., and J. G. Hirsch. 1964. Electron microscope studies on the

degranulation of rabbit peritoneal leukocytes during phagocytosis. *J. Exp. Med.* **120**:569.

23. Gerlings-Peterson, B. T., and K. W. Pondman. 1962. Erythrophagocytosis: a study of the antigen-antibody-complement reaction. *Vox Sang.* **7**:655.

24. Nelson, D. S. 1965. Immune adherence. *Complement, Ciba Found. Symp.* 222.

25. Lay, W. H., and V. Nussenzweig. 1968. Receptors for complement on leukocytes. *J. Exp. Med.* **128**:991.

26. Henson, P. M. 1969. The adherence of leukocytes and platelets induced by fixed IgG antibody or complement. *Immunology.* **16**:107.

27. Phillips-Quagliata, J. M., B. B. Levine, and J. W. Uhr. 1969. Studies on the mechanism of binding of immune complexes to phagocytes. *Nature (London).* **222**:1290.

28. Henson, P. M. 1971. Complement dependent adherence of cells to antigen and antibody: mechanisms and consequences. *In* Biological Activities of Complement. D. G. Ingram, editor. S. Karger AG., Basel. In press.

29. Gigli, I., and R. A. Nelson. 1968. Complement dependent immune phagocytsis I. Requirements for C′₁, C′₄, C′₂, C′₃. *Exp. Cell Res.* **51**:45.

30. Huber, H., M. J. Polley, W. D. Linscott, H. H. Fudenberg, and H. J. Müller-Eberhard. 1968. Human monocytes: distinct receptor sites for the third component of complement and for immunoglobulin G. *Science (Washington).* **162**:1281.

31. Ishizaka, T., K. Ishizaka, S. Salmon, and H. H. Fudenberg. 1967. Biologic activities of aggregated γ-globulin. VIII. Aggregated immunoglobulins of different classes. *J. Immunol.* **99**:82.

32. Messner, R. P., and J. Jelinek. 1970. Receptors for human γG globulin on human neutrophils. *J. Clin. Invest.* **49**:2165.

The Immunoglobulin Origin of Amyloid

GEORGE G. GLENNER, M.D.
DANIEL EIN, M.D.
WILLIAM D. TERRY, M.D.

Since the first description of amyloid infiltration in 1842 by
Rokitansky [1], the chemical composition and pathogenesis of
amyloid deposits have been in dispute. Virchow originally coined
the name "amyloid" (starch-like), since he was convinced the
deposits consisted primarily of carbohydrates. Virchow also
concluded that "only when we have discovered the means of
isolating the amyloid substance, shall we be able to come to any
definite conclusion with regard to its nature" [2]. Although the
first chemical analysis of amyloid by Friedreich and Kekulé [3]
in 1859 indicated amyloid to be a protein, controversy as to its
origin and chemical composition resulted in an abundant and
conflicting literature [4]. Only recently has it become clear that
in many, if not all instances, amyloid represents the tissue
deposition of fragments of immunoglobulin proteins. Possible
relationships between amyloid and the immune system were
suggested as early as 1902 [4–7], and in 1931, Magnus-Levy
commented on the frequent association of amyloidosis with
Bence Jones proteinuria in patients with multiple myeloma
[8,9]. He postulated that amyloid tissue infiltrates might be directly related to these Bence Jones proteins. Two other classic
observations implicated the immune system in the etiology of
amyloidosis. These were the demonstration by Apitz [10] of
abnormal plasma cells and plasmacytosis in the bone marrow
of some patients with "primary" amyloidosis [11] and the
association between chronic antigenic stimulation and so-called
"secondary" amyloidosis [5,12–14]. Extensive evidence of

a significant association between amyloidosis and myeloma-type proteins, particularly Bence Jones proteins, has been provided by the observations of Osserman and his associates [15–17] over the past several years. By electrophoretic and immunoelectrophoretic analyses, these investigators have consistently demonstrated the presence of characteristically homogeneous, monoclonal globulins and/or Bence Jones proteins indicative of an underlying plasma cell dyscrasia in the overwhelming majority of a large series of cases of amyloidosis of either the so-called "primary" or "secondary" type.

Although these studies implicated immunoglobulins as being an important element in amyloid deposits, many other investigations failed to substantiate this relationship [18–20]. Immunofluorescent and other immunochemical methods occasionally revealed immunoglobulins or immunoglobulin components in amyloid [21–24], but more often these findings were considered irrelevant or could not be confirmed [24–26]. In addition, studies of amyloid deposits often demonstrated the presence of a number of serum proteins including fibrinogen, complement components and lipoproteins [27–31], thus casting doubt on the significance of those observations reporting immunoglobulins in these lesions.

The identity of the components of human amyloid was not resolved by these investigations. Electron microscopic investigations, however, defined a fibrillar component [32–34], which was shown to be the structure responsible for amyloid's unique Congo red staining and polarization birefringence [35–37]. These fibrils had a distinctive appearance when examined in the electron microscope [38–40] and an x-ray diffraction picture characteristic of a β-pleated sheet conformation [41].

Ultracentrifugation procedures [26,39,40] provided a concentrated amyloid fibril preparation, but the marked insolubility of the fibrils in aqueous buffers made further purification impossible. Recently, however, fibrils were solubilized with 6 M

TABLE I   Chemical Analyses

Amino Acid*	Patient's Purified Amyloid Protein					
	III	IV	VI	VIII	X	XIV
Aspartic acid	75.5	154.9	55.5	103.1	97.3	24.6
Threonine	80.1	0	68.4	76.4	84.7	66.4
Serine	112.2	70.9	122.7	103.4	109.3	118.3
Glutamic acid	106.4	50.3	98.1	111.9	107.0	97.4
Proline	78.1	0	62.6	55.8	76.7	79.1
Glycine	83.5	103.2	107.8	69.1	96.2	20.2
Alanine	91.9	156.1	83.3	63.0	59.5	89.2
Half cystine	23.4	0	23.2	20.3	20.6	17.7
Valine	74.5	0	58.1	59.2	44.1	67.0
Methionine	3.1	43.7	0	8.4	10.9	0
Isoleucine	29.9	19.0	40.7	45.5	47.5	50.6
Leucine	83.9	25.2	80.7	80.0	59.5	84.1
Tyrosine	31.6	82.7	43.9	39.2	51.5	39.8
Phenylalanine	21.9	114.5	23.9	45.8	45.2	34.8
Lysine	53.3	25.2	60.0	55.4	43.5	24.7
Histidine	11.6	20.5	16.8	12.9	0	13.3
Arginine	24.8	110.9	41.3	39.2	32.6	12.0
Tryptophan	13.7	23.1	12.9	11.2	13.7	10.8
Total	999.9	999.9	999.9	999.8	999.8	1000.0
N-terminus	U†	Arg	U	Asp	Asp	U
Molecular weight	13,700	5,000	15,400	18,300	7,500	14,600

* Residues/1,000 residues.
† Unreactive to fluorodinitrobenzene.

guanidine hydrochloride in the presence of a reducing agent [42]. This permitted purification of fibrillar proteins in high yield [42,43] as well as their physical, chemical and immunochemical characterization [44,45]. These studies indicated that the major protein constituents of amyloid fibrils are fragments of immunoglobulin polypeptide chains [44,45], providing additional support for the hypothesis that immunoglobulins are involved in the pathogenesis of amyloidosis.

Immunoglobulin molecules are composed of light and heavy polypeptide chains. Chemical studies have shown that both kinds of polypeptide chains have amino-terminal variable regions which differ from chain to chain. The remainder of these polypeptide chains (constant regions) are nearly identical from molecule to molecule within a particular light chain type (kappa or lambda) or heavy chain class or subclass (IgG, IgA, IgM, etc.). These structural features are also demonstrable by immunochemical analysis. Antiserums prepared against homogeneous immunoglobulin polypeptide chains, such as Bence Jones proteins, react with common antigens shared by polypeptide chains of the same type (i.e., kappa-light chains). Each kappa-light chain has in addition unique (idiotypic) antigenic determinants [46–49]. Chemical and antigenic analysis of a kappa-type Bence Jones protein isolated from the serum and urine of the same patient usually will show the proteins to be identical, whereas kappa-type Bence Jones proteins isolated from two different patients will show differences due to different variable regions. Another characteristic finding is that the amino-terminal amino acid of kappa chains is either aspartic or glutamic acid, whereas that of lambda chains is usually pyrrolidone carboxylic acid (PCA).

The similarity of these properties with those of isolated amyloid fibrils is clearly shown by the following observations. Amyloid fibril proteins from different tissues of the same subject have identical amino acid compositions and peptide maps, whereas fibrillar proteins from different subjects vary (Table I). The amino-terminal amino acid of most of the fibrillar proteins is either aspartic acid or PCA [44,45]. Immunochemical studies indicate that, although the major protein of fibrils from different patients are antigenically related to one another, each patient's fibrillar protein possesses unique antigens [45]. Amyloid protein, like immunoglobulin protein, therefore, appears to have constant (shared) as well as variable (idiotypic) portions.

Additional support for the concept that there is a close relationship between amyloid fibrils and immunoglobulins comes from immunodiffusion experiments [50]. Antiserums to amyloid proteins with aspartic acid amino-termini react with other aspartic acid amino-terminal amyloid proteins and with 23 of 26 kappa Bence Jones proteins. These antiserums do not react with blocked (PCA) amino-terminal amyloid proteins or with lambda Bence Jones proteins. Antiserum to an amyloid fibril protein with a blocked amino-terminus reacts with other blocked amyloid proteins, as well as 7 of 23 lambda Bence Jones proteins, but does not react with kappa Bence Jones proteins or amyloid proteins with aspartic acid at the amino-terminus [50]. The fact that Bence Jones proteins and chemically related amyloid fibril proteins share antigenic determinants is further evidence that the protein moiety of amyloid fibrils is an immunoglobulin and indicates the existence of at least two types of amyloid proteins, a lambda and a kappa type.

The strongest support for the immunoglobulin origin of amyloid fibrils has come with the determination of the amino acid sequence of the major protein component of two amyloid fibril proteins with aspartic acid amino-termini. These highly purified proteins are obtained in 70 per cent yield from the starting fibrillar preparation. In the automatic amino acid sequence procedure used, the yield of the amino-terminal residues of these proteins is about 50 per cent. A similar yield is obtained when Bence Jones proteins of high purity are subjected to similar preparative procedures and sequenced with the automatic sequencer. The amino acid sequence of these two amyloid proteins is compared in Table II with the known amino acid sequence of a kappa Bence Jones protein, Ker [51,52]. It is evident that these sequences are similar, and the minor differences are no greater than those seen between any two kappa Bence Jones proteins. These results prove conclusively that the major protein component of these two amyloid fibril preparations is derived from kappa light polypeptide chains. As is true of Bence Jones proteins, each amyloid protein sequence is homogeneous indicating its probable origin from a single clone of immunoglobulin synthesizing cells.

This finding has relevance to possible patho-

TABLE II Sequence Analyses of Amyloid Protein X and VIII-b as Compared to the Sequence of the Prototype V_{KI}, Ker. (Variant residues are in bold type; undetermined or equivocal residues are indicated by brackets.)

	1	2	3	4	5	6	7	8	9	10	11	12	13	14	15	16	17	18
Ker	Asp	Ile	Gln	Met	Thr	Gln	Ser	Pro	Ser	Ser	Leu	Ser	Ala	Ser	Val	Gly	Asp	Arg
Amyloid X	Asp	Ile	Gln	Met	Thr	Gln	Ser	**Ala**	Ser	Ser	Leu	Ser	Ala	Ser	Val	Gly	Asp	Arg
Amyloid VIII	Asp	Ile	Gln	Met	Thr	Gln	Ser	Pro	Ser	Ser	Leu	Ser	Ala	Ser	Val	Gly	Asp	Arg

	19	20	21	22	23	24	25	26	27	28	29	30	31	32	33	34	35	36
Ker	Val	Thr	Ile	Thr	Cys	Gln	Ala	Ser	Gln	Asp	Ile	Lys						
Amyloid X	Val	**Ile**	Ile	[ ]	Cys	Glx	Ala	[ ]	Glx	Asx	Ile	[ ]	Pro	Tyr	Leu	[ ]	[ ]	Tyr
Amyloid VIII	Val	Thr	Ile	Thr	Cys	Gln	Ala	Ser	Gln	Asx	Ile	**Gly**	[ ]	Tyr	Leu	[ ]	Trp	

NOTE: Table from Glenner et al. [52].

genetic mechanisms in amyloidosis. One of these proteins comes from a patient with so-called "primary" amyloidosis, indicating the close relation of this disorder to the plasma cell dyscrasias, as previously emphasized by Osserman [53]. The second fibril protein with a kappa light chain sequence is from a patient with "secondary" amyloidosis. It is apparent that regardless of clinical classification, amyloid fibrils may consist of immunoglobulin protein. The origin of amyloid fibrils associated with overt multiple myeloma or plasma cell dyscrasia has also been established. The amyloid fibril and urinary Bence Jones protein of one such patient are identical by limited amino acid sequence and peptide map criteria [54]. This demonstrates that at least in some patients with amyloidosis, plasma cell dyscrasia and Bence Jones proteinuria, the amyloid fibril is derived from the homogeneous light polypeptide chain.

The molecular weights of amyloid fibril proteins are variable [44,45] and generally lower (5,000 to 18,300) than those of intact light chains (normally 22,500). Thus in most cases only a fragment of a light chain is contained in amyloid deposits. Amino acid sequence and peptide map studies indicate that most amyloid proteins contain the amino-terminal variable region of the light chain. The light chain variable region accounts for half the total light chain and has, therefore, a molecular weight of about 11,000. Since several amyloid fibril proteins have molecular weights slightly greater than this, these proteins either contain a portion of the common region or nonprotein components. The amino acid sequence data suggest, however, that it is the variable region of the light chain which plays an essential role in the formation of an amyloid fibril.

This assertion is further strengthened by the creation of "amyloid" fibrils in vitro. Under specific conditions of enzymatic digestion, Bence Jones proteins are cleaved into variable and constant halves [55]. Using a modified method, Bence Jones proteins have been subjected to proteolytic digestion under nearly physiologic conditions. With some proteins a precipitate results which has the typical Congo red birefringence, the electron microscopic fibrillar appearance and the x-ray diffraction pattern characteristic of all amyloid fibrils [56]. The molecular weight of the protein of one of these artificially created fibrils is 4,600 and, by partial amino acid sequence analysis, it is proved to derive entirely from the amino-terminal variable region of the Bence Jones protein. Peptide maps show that no common region peptides are present in the fibril protein. These studies clearly demonstrate that variable regions of light chains may become amyloid fibrils under conditions that are reasonably physiologic. Some of the Bence Jones proteins from which fibrils can be created come from patients without known amyloidosis. This suggests that although an appropriate variable region may be a necessary condition to the formation of amyloid fibrils it may not be sufficient. Other factors may operate in vivo to determine if a particular light chain will become an amyloid fibril. Some whole Bence Jones proteins can be converted directly to "amyloid" fibrils by thermal treatment [57]. Thus, several facts emerge from recent investigations on the nature of amyloid fibrils: (1) Amyloid fibrils can derive from the variable regions of immunoglobulin light chains. (2) Light chains may be digested in vitro to form "amyloid" fibrils. (3) Whole light chains can be converted by thermal treatment to "amyloid" fibrils.

The basis for the preponderance of light chain fragments in amyloid is unknown. It may reside in the mechanism of light chain catabolism [58] or in the fact that light chains are synthesized in excess of heavy chains [59,60]. A more attractive hypothesis is that certain light chain variable regions possess an "amyloidogenic" structure whereas other light chain variable regions and heavy chains do not. The following evidence favors this hypothesis: (1) The ratio of kappa to lambda light chains in paraproteins associated with amyloidosis [61] and in our series of amyloid proteins [44,45,50] is 1 to 2. This is the reverse of

the ratio in multiple myeloma without amyloidosis
and in normal immunoglobulins, suggesting that
lambda light chains have a structure more prone
to becoming amyloid fibrils than do kappa chains.
(2) Kappa-type amyloid proteins share antigens
with each other and with some, but not all, kappa
Bence Jones proteins. Lambda-type amyloid proteins share antigens with each other and with some
Bence Jones proteins primarily of one variable
region subclass [50]. These immunochemical findings suggest that specific variable region sequences are required for amyloid fibril formation.
(3) Osserman and associates [17] have reported
that Bence Jones proteins from patients with
amyloidosis exhibit a greater tendency to bind to
certain normal tissues (e.g., heart muscle, small
intestine, kidney and liver) than Bence Jones proteins from cases of plasma cell dyscrasia without amyloidosis, implying that "amyloidogenic"
light chains have greater tissue affinity than "non-
amyloidogenic" light chains. If confirmed, this
must be a property of the variable region.

The polysaccharide component usually found
in amyloid deposits is in most cases not a constituent of the fibril nor causally related to fibril
formation or deposition. It apparently accumulates
as a secondary phenomenon. This is indicated by
three findings: (1) the ability to form "amyloid"
fibrils from Bence Jones proteins in vitro in the
absence of polysaccharides [56]; (2) the dissociation of the "mucopolysaccharide" components of
amyloid fibril concentrates from the amyloid fibrils
themselves [62]; and (3) the demonstration that
only two of six amyloid proteins have a significant
polysaccharide component [44], a finding consistent with the low percentage of light chains having covalently linked carbohydrates [63]. Thus,
the term "amyloid" as coined by Virchow [2] to
signify its starch-like characteristic of iodine staining appears now to be misleading as does the in-
variable designation of amyloid fibrils as glycoproteins.

The next important advance in the understanding of the pathogenesis of amyloidosis will un-

doubtedly come from the characterization of the precursor of the amyloid fibril. There are four possible immunoglobulin precursor forms of the amyloid fibril, three of which are immunoglobulin fragments. (1) Antigen-antibody complexes may be catabolized by macrophages [58], and the immunoglobulin degraded in a manner leading to fibril formation and deposition in macrophage-rich organs such as liver and spleen, producing a distribution characteristic of "secondary" amyloidosis. (2) Free whole immunoglobulins or free light polypeptide chains circulating at increased concentrations in conditions such as multiple myeloma [59] may be the direct source of the fibrils in the vascular system as in "primary" amyloidosis. (3) Deletions in the light chain gene might result in light chain fragments analogous to the heavy chain fragments produced in heavy chain disease [64]. (4) Under certain circumstances there might be separate synthesis of variable and constant regions of light chains [55,65] leading to fibril formation.

Further chemical analyses may show that not all amyloid fibrils are derived from immunoglobulin light chains. Our definition of amyloid is, after all, based on certain derivative properties. It is a material deposited in tissues which exhibits Congo red polarization birefringence, has a fibrillar appearance by electron microscopy and a characteristic x-ray diffraction pattern indicating a β-pleated sheet conformation. Under appropriate conditions, proteins other than light chains could assume these same properties. An anti-parallel chain β-pleated sheet conformation has been found by infra-red studies in the Fd fragment of immunoglobulin heavy chains [57]. Studies of amino acid polymers show that poly-l-lysine in its β-conformation [66] has many of the properties of amyloid fibrils except for some difference in the spacing of the polypeptide chains of the β-sheet. Partial amino acid sequence determination of amyloid IV from a patient with classic "secondary" amyloidosis does not correspond, as of this writing, to any known protein sequence [67]. Thus, some cases of amyloidosis may result from tissue deposition of portions of immunoglobulins other than light chains or of proteins other than immunoglobulins.

The elucidation of the immunoglobulin origin of amyloid has profound clinical significance. In so-called "secondary" amyloidosis, the therapeutic removal or elimination of an antigenic stimulus can result in the resolution of amyloid deposits [68,69]. The finding of immunoglobulin fragments in "primary" as well as "secondary" amyloidosis emphasizes the importance of ruling out chronic inflammatory disease and investigating each case for the possible presence of exogenous or endogenous [70] antigenic stimuli. Furthermore, the well documented mobilization of amyloid deposits [68,69] implies that the fibrils exist in equilibrium with the surrounding medium. Preliminary data suggest that in some cases the fibril or its precursor circulates in the serum [45]. It might be possible to remove this material from the serum by selective absorption and thereby mobilize deposits.

A more immediate approach exists with agents already available. Remissions in cases of multiple myeloma can be produced by the administration of alkylating agents such as Melphalan® and Cytoxan® [71–73] suggesting that clinical trials with such drugs in amyloidosis may be of value. Preliminary use of similar drugs in small groups of patients with amyloidosis have not been of striking benefit [72,74], but therapy was admittedly not pursued vigorously. The theoretic basis for such antineoplastic and immunosuppressive therapy is now much stronger and further efforts seem justified.

REFERENCES

1. Rokitansky K: Handbuch der pathologischen Anatomie, vol 3. Vienna, Braumuller and Seidel, 1842.

2. Virchow R: Cellular Pathology, Philadelphia, JB Lippincott & Co, 1863, p 409.

3. Friedreich N, Kekulé A: Zur amyloidfrage. Virchow Arch Path Anat 16: 50, 1859.

4. Letterer E: History and development of amyloid research, Amyloidosis (Mandema E, Ruinen L, Scholten JH. Cohen AS, eds), Amsterdam, Excerpta Medica Foundation, 1968, p 3.

5. Zenoni C: Toxische Amyloidosis bei der antidiphtherischen Immunisation des Pferdes. Zbl Allg Path 13: 334, 1902.

6. Letterer E: Studien über Art und Entstehung des Amyloids. Zbl Allg Path 75: 487, 1926.

7. Loeschcke H: Vorstellungen über das Wesen von Hyalin und Amyloid auf Grund von serologischen Versuchen. Beitr Path Anat 77: 231, 1927.

8. Magnus-Levy A: Bence-Jones-Eiweiss und amyloid. Z Klin Med 116: 510, 1931.

9. Magnus-Levy A: Amyloidosis in multiple myeloma: progress noted in 50 years of personal observation. J Mount Sinai Hosp NY 19: 8, 1952.

10. Apitz K: Die Paraproteinosin. Über die Storung des Eiweisstoffwechsels bei Plasmocytom. Virchow Arch Path Anat 306: 631, 1940.

11. Randerath E: Über die Morphologie der Paraproteinosen. Verh Deutsch Ges Path 32: 27, 1948.

12. Arndt-Marburg HJ: Reticuloendothel und Amyloid. Verh Deutsch Ges Path 26: 243, 1931.

13. Reimann HA, Eklund CM: Long-continued vaccine therapy as a cause of amyloidosis. Amer J Med Sci 190: 88, 1935.

14. Jacobi M, Grayzel H: Generalized secondary amyloidosis. A clinicopathologic study of 84 cases. J Mount Sinai Hosp NY 12: 339, 1945.

15. Osserman EF: Plasma-cell myeloma. II. Clinical aspects. New Eng J Med 261: 3, 1959.

16. Osserman EF, Talal N, Takatsuki K: Amyloidosis: tissue proteinosis: gammaloidosis (editorial). Ann Intern Med 55: 1033, 1961.

17. Osserman EF, Takatsuki K, Talal N: The pathogenesis of "amyloidosis." Seminars Hemat 1: 3, 1964.

18. Sellin D, Haferkamp O: Bence Jones protein und amyloid. Z Ges Exp Med 147: 173, 1968.

19. Cathcart ES, Ritchie FR, Brandt K, Cohen AS: Serologic and urinary studies in patients with amyloidosis, Amyloidosis (Mandema E, Ruinen L, Scholten JH, Cohen AS, eds), Amsterdam, Excerpta Medica Foundation, 1968, p 110.

20. Aly FW, Braun HJ, Missmahl HP: Amyloid involvement and monoclonal immunoglobulins, Current Problems in Immunology, Bayer-Symposium I (Westphal O, Bock H-E, Grundmann E, eds), Berlin, Springer-Verlag, 1969, p 295.

21. Mellors RC, Ortega LG: Analytical pathology. III. New observations on the pathogenesis of glomerulonephritis, lipid nephrosis, periarteritis nodosa and secondary amyloidosis in man. Amer J Path 32: 455, 1956.

22. Vazquez JJ, Dixon FJ: Immunohistochemical analysis of amyloid by the fluorescent technic. J Exp Med 194: 727, 1956.
23. Lackman PJ, Muller-Eberhard HJ, Kunkel HG, Paronetto F: The localization of in vivo bound complement in tissue sections. J Exp Med 115: 63, 1962.
24. Schultz RT, Calkins E, Milgrom F, Witebsky E: Association of gamma globulin with amyloid. Amer J Path 48: 1, 1966.
25. Benditt EP, Lagunoff D, Eriksen N, Iseri OA: Amyloid. Extraction and preliminary characterization of some proteins. Arch Path (Chicago) 74: 323, 1962.
26. Cohen AS: High resolution ultrastructure, immunology and biochemistry of amyloid, Amyloidosis (Mandema E, Ruinen L, Scholten JH, Cohen AS, eds), Amsterdam, Excerpta Medica Foundation, 1968, p 149.
27. Muckle TJ: Protein components of amyloid. Nature (London) 203: 773, 1964.
28. Milgrom F, Kasukawa R, Calkins E: Studies on antigenic composition of amyloid. J Immun 96: 245, 1966.
29. Cathcart ES, Wollheim FA, Cohen AS: Plasma protein constituents of amyloid fibrils. J Immun 99: 376, 1967.
30. Horowitz RE, Stuyvesant VW, Wigmore W, Tatter D: Fibrinogen as a component of amyloid. Arch Path (Chicago) 79: 238, 1965.
31. Schultz RT, Calkins E, Milgrom F: Antigenic components of human amyloid. Amer J Path 50: 957, 1967.
32. Spiro D: The structural basis of proteinuria in man. Electron microscopic studies of renal biopsy specimens from patients with lipid nephrosis, amyloidosis, and subacute and chronic glomerulonephritis. Amer J Path 35: 47, 1959.
33. Cohen AS, Calkins E: Electron microscopic observations on a fibrous component in amyloid of diverse origins. Nature (London) 183: 1202, 1959.
34. Caesar R: Die Feinstruktur von Milz und Leber bei experimenteller Amyloidose. Z Zellforsch 52: 653, 1960.
35. Bennhold H: Ein spezifische Amyloidfarbung mit Kongorot. Munchen Med Wschr 69: 1537, 1932.
36. Puchtler H, Sweat F, Levine M: On the binding of Congo red by amyloid. J Histochem Cytochem 10: 355, 1962.
37. Missmahl HP, Hartwig M: Polarizationoptische Untersuchungen an der Amyloidsubstanz. Virchow Arch Path Anat 324: 480, 1953.
38. Shirahama T, Cohen AS: High resolution electron microscopic analysis of the amyloid fibril. J Cell Biol 33: 679, 1967.
39. Glenner GG, Keiser HR, Bladen HA, Cuatrecasas P, Eanes ED, Ram JS, Kanfer JN, DeLellis RA: Amyloid. VI. A comparison of two morphologic com-

ponents of human amyloid deposits. J Histochem Cytochem 16: 633, 1968.

40. Pras M, Zucker-Franklin D, Rimon A, Franklin EC: Physical, chemical and ultrastructural studies of water-soluble human amyloid fibrils. J Exp Med 130: 777, 1969.

41. Eanes ED, Glenner GG: X-ray diffraction studies on amyloid filaments. J Histochem Cytochem 16: 673, 1968.

42. Glenner GG, Cuatrecasas P, Isersky C, Bladen HA, Eanes ED: Physical and chemical properties of amyloid fibers. II. Isolation of a unique protein constituting the major component from human splenic amyloid fibril concentrates. J Histochem Cytochem 17: 769, 1969.

43. Glenner GG, Harada M, Isersky C: The purification of amyloid fibril proteins. Prep Biochem, in press.

44. Harada M, Isersky C, Cuatrecasas P, Page D, Bladen HA, Eanes ED, Keiser HR, Glenner GG: Human amyloid protein: chemical variability and homogeneity. J Histochem Cytochem 19: 1, 1971.

45. Glenner GG, Harada M, Isersky C, Cuatrecasas P, Page D, Keiser HR: Human amyloid protein: diversity and uniformity. Biochem Biophys Res Commun 41: 1013, 1970.

46. Oudin J: The genetic control of immunoglobulin synthesis. Proc Roy Soc Biol 116: 207, 1966.

47. Kunkel HG: Individual antigenic specificity, cross specificity and diversity of human antibodies. Fed Proc 29: 55, 1970.

48. Tan M, Epstein W: Antigenic analysis of an N-terminal fragment of a type κ Bence Jones protein. J Immun 98: 568, 1967.

49. Ruffilli A, Baglioni C: Subgroups of L type Bence-Jones proteins. J Immun 98: 874, 1967.

50. Isersky C, Ein D, Page DL, Harada M, Glenner GG: Immunochemical cross-reactions of human amyloid proteins with immunoglobulin light polypeptide chains. J Immun, in press.

51. Glenner GG, Harbaugh J, Ohms JI, Harada M, Cuatrecasas P: An amyloid protein: the aminoterminal variable fragment of an immunoglobulin light chain. Biochem Biophys Res Commun 41: 1287, 1970.

52. Glenner GG, Terry W, Harada M, Isersky C, Page D: Amyloid fibril proteins: proof of homology with immunoglobulin light chains by sequence analysis. Science 171: 1150, 1971.

53. Osserman EF: The plasmacytic dyscrasias. Amer J Med 31: 671, 1961.

54. Terry W, Page D, Osserman EF, Glenner GG: in preparation.

55. Solomon A, McLaughlin CL: Bence-Jones proteins and light chains of immunoglobulins. I. Formation and characterization of amino-terminal (variant) and carboxyl-terminal (constant) halves. J Biol Chem 244: 3393, 1960.

56. Glenner GG, Ein D, Eanes ED, Bladen HA, Terry W, Page D: The creation of "amyloid" fibrils from Bence Jones proteins in vitro. Science 714: 712, 1971.

57. Termine J, Eanes ED, Ein D, Glenner GG: In preparation.

58. Waldmann TA, Strober W: Metabolism of immunoglobulins. Progr Allergy 13: 1, 1969.

59. Askonas BA, Williamson AR: Balanced heavy and light chain synthesis in immune tissue and disulphide bond formation in IgG assembly in gamma globulins, Gamma Globulins, Nobel Symposium 3 (Killander J, ed) New York, Interscience, 1967, p 369.

60. Matsuoka Y, Yagi Y, Moore GE, Pressman D: Isolation and characterization of free λ-chain of immunoglobulin produced by an established cell line of human myeloma cell origin. II. Identity of λ-chains in cells and in medium. J Immun 103: 962, 1969.

61. Pick AI, Osserman EF: Amyloidosis associated with plasma cell dyscrasias, Amyloidosis (Mandema E, Ruinen L, Scholten JH, Cohen AS, eds), Amsterdam, Excerpta Medica Foundation, 1968, p 100.

62. Pras M, Nevo Z, Schubert M, Rotman J, Matalon R: The significance of mucopolysaccharides in amyloid. J Histochem Cytochem 19: 443, 1971.

63. Sox HC, Hood L: Attachment of carbohydrate to the variable region of myeloma immunoglobulin light chains. Proc Nat Acad Sci USA 66: 975, 1970.

64. Franklin EC, Frangione B: The molecular defect in a protein (CRA) found in $\lambda 1$ heavy chain disease, and its genetic implications. Proc Nat Acad Sci USA 68: 187, 1971.

65. Schubert D, Cohn M: Immunoglobulin biosynthesis V. Light chain assembly. J Molec Biol 53: 305, 1970.

66. Fasman GD: Factors responsible for conformation stability, Poly-α-Amino Acids (Fasman GD, ed), New York, Marcel Dekker, 1967, p 499.

67. Ein D, Kimura S, Glenner GG: An amyloid fibril protein of unknown origin: partial amino acid sequence analysis. Biochem Biophys Res Commun (in press).

68. Waldenstrom H: On the formation and disappearance of amyloid in man. Acta Chir Scand 63: 479, 1928.

69. Lowenstein J, Gallo G: Remission of the nephrotic syndrome in renal amyloidosis. New Eng J Med 282: 128, 1970.

70. Andrade C, Araki S, Block WD, Cohen AS, Jackson CE, Kuroiwa Y, McKusick VA, Nissim J, Sohar E, Van Allen MW: Hereditary amyloidosis. Arthritis Rheum 13: 902, 1970.

71. Karnofsky DA: Drugs for cancer and allied diseases, Drugs of Choice (Modell W, ed), St. Louis, CV Mosby, 1971, p 553.

72. Osserman EF: Plasma cell dyscrasias, Cecil-Loeb Textbook of Medicine, 13th ed (Beeson PB, Mc-

Dermott W, eds), New York, WB Saunders, 1971, p 1574.

73. Grollman A, Grollman EF: Antineoplastic and immunosuppressive drugs, Pharmacology and Therapeutics, 7th ed (Grollman A, Grollman EF, eds), Philadelphia, Lea & Febiger, 1970, p 665.

74. Barth WF, Willerson JT, Waldmann TA, Decker JL: Primary amyloidosis. Clinical, immunochemical and immunoglobulin metabolism studies in fifteen patients. Amer J Med 47: 259, 1969.

AUTHOR INDEX

KEY-WORD TITLE INDEX